THROWING THE SALT SHAKER AWAY IS ONLY THE BEGINNING. . . .

Everyone knows that a piece of chocolate cake is high in calories whether it's homemade or store-bought, and no matter what brand it is. But what many people don't realize is that there can be huge variations in sodium among the various brands of a particular food item. For instance, one leading brand of tomato paste has more than five times as much sodium as another leading brand. One brand of English muffins has twice the sodium of one of its competitors. And while a cup of fresh corn has about 1 mg. of sodium, a cup of canned corn could contain over 300 mg.

As public concern over the damaging effects of too much sodium in the diet has grown, so, too, has the need to discover the actual sodium content of the foods we eat. And here is the one guide that fully answers that need, your essential handbook to good health through good nutrition.

BARBARA KRAUS
COMPLETE GUIDE TO
SODIUM

Barbara Kraus Complete Guide to Sodium

FOURTH EXPANDED EDITION

With *A Note on Sodium* by
Reva T. Frankle, Ed.D., R.D.,
Director of Nutrition,
Weight Watchers International, Inc.

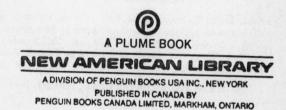

A PLUME BOOK

NEW AMERICAN LIBRARY

A DIVISION OF PENGUIN BOOKS USA INC., NEW YORK
PUBLISHED IN CANADA BY
PENGUIN BOOKS CANADA LIMITED, MARKHAM, ONTARIO

Excerpted from *The Dictionary of Sodium, Fats, and Cholesterol*

SIGNET, SIGNET CLASSIC, MENTOR, ONYX, PLUME, MERIDIAN and
NAL BOOKS are published *in the United States* by New American
Library, a division of Penguin Books USA, Inc., 1633 Broadway,
New York, New York 10019, *in Canada* by Penguin Books
Canada Limited, 2801 John Street, Markham, Ontario L3R 1B4

First Printing, Fourth Expanded Edition, February, 1990

1 2 3 4 5 6 7 8 9

PRINTED IN THE UNITED STATES OF AMERICA

PJ Johnson and
Dan Murphy

Contents

A Note on Sodium
  by Reva T. Frankle, Ed.D, R.D.   ix

Introduction   xiii

Abbreviations and Symbols   xvii

Equivalents   xvii

Dictionary of Brand Names and Basic Foods   1

Canadian Supplement: Dictionary of Brand Names
  and Basic Foods   343

A Note on Sodium

by Reva T. Frankle, Ed.D., R.D.
Director of Nutrition,
Weight Watchers International, Inc.

"Excess of salty flavor hardens the pulse."
The Yellow Emperor's Classic
of Internal Medicine, circa 1000 B.C.

Salt has always been considered the king of seasonings. Historically, it has been associated with social status and wealth. In previous centuries, the most important guests at the table were seated "above the salt," and salt provided the root for the word "salary" (literally, money earned for the purchase of salt).

Today, however, salt's age-old preeminence is being challenged. Research has linked excessive salt consumption with hypertension (high blood pressure), an important risk factor in cardiovascular disease. For this reason, the government's "Dietary Guidelines for Americans," published by the Department of Agriculture in 1980, recommends avoiding too much sodium.

It has been estimated that Americans consume about 10 to 12 grams of salt daily, which amounts to about 2 to 2½ teaspoons. Since salt (sodium chloride) is about 40 percent sodium, this level of salt intake is equal to between 4 and 4½ grams of sodium per day. Where does this salt come from? Of the 10 to 12 grams of salt consumed daily, approximately one-third occurs naturally in foods, one-third comes from salt-containing ingredients added to foods during processing, and one-third represents discretionary salt added by the consumer (from the salt shaker during cooking and at the table). Drinking water also contains sodium, the amount varying from locale to locale.

Though there has been much discussion recently about the dangers of salt, let's not lose sight of the fact that sodium, a naturally occurring constituent of all foods, is an essential nutrient. Sodium is a key element in the regulation of body water and plays a vital role in the acid-base balance of the body. In fact, sodium, like chloride, is indispensable for many body processes, including the conduction of nerve impulses, heart action, and the function of certain enzyme systems. It's the *excessive* intake of salt that is being questioned.

Today, about 20 percent of the American population has high blood pressure—a primary cause of the 500,000 cases of stroke and the 1.2 million heart attacks that occur each year. High blood pressure is painless, "silent," and therefore often ignored until a complicating event causes it to manifest itself. Yet with proper diet and medical treatment, high blood pressure can be controlled and its complications prevented. For many Americans who suffer this silent disease, a reduced sodium intake is critical. In addition, those people who tend to retain body fluids due to kidney, heart, and liver conditions may want to check with their physicians about a decreased sodium intake. Available evidence indicates that restricting sodium to approximately 3.5 grams of salt per day will effect a slight reduction in blood pressure among moderately hypertensive adults. Several very carefully controlled studies of severely hypertensive adults have shown that sodium must be restricted to 200 milligrams (0.5 grams of salt) per day in order to achieve a significant reduction in blood pressure.

Although efforts to correlate salt intake with the incidence of hypertension have not provided definitive evidence of a causal relationship, nonetheless, evidence seems to indicate there is no risk in lowering present intakes of dietary sodium. The possible link between sodium intake and hypertension has become an issue of increased concern in the United States. Since hypertension is a potent risk factor for coronary heart disease and stroke, its control is a major health concern. Current treatment of hypertension requires a change in lifestyle—particularly in terms of dietary habits.

A discussion of dietary sodium is complicated. As you will learn as you use this book, some high-sodium foods do not taste salty or are not thought of as salty. For example, an analysis of a serving of fast-food french fries shows about 115 milligrams of sodium per serving, whereas a serving of cherry pie has nearly four times this amount, or about 450 milligrams.

As a public health nutritionist and a clinical dietitian, may I suggest that in place of salt you sometimes try seasoning foods with some of the following condiments and spices. Onion, garlic, lemon, lime, and vinegar are particularly useful, as are herbs and spices like allspice, aniseed, basil, bay leaf, caraway seed, cardamom, cayenne pepper, celery seed, chili powder, cinnamon, cloves, curry powder, dill seed, fennel seed, garlic, ginger, mace, marjoram, mint, mustard (dry), mustard seed, nutmeg, onion powder, oregano, parsley, pepper, poppy seed, poultry seasoning, rosemary, saffron, sage, sesame seed, tarragon, thyme, turmeric, and vanilla.

Agreed, the sodium intake of Americans is excessive. Since there is no reason to believe that reducing sodium chloride intake would be harmful for healthy persons, and it may even help prevent hypertension in some people, it is time to evaluate our sodium intake. The consumer can meet the challenge of decreasing sodium intake by being aware of the sodium content of foods and using discretion with the salt shaker. There is no specific recommended amount or safety level, but the National Research Council suggests that the estimated safe and adequate daily dietary intake of sodium is about 1100 to 3300 milligrams (1.1 to 3.3 grams). Limiting salt intake to 3 grams per day would allow for some salt to be used in cooking but none at the table.

Industry is responding. Sodium-containing substances such as salt are added to foods for three basic reasons: 1) to provide and enhance flavors in foods, 2) to develop and maintain expected characteristics of foods such as texture and freshness, and 3) as a preservative. Gradual reduction, appropriate for some foods, is taking place. Industry is experimenting with safe new processes for the use of salt, with reduced sodium formulas, and with the use of alternatives to sodium-containing ingredients. Gradual reduction will allow time for industry to determine the microbiologic safety of certain reduced-sodium products.

FDA is working with the processed-food industry on a voluntary basis to lower the sodium content of foods they produce. (Sodium is used almost universally in the preserving and processing of food.) The Department of Health and Human Services is working to give consumers more information about the sodium content of foods they buy, and has said it "would like to see more public awareness in general about sodium and health."

Dietary change is the cornerstone of safe, effective, long-term blood pressure control. How fortunate that we now have the *Barbara Kraus Complete Guide to Sodium*, a comprehensive and easy-to-use book that enables readers to estimate their daily salt intake and to plan a diet that is lower in sodium.

Introduction

ARRANGEMENT OF THIS BOOK

This dictionary of foods lists several thousand brand-name products and basic foods with their sodium counts. Foods are listed alphabetically by brand name or by the name of the food. The singular form is used for entries, that is, blackberry instead of blackberries. Most items are listed individually although a few are grouped (see p. xvi). For example, all candies are listed together so that if you are looking for *Mars* bar, you look first under Candy, then under *M* in alphabetical order. But, if you are looking for a breakfast food such as Oatmeal, you will find it under *O* in the main alphabet. Many cross references are included to assist you in finding items known by different names.

Under the main headings, it was often not possible nor even desirable to follow an alphabetical arrangement. For basic foods, such as apricots, the first entries are for the fresh product weighed with seeds as it is purchased from the store, then the fruit in small portions as they may be eaten or measured. These entries are followed by the processed products, canned (although it may actually be a bottle or a jar), dehydrated, dried, and frozen items. This basic plan, with adaptations where necessary, was followed for fruits, vegetables, and meats.

In almost all entries, where data were available, the U.S. Department of Agriculture figures are shown first. The Department values represent averages from several manufacturers and are shown for comparison with the values from individual companies or for use where particular brands are not available.

All brand-name products have been italicized and company names appear in parentheses.

Portions Used

The portion column is a most important one to read and note. Common household measures are used wherever possible. For some items, the amounts given are those commonly purchased in the store, such as one pound of meat, or a 15-ounce package of cake mix. These quantities can be divided into the number of servings used in the home and the nutritive values in each portion can then be readily determined. Any ingredients added in preparing such products must also be taken into account.

The smaller portions given are for foods as served or measured in moderate amounts, such as one-half cup of reconstituted juice, or four ounces of meat. Be sure to adjust the amount of the nutrients to the actual portions you use. For example, if you serve one cup of juice instead of one-half cup, multiply the amount of nutrients shown for the smaller amount by two.

The size of portions you use is extremely important in controlling the intake of any nutrient. The amount of a nutrient is directly related to the weight of the food served. The weight of a volumetric measure, such as a cup or a pint, may vary considerably depending on many factors; four ounces by weight may be very different from one-half cup or four fluid ounces. Ounces in the tables are always ounces by weight unless specified as fluid ounces, fractions of a cup, or other volumetric measure. Foods that are fluffy in texture such as flaked coconut and bean sprouts vary greatly in weight per cup, depending on how tightly they are packed. Such foods as canned green beans also vary when measured with and without liquid; for instance, canned beans with liquid weigh 4.2 ounces for one-half cup, but drained beans weigh 2.5 ounces for the same half cup. Check the weights of your serving portions regularly. Bear in mind that you can reduce or increase the intake of any nutrient by changing the serving size.

It was impossible to convert all the portions to a uniform

basis. Some sources were able to report data only in terms of weights with no information on cup or other volumetric measures. We have shown small portions in quantities that might reasonably be expected to be served or measured in the home or institution.

You will find in the portion column the phrases "weighed with bone," and "weighed with skin and seeds." These descriptions apply to the products as you purchase them in the markets, but the nutritive values as shown are for the amount of edible foods after you discard the bone, skin, seed, or other inedible part. The weight given in the "measure" or "quantity" column is to the nearest gram or fraction of an ounce.

Data on the composition of foods are constantly changing for many reasons. Better sampling and analytical methods, improvements in marketing procedures, and changes in formulas of mixed products may alter values for all of the nutrients. Weights of packaged foods are frequently changed. It is essential to read label information in order to be knowledgeable about these matters and to make intelligent use of food tables.

Sources of Data

Values in this dictionary are based on publications issued by the U.S. Department of Agriculture and on data submitted by manufacturers and processors. The U.S. Department of Agriculture issues basic tables on food composition for use in the United States. The commercial products from U.S.D.A. publications represent average values obtained on products of more than one company. The figures designated as "home recipe" are based on recipes on file with the Department of Agriculture. Data on commercial products listed by brand name in this publication are based on values supplied by manufacturers and processors for their own individual products. Supermarket brand names, such as the A & P's *Ann Page*, or private labels could not be included in this book inasmuch as they are not usually analyzed under these trade names. Every care has been taken to interpret the data and the descriptions supplied by the companies as fully and as accurately as possible. Many values have been recalculated to different portions from those submitted, in order to bring about greater uniformity among similar items.

Analyses of foods to provide information on nutritive values are extremely expensive to conduct. Many small companies cannot afford to have their products analyzed and were unable to provide data. Other companies have simply never gotten around to having the analyses done. New requirements for labeling nutritive values for products may provide information on additional items in the future.

Foods Listed by Groups

Foods in the following classes are reported together rather than as individual items in the main alphabet: baby food, bread, cake, cake icing, cake icing mix, candy, cheese, cookies, cookie mix, crackers, gravy, pie, pie filling, salad dressing, sauce, soft drinks, soup, and yogurt.

BARBARA KRAUS

Abbreviations and Symbols

(USDA) = United States Department of Agriculture

(HEW/FAO) = Health, Education and Welfare/Food and Agriculture Organization

* = prepared as package directs[1]

< = less than

& = and

" = inch

canned = bottles or jars as well as cans

dia. = diameter

fl. = fluid

g. = gram

liq. = liquid

lb. = pound

med. = medium

oz. = ounce

pkg. = package

pt. = pint

qt. = quart

sq. = square

T. = tablespoon

Tr. = trace

tsp. = teaspoon

wt. = weight

italics or name in parentheses = registered trademark,™

The letters DNA indicate that no data are available.

Equivalents

By Weight

1 pound = 16 ounces

1 ounce = 28.35 grams

3.52 ounces = 100 grams

1 gram = 1,000 milligrams

By Volume

1 quart = 4 cups

1 cup = 8 fluid ounces

1 cup = ½ pint

1 cup = 16 tablespoons

2 tablespoons = 1 fluid ounce

1 tablespoon = 3 teaspoons

[1] If the package directions call for whole or skim milk, the data given here are for whole milk, unless otherwise stated.

Food and Description	Measure or Quantity	Sodium (milligrams)

A

AC'CENT	¼ tsp. (1 g.)	129
ACEROLA, fresh (USDA)	½ lb. (weighed with seeds)	15
AGNOLETTI, frozen (Buitoni)		
Cheese filling	2 oz.	158
Meat filling	2 oz.	237
ALBACORE, raw, meat only (USDA)	4 oz.	45
ALCOHOLIC BEVERAGES (See individual listings)		
ALE (See **BEER**)		
ALLSPICE (French's)	1 tsp. (1.7 g.)	1
ALMOND:		
Shelled:		
(USDA):		
Whole	½ cup (2½ oz.)	3
Whole	1 oz.	Tr.
Whole	13–15 almonds (.6 oz.)	Tr.
Chopped	1 cup (4½ oz.)	5
Blanched (USDA) salted	½ cup	155
Chocolate-covered (See **CANDY**)		
Roasted:		
(USDA) salted	½ cup (2.8 oz.)	155
(Blue Diamond) diced	1 oz.	56
(Fisher):		
Dry, smoked	1 oz.	220
Honey roasted	1 oz.	75
(Planters) dry roasted, salted	1 oz.	200
(Tom's) salted	1 oz.	120

Food and Description	Measure or Quantity	Sodium (milligrams)
ALMOND EXTRACT, pure (Durkee or Virginia Dare)	1 tsp.	0
ALPHA-BITS, cereal (Post)	1 cup (1 oz.)	224
ANCHOVY, PICKLED (Granadaisa)	1 oz.	1587
ANISE EXTRACT (Durkee) imitation	1 tsp.	0
APPLE, any variety:		
Fresh (USDA):		
Eaten with skin	1 lb. (weighed with skin & core)	4
Eaten with skin	1 med., 2½″ dia. (about 4 per lb.)	1
Eaten without skin	1 lb. (weighed with skin & core)	4
Eaten without skin	1 med., 2½″ dia. (about 4 per lb.)	1
Pared, diced or sliced	1 cup (3.9 oz.)	1
Pared, quartered	1 cup (4.4 oz.)	1
Canned:		
(Comstock) rings, drained	1 ring (1.1. oz.)	8
(White House):		
Rings, spiced, drained	1 ring (.5 oz.)	5
Sliced	½ cup (4 oz.)	10
Dehydrated (USDA):		
Uncooked	1 oz.	2
Cooked, sweetened	½ cup (4½ oz.)	1
Dried:		
(USDA)		
Uncooked	1 cup (3 oz.)	4
Cooked, unsweetened	½ cup (4½ oz.)	1
Cooked, sweetened	½ cup (4.9 oz.)	1
(Del Monte) uncooked	1 cup (2 oz.)	57
Frozen, sweetened, slices, not thawed (USDA)	10-oz. pkg.	40
APPLE BROWN BETTY, home recipe (USDA)	1 cup (7.6 oz.)	330
APPLE BUTTER:		
(USDA)	1 T. (.6 oz.)	<1

Food and Description	Measure or Quantity	Sodium (milligrams)
(Bama)	1 T.	7
(Home Brands)	1 T.	8
(White House)	1 T.	7
APPLE CHERRY BERRY DRINK, canned (Lincoln)	6 fl. oz.	30
APPLE CIDER:		
(USDA)	½ cup (4.4 oz)	1
Canned:		
(Johanna Farms) sweet	½ cup	1
(Tree Top)	6 fl. oz.	10
*Mix *Country Time*	8 fl. oz.	94
APPLE-CRANBERRY DRINK (Hi-C):		
Canned	6 fl. oz.	23
*Mix	6 fl. oz.	11
APPLE DRINK:		
Canned:		
Capri Sun, natural	6¾ fl. oz.	2
(Hi-C)	6 fl. oz.	12
Ssips (Johanna Farms)	8.45-fl.-oz. container	<10
*Mix (Hi-C)	6 fl. oz.	20
APPLE DUMPLING, frozen (Pepperidge Farm)	1 dumpling	240
APPLE, ESCALLOPED:		
Canned (White House)	½ cup (4.5 oz.)	60
Frozen (Stouffer's)	4 oz.	50
APPLE-GRAPE JUICE, canned (Red Cheek)	6 fl. oz.	2
APPLE JACKS, cereal (Kellogg's)	1 cup (1 oz.)	125
APPLE JELLY:		
Sweetened:		
(Bama)	1 T.	7
(Home Brands)	1 T.	8
Dietetic (See **APPLE SPREAD**)		
APPLE JUICE:		
Canned:		
(USDA)	1 cup (8.7 oz.)	2

Food and Description	Measure or Quantity	Sodium (milligrams)
(Borden) *Sippin' Pak*	8.45-fl.-oz. container	25
(Johanna Farms):		
Florida citrus	6 fl. oz.	3
Tree Ripe	8.45-fl.-oz. container	2
(Minute Maid)	6 fl. oz.	2
(Mott's) regular or McIntosh	6 fl. oz.	<10
(Ocean Spray)	6 fl. oz.	14
(Red Cheek)	6 fl. oz.	2
(Thank You Brand):		
Regular	6 fl. oz.	37
With Vitamin C	6 fl. oz.	28
(Tree Top) regular	6 fl. oz.	10
(White House)	6 fl. oz.	5
Chilled (Minute Maid)	6 fl. oz.	2
*Frozen:		
(Minute Maid)	6 fl. oz.	2
(Seneca Foods) natural	6 fl. oz.	1
(Tree Top) regular	6 fl. oz.	10
APPLE JUICE DRINK, canned		
(Sunkist)	8.45-fl.-oz. container	0
APPLE RAISIN CRISP, cereal		
(Kellogg's)	⅔ cup (1 oz.)	200
APPLESAUCE, canned:		
Sweetened:		
(USDA)	½ cup (4.5 oz.)	3
(Comstock)	½ cup (4.4 oz.)	90
(Del Monte)	½ cup (4.0 oz.)	1
(Hunt's) any flavor	4¼ oz.	0
(Mott's):		
Regular, jarred:		
Plain or cinnamon	6 oz.	<1
Chunky	6 oz.	11
Single-serve cups:		
Plain or cinnamon	4-oz. container	<1
Cherry	3¾-oz. container	8
Peach	3¾-oz. container	7
Strawberry	3¾-oz. container	10

Food and Description	Measure or Quantity	Sodium (milligrams)
(Thank You Brand)	½ cup (4.5 oz.)	26
(Tree Top)	½ cup	0
(White House) regular or chunky	½ cup (5 oz.)	5
Unsweetened, dietetic or low calorie:		
(USDA)	½ cup (4.3 oz.)	2
(Diet Delight)	½ cup (4.3 oz.)	2
(Featherweight) water pack	½ cup	<10
(Hunt's) natural	4¼ oz.	0
(Mott's):		
Jarred	6 oz.	3
Single-serve cups	4-oz. container	2
(Thank You Brand)	½ cup (4.3 oz.)	12
(White House) regular or with added apple juice	½ cup (4.7 oz.)	5
APPLE SPREAD, low sugar:		
(Diet Delight)	1 T. (.6 oz.)	9
(Slenderella)	1 T. (.6 oz.)	19
(Smucker's)	1 T. (.6 oz.)	19
APRICOT:		
Fresh (USDA):		
Whole	1 lb. (weighed with pits)	4
Whole	3 apricots (about 12 per lb.)	1
Halves	1 cup (5½ oz.)	2
Canned, regular pack, solids & liq.:		
(USDA):		
Juice pack	4 oz.	1
Light syrup	4 oz.	1
Heavy syrup, halves	½ cup (4.6 oz.)	1
Heavy syrup, halves	3 med. halves with 1¾ T. syrup (3 oz.)	1
Extra heavy syrup	4 oz.	1
(Del Monte):		
Halves, unpeeled	½ cup (4¼ oz.)	7
Whole, peeled	½ cup (4¼ oz.)	18

Food and Description	Measure or Quantity	Sodium (milligrams)
(Libby's) heavy syrup, halves	½ cup (4½ oz.)	7
(Stokely-Van Camp)	½ cup (4.6 oz.)	22
Canned, unsweetened or dietetic, solids & liq.:		
(USDA) water pack, halves	½ cup (4.4. oz.)	1
(Del Monte) *Lite*, unpeeled, extra light syrup	½ cup (4.3 oz.)	2
(Diet Delight) juice pack	½ cup (4.4 oz.)	5
(Featherweight):		
Juice pack	½ cup	<10
Water pack	½ cup	<10
Dehydrated (USDA):		
Uncooked, sulfured	4 oz.	37
Cooked, sugar added, solids & liq.	4 oz.	9
Dried:		
(USDA):		
Uncooked	1 cup (4.6 oz.)	34
Uncooked	10 large halves (¼ cup or 1.7 oz.)	13
Cooked, sweetened	½ cup with liq. (4.7 oz.)	9
Cooked, unsweetened	½ cup with liq. (4.4 oz.)	10
(Del Monte)	½ cup (2.3 oz.)	4
(Sun-Maid)	½ cup (3.5 oz.)	52
(Sunsweet)	½ cup (3½ oz.)	52
Frozen, unthawed, sweetened (USDA)	10-oz. pkg.	11
APRICOT NECTAR, canned, sweetened:		
(USDA)	½ cup (4.4 oz.)	Tr.
(Del Monte)	6 fl. oz. (6.6 oz.)	<10
APRICOT & PINEAPPLE PRESERVE, sweetened (Smucker's)	1 T. (.7 oz.)	3
APRICOT & PINEAPPLE SPREAD, low sugar (Diet Delight)	1 T. (.6 oz.)	45

Food and Description	Measure or Quantity	Sodium (milligrams)
APRICOT PRESERVE:		
Sweetened (Home Brands)	1 T.	7
Dietetic:		
(Estee)	1 T.	<3
(Featherweight)	1 T.	40–50
(Louis Sherry)	1 T.	Tr.
ARBY'S:		
Bac'n Cheddar Deluxe	7.8-oz. sandwich	1385
Beef'n Cheddar	6-oz. sandwich	1520
Chicken breast sandwich	7¼-oz. sandwich	1340
Croissant:		
Bacon & egg	4.5-oz. croissant	550
Butter	2-oz. croissant	225
Chicken salad	5-oz. croissant	725
Ham & Swiss	4-oz. croissant	995
Mushroom & Swiss	4-oz. croissant	630
Sausage & egg	5¾-oz. croissant	745
Ham & cheese	1 sandwich	1655
Potato:		
Cake	3-oz. serving	425
Fried, French	2½-oz. serving	30
Stuffed:		
Broccoli & cheese	12-oz. potato	475
Deluxe	11.1-oz. potato	475
Mushroom & cheese	10.6-oz. potato	635
Taco	15-oz. potato	1065
Roast beef sandwich:		
Regular	5.2-oz. sandwich	590
Junior	3-oz. sandwich	345
Super	8.3-oz. sandwich	800
Shake:		
Chocolate	10.6-oz. shake	300
Jamocha	10.6-oz. shake	280
Vanilla	8.8-oz. shake	245
ARTICHOKE, Globe or French:		
Raw (USDA) whole	1 lb. (weighed untrimmed)	78
Boiled (USDA) without salt, drained	4 oz.	34

Food and Description	Measure or Quantity	Sodium (milligrams)
Canned (Cara Mia) marinated, drained	6-oz. jar	94
Frozen (Birds Eye) deluxe hearts	⅓ of 9-oz. pkg.	40
ASPARAGUS:		
Raw (USDA) whole spears	1 lb. (weighed untrimmed)	5
Boiled (USDA) without salt, drained:		
Whole spears	4 spears (½" at base, 2.1 oz.)	<1
Cut spears, 1½"-2" pieces	1 cup (5.1 oz.)	1
Canned, regular pack:		
(USDA):		
Green spears, solids & liq.	1 cup (8.6 oz.)	576
Green spears, drained	1 cup (8.3 oz.)	536
Green spears only	4 med. spears (2.8 oz.)	188
Green, liquid only	2 T. liquid	71
White spears, solids & liq.	1 cup (8.6 oz.)	577
White spears only	4 med. spears (2.8 oz.)	188
White, liquid only	2 T. liquid	71
(Del Monte):		
Green tips & spears, solids & liq.	½ cup	355
Green or white spears, solids & liq.	½ cup	355
(Green Giant) green, cut spears, solids & liq.	½ of 8-oz. can	450
(Kounty Kist) green spears, solids & liq.	⅓ of 14-oz. can	483
(Lindy) green, cut spears, solids & liq.	⅓ of 10½-oz. can	360
(Stokely-Van Camp):		
Green, spears, solids & liq.	1 cup (8.4 oz.)	896
Green, cut spears, solids & liq.	1 cup (8.4 oz.)	896

Food and Description	Measure or Quantity	Sodium (milligrams)
Canned, dietetic or low calorie: (USDA):		
Green, spears, solids & liq.	4 oz.	3
Green, spears, drained solids	4 oz.	3
Green, liquid only	4 oz. liquid	3
White, spears, drained solids	4 oz.	5
(Diet Delight) solids & liq.	½ cup (4.2 oz.)	5
(S&W) *Nutradiet*, green spears, solids & liq.	½ cup	<10
Frozen:		
(USDA):		
Cuts & tips, boiled, drained	½ cup (3.2 oz.)	<1
Spears, unthawed	4 oz.	2
Spears, boiled, drained	4 oz.	1
(Birds Eye):		
Cuts, 5-minute style	⅓ of 10-oz. pkg.	<1
Spears, regular or jumbo	⅓ of 10-oz. pkg.	4
(Frosty Acres) cuts & tips or spears	3.3 oz.	4
(Green Giant) cut spears in butter sauce	½ cup	725
(McKenzie) spears	3⅓-oz. serving	19
(Stouffer's) souffle	⅓ of 12-oz. pkg.	440
ASPARAGUS PUREE, canned (Larsen) no salt added	½ cup (4.4 oz.)	6
AUNT JEMIMA SYRUP (See SYRUP)		
AVOCADO, peeled, pitted, all commercial varieties (USDA):		
Whole	1 fruit (10.7 oz., weighed with seed & skin)	12
Cubed	1 cup (5.3 oz.)	6
Puree	1 cup (8.1 oz.)	9
***AWAKE** (Birds Eye)	6 fl. oz.	14

Food and Description	Measure or Quantity	Sodium (milligrams)
AYDS:		
Butterscotch, chocolate or chocolate mint	1 piece (.2 oz.)	9
Vanilla	1 piece (.2 oz.)	12

B

Food and Description	Measure or Quantity	Sodium (milligrams)
BABY FOOD:		
Advance (Similac)	1 fl. oz.	Tr.
Apple-banana juice (Gerber) strained	4.2 fl. oz.	4
Apple betty (Beech-Nut):		
Junior	7¾-oz. jar	1
Strained	4¾-oz. jar	<1
Apple-blueberry (Gerber):		
Junior	7½-oz. jar	6
Strained	4½-oz. jar	4
Apple-cherry juice:		
Strained:		
(Beech-Nut)	4⅕ fl. oz.	6
(Gerber)	4.2 fl. oz.	Tr.
Toddler (Gerber)	4 fl. oz.	2
Apple-cranberry juice (Beech-Nut) Strained	4½ fl. oz.	6
Apple dessert, Dutch (Gerber):		
Junior	7¾-oz. jar	46
Strained	4¾-oz. jar	27
Apple-grape juice:		
Strained:		
(Beech-Nut)	4⅕ fl. oz.	6
(Gerber)	4.2 fl. oz.	2
Toddler (Gerber)	4 fl. oz.	2
Apple juice:		
Strained:		
(Beech-Nut)	4.2 fl. oz.	5

Food and Description	Measure or Quantity	Sodium (milligrams)
(Gerber)	4.2 fl. oz.	2
Toddler (Gerber)	4 fl. oz.	1
Apple-peach juice, strained:		
(Beech-Nut)	4⅕ fl. oz.	6
(Gerber)	4.2 fl. oz.	4
Apple-plum juice (Gerber) strained	4.2 fl. oz.	4
Apple-prune juice (Gerber) strained	4.2 fl. oz.	5
Applesauce:		
Junior:		
(Beech-Nut)	7¾-oz. jar	5
(Gerber)	7½-oz. jar	2
Strained:		
(Beech-Nut)	4¾-oz. jar	0
(Gerber)	4½-oz. jar	3
Applesauce & apricots (Gerber):		
Junior	7½-oz. jar	6
Strained	4½-oz. jar	3
Applesauce & bananas (Beech-Nut) strained	4¾-oz. jar	<1
Applesauce & cherries (Beech-Nut):		
Junior	7¾-oz. jar	5
Strained	4¾-oz. jar	3
Applesauce with pineapple (Gerber) strained	4½-oz. jar	3
Applesauce & raspberries (Beech-Nut):		
Junior	7¾-oz. jar	5
Strained	4¾-oz. jar	3
Apple & yogurt (Gerber) strained	4½-oz. jar	22
Apricot with tapioca:		
Junior:		
(Beech-Nut)	7½-oz. jar	15
(Gerber)	7¾-oz. jar	22
Strained (Gerber)	4¾-oz. jar	8
Apricot with tapioca & apple juice (Beech-Nut) strained	4¾-oz. jar	9

Food and Description	Measure or Quantity	Sodium (milligrams)
Banana-apple dessert (Gerber):		
Junior	7¾-oz. jar	9
Strained	4¾-oz. jar	3
Banana dessert (Beech-Nut) junior	7½-oz. jar	10
Banana with pineapple & tapioca (Gerber):		
Junior	7½-oz. jar	8
Strained	4½-oz. jar	6
Banana & pineapple with tapioca & apple juice (Beech-Nut):		
Junior	7¾-oz. jar	20
Strained	4¾-oz. jar	12
Banana with tapioca:		
Junior:		
(Beech-Nut)	7¾-oz. jar	10
(Gerber)	7½-oz. jar	8
Strained:		
(Beech-Nut)	4¾-oz. jar	6
(Gerber)	7½-oz. jar	9
Banana & yogurt (Gerber) strained	4½-oz. jar	22
Bean, green:		
Junior (Beech-Nut)	7¼-oz. jar	5
Strained:		
(Beech-Nut)	4½-oz. jar	3
(Gerber)	4½-oz. jar	4
Bean, green, creamed (Gerber) junior	7½-oz. jar	19
Bean, green, potatoes & ham casserole (Gerber) toddler	6¼-oz. jar	538
Beef (Gerber):		
Junior	3½-oz. jar	52
Strained	3½-oz. jar	52
Beef & beef broth (Beech-Nut):		
Junior	7½-oz. jar	162
Strained	4½-oz. jar	88
Beef with beef heart (Gerber) Strained	3½-oz. jar	58

Food and Description	Measure or Quantity	Sodium (milligrams)
Beef dinner, high meat, with vegetables (Gerber):		
Junior	4½-oz. jar	36
Strained	4½-oz. jar	31
Beef & egg noodle (Beech-Nut):		
Junior	7½-oz. jar	54
Strained	4½-oz. jar	32
Beef & egg noodles with vegetables (Gerber):		
Junior	7½-oz. jar	36
Strained	4½-oz. jar	19
Beef lasagna (Gerber) toddler	6¼-oz. jar	685
Beef liver (Gerber) strained	3½-oz. jar	47
Beef & rice with tomato sauce (Gerber) toddler	6¼-oz. jar	680
Beef stew (Gerber) toddler	6-oz. jar	593
Beef with vegetables & cereal, high meat (Beech-Nut):		
Junior	4½-oz. jar	38
Strained	4½-oz. jar	38
Beet (Gerber) strained	4½-oz. jar	119
Biscuit (Gerber)	11-gram piece	30
Carrot:		
Junior:		
(Beech-Nut)	7½-oz. jar	147
(Gerber)	7½-oz. jar	111
Strained:		
(Beech-Nut)	4½-oz. jar	88
(Gerber)	4½-oz. jar	47
Cereal, dry:		
Barley:		
(Beech-Nut)	½-oz. serving	4
(Gerber)	4 T. (½ oz.)	4
High protein:		
(Beech-Nut)	½-oz. serving	<20
(Gerber)	4 T. (½ oz.)	3
High protein with apple & orange (Gerber)	4 T. (½ oz.)	15
Mixed:		
(Beech-Nut)	½-oz. serving	<20

Food and Description	Measure or Quantity	Sodium (milligrams)
(Gerber)	4 T. (½ oz.)	4
Mixed with banana (Gerber)	4 T. (½ oz.)	13
Oatmeal:		
(Beech-Nut)	½-oz. serving	<20
(Gerber)	4 T. (½ oz.)	4
Oatmeal & banana (Gerber)	4 T. (½ oz.)	14
Rice:		
(Beech-Nut)	½-oz. serving	<20
(Gerber)	4 T. (½ oz.)	4
Cereal, dry:		
Rice with banana (Gerber)	4 T. (½ oz.)	11
Cereal or mixed cereal:		
With applesauce & banana:		
Junior (Gerber)	7½-oz. jar	8
(Beech-Nut)	4½-oz. jar	27
(Gerber)	4½-oz. jar	3
& egg yolk (Gerber):		
Junior	7½-oz. jar	26
Strained	4½-oz. jar	17
With egg yolks & bacon (Beech-Nut):		
Junior	7½-oz. jar	168
Strained	4½-oz. jar	88
Oatmeal with applesauce & banana (Gerber):		
Junior	7½-oz. jar	4
Strained	4½-oz. jar	3
Rice with applesauce & banana, strained:		
(Beech-Nut)	4¾-oz. jar	34
(Gerber)	4¾-oz. jar	34
Rice with mixed fruit (Gerber) junior	7¾-oz. jar	8
Cherry vanilla pudding (Gerber):		
Junior	7½-oz. jar	18
Strained	4½-oz. jar	17
Chicken (Gerber):		
Junior	3½-oz. jar	39
Strained	3½-oz. jar	39

Food and Description	Measure or Quantity	Sodium (milligrams)
Chicken & chicken broth (Beech-Nut):		
Junior	7½-oz. jar	147
Strained	4½-oz. jar	88
Chicken & noodles:		
Junior:		
(Beech-Nut)	7½-oz. jar	44
(Gerber)	7½-oz. jar	28
Strained:		
(Beech-Nut)	4½-oz. jar	26
(Gerber)	4½-oz. jar	20
Chicken & rice (Beech-Nut) strained	4½-oz. jar	20
Chicken with vegetables, high meat (Gerber) junior	4½-oz. jar	33
Chicken with vegetables & cereal (Beech-Nut):		
Junior	7½-oz. jar	61
Strained	4½-oz. jar	38
Chicken soup, cream of (Gerber) strained	4½-oz. jar	29
Chicken stew (Gerber) toddler	6-oz. jar	651
Chicken sticks (Gerber) junior	2½-oz. jar	323
Cookie (Gerber):		
Animal-shaped	6½-g. piece	13
Arrowroot	5½-g. piece	20
Corn, creamed:		
Junior:		
(Beech-Nut)	7½-oz. jar	34
(Gerber)	7½-oz. jar	21
Strained:		
(Beech-Nut)	4½-oz. jar	20
(Gerber)	4½-oz. jar	11
Cottage cheese with pineapple juice (Beech-Nut):		
Junior	7¾-oz. jar	46
Strained	4¾-oz. jar	28
Custard:		
Apple (Beech-Nut):		
Junior	7½-oz. jar	54

Food and Description	Measure or Quantity	Sodium (milligrams)
Strained	4½-oz. jar	32
Chocolate (Gerber) strained	4½-oz. jar	30
Vanilla:		
Junior:		
(Beech-Nut)	7½-oz. jar	69
(Gerber)	7¾-oz. jar	51
Strained:		
(Beech-Nut)	4½-oz. jar	41
(Gerber)	4½-oz. jar	31
Egg yolk (Gerber):		
Junior	3⅓-oz. jar	57
Strained	3⅓-oz. jar	45
Fruit dessert:		
Junior:		
(Beech-Nut):		
Regular	7¾-oz. jar	46
Tropical	7¾-oz. jar	35
(Gerber)	7¾-oz. jar	18
Strained:		
(Beech-Nut)	4½-oz. jar	26
(Gerber)	4¾-oz. jar	13
Fruit juice, mixed:		
Strained:		
(Beech-Nut)	4⅕ fl. oz.	6
(Gerber)	4.2 fl. oz.	2
Toddler (Gerber)	4 fl. oz.	1
Fruit, mixed, with yogurt:		
Junior (Beech-Nut)	7½-oz. jar	54
Strained:		
(Beech-Nut)	4¾-oz. jar	34
(Gerber)	4½-oz. jar	23
Guava (Gerber) strained	4½-oz. jar	.5
Guava & papaya (Gerber) strained	4½-oz. jar	.6
Ham (Gerber):		
Junior	3½-oz. jar	39
Strained	3½-oz. jar	40
Ham & ham broth (Beech-Nut) strained	4½-oz. jar	76

Food and Description	Measure or Quantity	Sodium (milligrams)
Ham with vegetables, high meat (Gerber):		
Junior	4½-oz. jar	24
Strained	4½-oz. jar	22
Ham with vegetable & cereal (Beech-Nut):		
Junior	4½-oz. jar	44
Strained	4½-oz. jar	44
Hawaiian Delight (Gerber):		
Junior	7¾-oz. jar	40
Strained	4½-oz. jar	23
Isomil Similac ready-to-feed	1 fl. oz.	Tr.
Lamb (Gerber):		
Junior	3½-oz. jar	53
Strained	3½-oz. jar	51
Lamb & lamb broth (Beech-Nut):		
Junior	7½-oz. jar	172
Strained	4½-oz. jar	97
Macaroni & cheese (Gerber):		
Junior	7½-oz. jar	168
Strained	4½-oz. jar	102
Macaroni & tomato with beef:		
Junior:		
(Beech-Nut)	7½-oz. jar	64
(Gerber)	7½-oz. jar	34
Strained:		
(Beech-Nut)	4½-oz. jar	32
(Gerber)	4½-oz. jar	38
Mango (Gerber) strained	4¾-oz. jar	5
MBF (Gerber)		
Concentrate	1 fl. oz. (2 T.)	16
Concentrate	15-fl.-oz. can	248
*Diluted, 1 to 1	1 fl. oz. (2 T.)	8
Meat sticks (Gerber) junior	2½-oz. jar	325
Orange-apple juice, strained:		
(Beech-Nut)	4½ fl. oz.	3
(Gerber)	4.2 fl. oz.	5
Orange-apricot juice (Beech-Nut) strained	4.2 fl. oz.	7

Food and Description	Measure or Quantity	Sodium (milligrams)
Orange-banana juice (Beech-Nut) strained	4⅕ fl. oz.	3
Orange juice, strained:		
(Beech-Nut)	4⅕ fl. oz.	3
(Gerber)	4.2 fl. oz.	4
Orange-pineapple dessert (Beech-Nut) strained	4¾-oz. jar	28
Orange-pineapple juice, strained·		
(Beech-Nut)	4⅕ fl. oz.	3
(Gerber)	4.2 fl. oz.	1
Orange pudding (Gerber) strained	4¾-oz. jar	28
Papaya & applesauce (Gerber) strained	4½-oz. jar	6
Pea:		
Junior:		
(Beech-Nut)	7¼-oz. jar	5
(Gerber)	7½-oz. jar	11
Strained:		
(Beech-Nut)	4½-oz. jar	3
(Gerber)	4½-oz. jar	11
Pea & carrot (Beech-Nut) strained	4½-oz. jar	50
Peach:		
Junior:		
(Beech-Nut)	7¾-oz. jar	15
(Gerber)	7½-oz. jar	6
Strained:		
(Beech-Nut)	4¾-oz. jar	0
(Gerber)	4½-oz. jar	4
Peach & apple with yogurt (Beech-Nut):		
Junior	7½-oz. jar	54
Strained	4½-oz. jar	32
Peach cobbler (Gerber):		
Junior	7¾-oz. jar	20
Strained	4¾-oz. jar	9
Peach melba (Beech-Nut):		
Junior	7¾-oz. jar	20
Strained	4¾-oz. jar	12

Food and Description	Measure or Quantity	Sodium (milligrams)
Pear:		
Junior:		
(Beech-Nut)	7½-oz. jar	5
(Gerber)	7½-oz. jar	6
Strained:		
(Beech-Nut)	4½-oz. jar	0
(Gerber)	7½-oz. jar	4
Pear & pineapple:		
Junior:		
(Beech-Nut)	7½-oz. jar	10
(Gerber)	7½-oz. jar	4
Strained:		
(Beech-Nut)	4½-oz. serving	6
(Gerber)	4½-oz. jar	3
Pineapple dessert (Beech-Nut) strained	4¾-oz. jar	12
Pineapple with yogurt (Beech-Nut):		
Junior	7½-oz. jar	64
Strained	4¾-oz. jar	40
Plum with tapioca (Gerber):		
Junior	7¾-oz. jar	11
Strained	4¾-oz. jar	5
Plum with tapioca & apple juice (Beech-Nut):		
Junior	7¾-oz. jar	15
Strained	4¾-oz. jar	9
Pork (Gerber) strained	3½-oz. jar	38
Pretzel (Gerber)	6-g. piece	15
Prune-orange juice (Beech-Nut) strained	4⅕ fl. oz.	6
Prune with tapioca:		
Junior:		
(Beech-Nut)	7¾-oz. jar	10
(Gerber)	7¾-oz. jar	20
Strained:		
(Beech-Nut)	4¾-oz. jar	6
(Gerber)	4¾-oz. jar	13

Food and Description	Measure or Quantity	Sodium (milligrams)
Similac:		
Ready-to-feed or concentrated liquid, with or without added iron	1 fl. oz.	9
*Powder, regular or with iron	1 fl. oz.	11
Spaghetti, & meatballs (Gerber) toddler	6½-oz. jar	63
Spaghetti, tomato & beef (Beech-Nut) junior	7½-oz. jar	74
Spaghetti with tomato sauce & beef (Gerber) junior	7½-oz. jar	58
Spinach, creamed (Gerber) strained	4½-oz. jar	49
Split pea & ham, junior:		
(Beech-Nut)	7½-oz. jar	55
(Gerber)	7½-oz. jar	36
Squash:		
Junior:		
(Beech-Nut)	7½-oz. jar	5
(Gerber)	7½-oz. jar	4
Strained:		
(Beech-Nut)	4½-oz. jar	3
(Gerber)	4½-oz. jar	5
Sweet potato:		
Junior:		
(Beech-Nut)	7¾-oz. jar	111
(Gerber)	7¾-oz. jar	51
Strained (Gerber)	4¾-oz. jar	24
Turkey (Gerber):		
Junior	3½-oz. jar	50
Strained	3½-oz. jar	56
Turkey & rice (Beech-Nut):		
Junior	7½-oz. jar	55
Strained	4½-oz. jar	33
Turkey & rice with vegetables (Gerber):		
Junior	7½-oz. jar	36
Strained	4½-oz. jar	23

Food and Description	Measure or Quantity	Sodium (milligrams)
Turkey & vegetables, high meat (Gerber):		
Junior	4½-oz. jar	40
Strained	4½-oz. jar	37
Turkey with vegetables & cereal (Beech-Nut) high meat:		
Junior	4½-oz. jar	65
Strained	4½-oz. jar	65
Turkey sticks (Gerber) junior	2½-oz. jar	33
Turkey & turkey broth (Beech-Nut) strained	4½-oz. jar	76
Veal (Gerber):		
Junior	3½-oz. jar	55
Strained	3½-oz. jar	52
Veal & vegetables (Gerber):		
Junior	4½-oz. jar	31
Strained	4½-oz. jar	27
Veal with vegetables & cereal, high meat (Beech-Nut) junior or strained	4½-oz. jar	44
Veal & veal broth (Beech-Nut) strained	4½-oz. jar	88
Vegetable & bacon:		
Junior (Gerber)	7½-oz. jar	121
Strained:		
(Beech-Nut)	4½-oz. jar	141
(Gerber)	4½-oz. jar	79
Vegetable & beef:		
Junior:		
(Beech-Nut)	7½-oz. jar	55
(Gerber)	7½-oz. jar	26
Strained:		
(Beech-Nut)	4½-oz. jar	33
(Gerber)	4½-oz. jar	17
Vegetable & chicken:		
Junior:		
(Beech-Nut)	7½-oz. jar	44
(Gerber)	7½-oz. jar	21
Strained:		
(Beech-Nut)	4½-oz. jar	38

Food and Description	Measure or Quantity	Sodium (milligrams)
(Gerber)	4½-oz. jar	14
Vegetable & ham, strained:		
(Beech-Nut)	4½-oz. jar	33
(Gerber)	4½-oz. jar	15
Vegetable & lamb (Gerber):		
Junior	7½-oz. jar	26
Strained	4½-oz. jar	15
Vegetable & lamb with rice & barley (Beech-Nut):		
Junior	7½-oz. jar	44
Strained	4½-oz. jar	26
Vegetable & liver (Gerber):		
Junior	7½-oz. jar	28
Strained	4½-oz. jar	19
Vegetable & liver with rice & barley (Beech-Nut):		
Junior	7½-oz. jar	44
Strained	4½-oz. jar	26
Vegetable & ham (Gerber)		
Junior	7½-oz. jar	30
Vegetable, mixed:		
Junior:		
(Beech-Nut)	7½-oz. jar	64
(Gerber)	7½-oz. jar	77
Strained:		
Regular	4½-oz. jar	38
Garden	4½-oz. jar	50
(Gerber):		
Regular	4½-oz. jar	27
Garden	4½-oz. jar	28
Vegetable & turkey:		
Junior (Gerber)	7½-oz. jar	32
Strained:		
(Beech-Nut)	4½-oz. jar	26
(Gerber)	4½-oz. jar	20
Vegetable & turkey casserole (Gerber) toddler	6¼-oz. jar	58
BACON, cured:		
Raw (USDA):		
Slab	1 oz. (weighed with rind)	181

Food and Description	Measure or Quantity	Sodium (milligrams)
Sliced	1 oz.	193
Broiled or fried crisp, drained:		
(USDA):		
Medium slice	1 slice (7½ g.)	77
Thick slice	1 slice (12 g.)	123
Thin slice	1 slice (5 g.)	51
(Hormel):		
Black Label	1 slice	149
Range Brand	1 slice	186
(Oscar Mayer):		
Regular	.2-oz. slice	118
Center cut	.2-oz. slice	96
Thick slice	.4-oz. slice	208
BACON BITS:		
(Durkee) imitation	1 tsp. (2 g.)	229
(Estee) imitation	1 tsp.	30
(French's) imitation, crumbles	1 tsp. (2 g.)	55
(General Mills) *Bac*Os*	1 T. (7.6 g.)	230
(Hormel)	1 tsp.	104
(Oscar Mayer) real	1 tsp. (.1 oz.)	56
BACON, CANADIAN:		
Unheated:		
(USDA)	1 oz. (3⅜" dia., ³⁄₁₆" thick)	536
(Eckrich)	1-oz. slice	460
(Hormel) regular	1 oz.	315
(Oscar Mayer) 93% fat free:		
Sliced	.7-oz. slice	272
Sliced	.8-oz. slice	311
Sliced	1-oz. slice	389
Broiled or fried (USDA) drained	1 oz.	726
BACON, SIMULATED, cooked:		
(Oscar Mayer) *Lean 'N Tasty:*		
Beef	1 strip	190
Pork	1 strip	207
(Swift) *Sizzlean*, pork	.4-oz. strip	159
BAGEL:		
(USDA):		
Egg	3" dia. (1.9 oz.)	245
Water	3" dia. (1.9 oz.)	205

Food and Description	Measure or Quantity	Sodium (milligrams)
(Lender's):		
Plain:		
Regular	2-oz. piece	350
Bagelettes	.9-oz. piece	Tr.
Onion	1 bagel	290
Raisin & honey or wheat & raisin with honey	2½-oz. bagel	310
BAKING POWDER:		
(USDA):		
Low sodium	1 tsp (3.7 g.)	<1
Phosphate	1 tsp. (3.8 g.)	312
SAS	1 tsp. (3 g.)	329
Tartrate	1 tsp. (2.8 g.)	204
(Calumet)	1 tsp. (3.8 g.)	396
(Davis)	1 tsp. (.1 oz.)	326
(Featherweight) low sodium	1 tsp.	2
BALSAMPEAR, fresh		
(HEW/FAO):		
Whole	1 lb. (weighed with cavity contents)	7
Flesh only	4 oz.	2
BAMBOO SHOOT, canned:		
(Chun King) drained	8½-oz. can	0
(La Choy) drained	¼ cup (1½ oz.)	0
BANANA (USDA):		
Common yellow:		
Fresh:		
Whole	1 lb. (weighed with skin)	3
Small size	5.9-oz. banana (7¾″ × 11/32″)	1
Medium size	6.2-oz. banana (8 ¾″ × 1 13/32″)	1
Large size	7-oz. banana (9¾″ × 1 7/16″)	1
Mashed	1 cup (about 2 med.)	2
Sliced	1 cup (about 1¼ med.)	1
Dehydrated flakes	½ cup (1.8 oz.)	2

Food and Description	Measure or Quantity	Sodium (milligrams)
Red, fresh, whole	1 lb. (weighed with skin)	3
BANANA NECTAR, canned (Libby's)	6 fl. oz.	5
BARBECUE SEASONING (French's)	1 tsp. (2½ g.)	70
BARLEY, pearled, dry:		
Light (USDA)	¼ cup (1.8 oz.)	2
Pot or Scotch (Quaker)	¼ cup (1.7 oz.)	5
BASIL:		
Fresh (HEW/FAO) sweet, leaves	½ oz.	2
Dried (French's) leaves	1 tsp. (1.1 g.)	Tr.
BASS (USDA) Black Sea, raw, whole	1 lb. (weighed whole)	120
BAY LEAF (French's) dried	1 tsp. (1.3 g.)	Tr.
B.B.Q. SAUCE & BEEF, frozen (Banquet) sliced, *Cookin' Bag*	5-oz. pkg.	885
BEAN, BAKED, canned:		
(USDA):		
With pork & molasses sauce	1 cup (9 oz.)	969
With pork & tomato sauce	1 cup (9 oz.)	1181
With tomato sauce	1 cup (9 oz.)	862
(Allen's) & pork, *Wagon Master*	1 cup (8 oz.)	1200
(B & M) *Brick Oven:*		
Pea bean with pork in brown sugar sauce	8-oz. serving	750
Red kidney in brown sugar sauce	½ of 16-oz. can	640
Yellow eye bean in brown sugar sauce	½ of 16-oz. can	770
(Campbell):		
Home style	8-oz. can	1130
Old fashioned, in molasses & brown sugar sauce	8-oz. can	1060
With pork & tomato sauce	8-oz. can	820

Food and Description	Measure or Quantity	Sodium (milligrams)
(Friend's):		
Pea	9-oz. can	1270
Red kidney	9-oz. can	1320
Yellow eye	9-oz. can	1470
(Furman's) & pork, in tomato sauce	8 oz.	718
(Hormel) *Short Orders:*		
With bacon	7½-oz. can	813
With ham	7½-oz. can	1182
(Hunt's) & pork	8 oz.	800
(Van Camp):		
& pork	8 oz.	1005
Vegetarian style	8 oz.	959
BEAN BARBECUE (Campbell)	7⅞-oz. can	1110
BEAN, BAYO, black or brown (USDA) dry	4 oz.	28
BEAN, BLACK (USDA) dry	4 oz.	28
BEAN, BROWN (USDA) dry	4 oz.	28
BEAN, CALICO (USDA) dry	4 oz.	11
BEAN, CHILI (See **CHILI**)		
BEAN & FRANKFURTER, canned:		
(USDA)	1 cup (9 oz.)	1374
(Campbell) in tomato & molasses sauce	7⅞-oz. serving	1140
(Hormel) & weiners, *Short Orders*	7½-oz. can	1342
BEAN & FRANKFURTER DINNER, frozen:		
(Banquet)	10¼-oz. dinner	1377
(Morton)	10¾-oz. dinner	1000
(Swanson)	12½-oz. dinner	1100
BEAN, GARBANZO, canned:		
Regular (Old El Paso) solids & liq.	½ cup	247
Dietetic (S&W) *Nutradiet,* solids & liq.	½ cup	<10
BEAN, GREEN or SNAP:		
Fresh (USDA):		
Whole	1 lb. (weighed untrimmed)	28

Food and Description	Measure or Quantity	Sodium (milligrams)
French style	½ cup (1.4 oz.)	3
Boiled (USDA):		
Whole, drained	½ cup (2.2 oz.)	2
Pieces, 1½" to 2", drained	½ cup (2.4 oz.)	3
Canned, regular pack:		
(USDA):		
Whole, solids & liq.	½ cup (4.2 oz.)	283
Whole, drained solids	4 oz.	268
Cut, drained solids	½ cup (2.5 oz.)	165
Drained, liquid only	4 oz.	268
(Allen's) solids & liq.:		
Regular, cut, french or whole	½ cup	350
Cut with dry, shelled beans	½ cup	230
(Comstock) cut or French style, solids & liq.	½ cup (4.2 oz.)	400
(Del Monte):		
Cut, solids & liq.	½ cup (4 oz.)	447
Cut, drained solids	½ cup (4 oz.)	445
(Green Giant) whole, cut or French style, solids & liq.	½ cup	270
(Larsen) any style, *Freshlike*, solids & liq.	½ cup	340
(Libby's):		
Cut, Blue Lake, solids & liq.	¼ of 16-oz. can	333
French style, Blue Lake, solids & liq.	¼ of 16-oz. can	335
Whole, Blue Lake, solids & liq.	¼ of 16-oz. can	351
(Stokely-Van Camp) cut, sliced or whole, solids & liq.	½ cup (4.2 oz.)	103
(Sunshine) solids & liq.	½ cup (4.2 oz.)	312
Canned, dietetic or low calorie:		
(USDA):		
Solids & liq.	4 oz.	2
Drained Solids	4 oz.	2
(Del Monte) no salt added, solids & liq.	½ cup	<10

Food and Description	Measure or Quantity	Sodium (milligrams)
(Diet Delight) solids & liq.	½ cup (4.2 oz.)	5
(Featherweight) cut or French style, solids & liq.	½ cup (4 oz.)	<10
(Larsen) *Fresh-Lite*, solids & liq.	½ cup	6
(S&W) *Nutradiet*, cut, solids & liq., green label	½ cup	<10
Frozen:		
(USDA):		
Cut or French style, unthawed	10-oz. pkg.	3
Cut or French style, boiled, drained	½ cup (2.8 oz.)	<1
(Birds Eye):		
Cut	⅓ of 9-oz. pkg.	0
French	⅓ of 9-oz. pkg.	0
French, with almonds	⅓ of 9-oz. pkg.	340
Whole, deluxe	⅓ of 9-oz. pkg.	0
(Frosty Acres)	3 oz.	0
(Green Giant):		
Cut or French, in butter sauce	½ cup	355
Cut, *Harvest Fresh*	½ cup	175
With mushrooms in cream sauce	½ cup	280
Polybag	½ cup	5
(Larsen) any style	3 oz.	5
(McKenzie) cut or French	3 oz.	17
(Southland)	⅕ of 16-oz. pkg.	0
BEAN, GREEN, MUSHROOM, CASSEROLE, frozen (Stouffer's)	4¾ oz.	675
BEAN, ITALIAN, frozen:		
(Birds Eye)	3 oz.	0
(Frosty Acres)	3 oz.	0
(Larsen)	3 oz.	5
BEAN, KIDNEY or RED:		
(USDA):		
Dry	1 lb.	45
Dry	½ cup (3.3. oz.)	9
Cooked	½ cup (3.3. oz.)	6

Food and Description	Measure or Quantity	Sodium (milligrams)
Canned, solids & liq.:		
Regular:		
(Allen's) dark or light	½ cup	290
(Comstock)	½ cup	410
(Hunt's):		
Regular	4 oz.	400
Small	½ cup (3½ oz.)	500
(Van Camp):		
Dark	8 oz.	732
Light	8 oz.	680
New Orleans style	8 oz.	793
Red	8 oz.	930
Dietetic (S&W) *Nutradiet*	½ cup	<10
BEAN, LIMA:		
Raw (USDA):		
Young, whole	1 lb. (weighed in pod)	4
Mature, dry	½ cup (3.4 oz.)	4
Young, without shell	1 lb. (weighed shelled)	9
Boiled (USDA) mature, drained	½ cup (3.4 oz.)	2
Canned, regular pack:		
(USDA) drained solids	½ cup (3 oz.)	201
(Allen's) solids & liq.:		
Regular	½ cup (4 oz.)	370
Large butter	½ cup (4 oz.)	330
(Comstock) solids & liq.:		
Regular	½ cup	400
Butter	½ cup	500
(Del Monte) solids & liq.	½ cup (4 oz.)	355
(Furman's) butter, solids & liq.	½ cup (3.9 oz.)	459
(Larsen's) *Freshlike*, solids & liq.	½ cup (4 oz.)	320
Canned, dietetic or low calorie:		
(USDA):		
Low sodium, solids & liq.	4 oz.	5
Low sodium, drained solids	4 oz.	5
(Featherweight) solids & liq.	½ cup	25

Food and Description	Measure or Quantity	Sodium (milligrams)
(Larsen) *Fresh-Lite*, solids & liq.	½ cup	6
Frozen:		
(USDA):		
Baby, unthawed	4 oz.	167
Fordhooks, unthawed	4 oz.	115
Boiled, drained solids	½ cup (3.1 oz.)	114
Boiled, Fordhooks, drained	½ cup (3 oz.)	86
(Birds Eye):		
Baby	⅓ of pkg.	115
Fordhooks	⅓ of pkg.	100
(Frosty Acres):		
Baby	3.3 oz.	125
Butter	3.2 oz.	213
Fordhook	3.3 oz.	70
(Green Giant):		
Baby, in butter sauce	½ cup	445
Harvest Fresh	½ cup	310
Polybag	½ cup	30
(Larsen) baby	3.3 oz.	100
(McKenzie):		
Baby	3.3 oz.	117
Fordhook	3.3 oz.	94
Speckled butter	3.3 oz.	28
(Southland) speckled butter bean	⅕ of 16-oz. pkg.	17
BEAN, MUNG (USDA) dry	½ cup (3.7 oz.)	6
BEAN, PINTO:		
Dry (USDA)	½ cup (3.4 oz.)	10
Canned (Gebhardt)	½ cup (4.3 oz.)	654
BEAN, RED MEXICAN, dry (USDA)	4 oz.	11
BEAN REFRIED, canned:		
(Del Monte):		
Regular	½ cup (4.3 oz.)	530
Spicy	½ cup (4.3 oz.)	480
(Gebhardt):		
Regular	4 oz.	490
Jalapeño	4 oz.	320
Little Pancho	½ cup	330

Food and Description	Measure or Quantity	Sodium (milligrams)
(Old El Paso):		
Plain	4 oz.	593
With green chili pepper	4 oz.	317
With sausage	4 oz.	355
(Rosarita):		
Regular or vegetarian	4 oz.	460
With green chiles	4 oz.	430
Spicy	4 oz.	440
BEAN SALAD, canned (Green Giant)	¼ of 17-oz. can	540
BEANS 'N FIXIN'S (Hunt's) canned, *Big John's:*		
Beans	3 oz.	370
Fixin's	1 oz.	125
BEAN SPROUT:		
Fresh (USDA) Mung:		
Raw	½ lb.	11
Raw	½ cup (1.6 oz.)	2
Boiled, drained	½ cup (2.2. oz.)	2
Canned (La Choy) drained	⅔ cup (2 oz.)	18
BEAN, WAX (*See* **BEAN, YELLOW**)		
BEAN, WHITE (USDA):		
Raw:		
Great Northern	½ cup (3.1 oz.)	17
Navy or pea	½ cup	20
White	1 oz.	5
Cooked:		
Great Northern	½ cup (3 oz.)	6
Navy or pea	½ cup (3.4 oz.)	7
All other white	4-oz. serving	8
BEAN, YELLOW OR WAX:		
Raw, whole (USDA)	1 lb. (weighed untrimmed)	28
Boiled, drained (USDA) 1″ pieces	½ cup (2.9 oz.)	2
Canned, regular pack:		
(USDA):		
Solids & liq.	½ cup (4.2 oz.)	283
Drained solids	½ cup (2.2 oz.)	146
Drained, liquid only	4 oz.	26

Food and Description	Measure or Quantity	Sodium (milligrams)
(Comstock) solids & liq.	½ cup	370
(Del Monte), solids & liq.	½ cup (4 oz.)	355
(Festal):		
Cut, solids & liq.	½ cup	332
French-style, solids & liq.	½ cup (4 oz.)	383
(Larsen) *Freshlike*, cut, solids & liq.	½ cup (4.2 oz.)	320
Canned, dietetic or low calorie:		
(USDA):		
Solids & liq.	4-oz. serving	2
Drained solids	4-oz. serving	2
(Blue Boy) solids & liq.	4-oz. serving	2
(Featherweight) cut, solids & liq.	½ cup	<10
(Larsen) *Fresh-Lite*, solids & liq.	½ cup	6
Frozen:		
(USDA) cut, unthawed	4-oz. serving	1
(Frosty Acres)	3 oz.	5
(Larsen) cut	3 oz.	5
(McKenzie) cut	3 oz.	1

BEEF. Values for beef cuts are given below for "lean and fat" and for "lean only." Beef purchased by the consumer at the retail store usually is trimmed to about one-half inch layer of fat. This is the meat described as "lean and fat." If all the fat that can be cut off with a knife is removed, the remainder is the "lean only." These cuts still contain flecks of fat known as 'marbling" distributed through the meat. Cooked meats are medium done. Choice grade cuts (USDA): Brisket:

Raw	1 lb. (weighed with bone)	248
Braised lean only	4 oz.	68

Food and Description	Measure or Quantity	Sodium (milligrams)
Chuck:		
Raw	1 lb. (weighed with bone)	248
Braised or pot-roasted lean only	4 oz.	68
Dried (See **BEEF CHIPPED**)		
Filet mignon. There are no data available on its composition. For dietary estimates, the data for sirloin, lean only, afford the closest approximation.		
Flank:		
Raw	1 lb.	295
Braised	4 oz.	68
Foreshank:		
Raw	1 lb. (weighed with bone)	165
Simmered:		
Lean & fat	4 oz.	68
Lean only	4 oz.	68
Ground:		
Lean:		
Raw	1 lb.	236
Raw	1 cup (8 oz.)	118
Broiled	4 oz.	54
Regular		
Raw	1 lb.	295
Raw	1 cup (8 oz.)	147
Broiled	4 oz.	53
Heel of round:		
Raw	1 lb.	295
Roasted:		
Lean & fat	4 oz.	68
Lean only	4 oz.	68
Hindshank:		
Raw	1 lb. (weighed with bone)	136
Simmered:		
Lean & fat	4 oz.	68
Lean only	4 oz.	68

Food and Description	Measure or Quantity	Sodium (milligrams)
Neck:		
Raw	1 lb. (weighed with bone)	236
Pot-roasted:		
Lean & fat	4 oz.	51
Lean only	4 oz.	68
Plate:		
Raw	1 lb. (weighed with bone)	263
Simmered lean & fat	4 oz.	68
Rib roast:		
Raw	1 lb. (weighed with bone)	271
Roasted, lean & fat	4 oz.	68
Round:		
Raw:		
Lean & fat	1 lb. (weighed with bone)	286
Lean & fat	1 lb. (weighed without bone)	295
Roasted:	1 lb. (weighed with bone)	286
Broiled:		
Lean & fat	4 oz.	68
Lean only	4 oz.	68
Steak, club:		
Raw	1 lb. (weighed without bone)	295
Broiled:		
Lean & fat	4 oz.	68
Lean only	4 oz.	68
Steak, porterhouse:		
Raw	1 lb. (weighed with bone)	268
Broiled:		
Lean & fat	4 oz.	68
Lean only	4 oz.	68
Steak, ribeye, broiled:		
One 10-oz. steak (weighed before cooking without bone) will give you lean & fat	7.3 oz	147

Food and Description	Measure or Quantity	Sodium (milligrams)
Steak, sirloin, double-bone:		
Raw	1 lb. (weighed with bone)	242
Broiled:		
Lean & fat	4 oz.	68
Lean only	4 oz.	68
One 16-oz. steak (weighed before cooking with bone) will give you:		
Lean & fat	8.9 oz.	151
Lean only	5.9 oz.	100
One 12-oz. steak (weighed before cooking with bone) will give you:		
Lean & fat	6.6 oz.	113
Lean only	4.4 oz.	74
Steak, sirloin, hipbone:		
Raw	1 lb. (weighed with bone)	251
Broiled:		
Lean & fat	4 oz.	68
Lean only	4 oz.	68
Steak, sirloin, wedge & round-bone:		
Raw	1 lb. (weighed with bone)	274
Broiled:		
Lean & fat	4 oz.	68
Lean only	4 oz.	68
Steak T-bone:		
Raw	1 lb. (weighed with bone)	263
Broiled:		
Lean & fat	4 oz.	68
Lean only	4 oz.	68
One 16-oz. steak (weighed before cooking with bone) will give you:		
Broiled:		
Lean & fat	4 oz.	167

Food and Description	Measure or Quantity	Sodium (milligrams)
Lean only	4 oz.	94
BEEFAMATO COCKTAIL,		
canned (Mott's)	6 fl. oz.	240
BEEF BOUILLON, cubes or powder:		
(Borden) *Lite-Line*, instant, low sodium	1 tsp.	5
(Featherweight) cube or instant, low sodium	1 cube or 1 tsp.	10
(Herb-Ox):		
Cube	1 cube (3.7 g.)	500
Powder	1 packet (4.5 g.)	1040
(Maggi)	1 cube (3½ g.)	743
MBT	1 packet (5½ g.)	755
(Wyler's) cube or instant	1 cube or 1 tsp.	930
BEEF, CHIPPED:		
Home recipe (USDA) creamed	½ cup (4.3 oz.)	877
Frozen, creamed:		
(Banquet)	4-oz. pkg.	818
(Stouffer's)	11-oz. entree	1800
(Swanson)	10½-oz. entree	1545
BEEF, CORNED (See **CORNED BEEF**)		
BEEF DINNER OR ENTREE, frozen:		
(Armour):		
Classic Lites		
Steak Diane	10-oz. meal	770
Dinner Classics:		
Burgundy	10½-oz. meal	990
Sirloin tips	11-oz. meal	1180
(Banquet):		
American favorites:		
Chopped	11-oz. dinner	1199
With gravy	10-oz. dinner	1009
Extra Helping:		
Regular	16-oz. dinner	1731
Chopped	18-oz. dinner	1792
(Blue Star) *Dining Lite*, teriyaki, with vegetables & rice	8⅝-oz. meal	980

Food and Description	Measure or Quantity	Sodium (milligrams)
(Conagra) *Light & Elegant*:		
Burgundy	9-oz. entree	1240
Julienne	8½-oz. entree	990
(Le Menu):		
Chopped sirloin	11½-oz. dinner	840
Sirloin tips	12¼-oz. dinner	1080
Yankee pot roast	11-oz. dinner	810
(Morton):		
Regular	11-oz. dinner	700
Light, sliced	11-oz. dinner	850
(Stouffer's) *Lean Cuisine*, oriental, in sauce with vegetable & rice	8⅝-oz. meal	1150
(Swanson) *Hungry Man:*		
Chopped	17¼-oz. dinner	1640
Sliced, dinner	16-oz. dinner	1150
Sliced, entree	12¼-oz. entree	1040
(Weight Watchers):		
Beefsteak	8¹⁵⁄₁₆-oz. meal	980
Oriental	10-oz. meal	1130
BEEF, DRIED, packaged (Hormel) sliced	1 oz.	822
BEEF, GROUND, SEASONING MIX:		
*(Durkee) regular or with onion	1 cup	1099
(French's) with onion	1⅛-oz. pkg.	1760
BEEF HASH, ROAST, canned, *Mary Kitchen* (Hormel):		
Regular	7½-oz. serving	1142
Short Orders	7½-oz. can	1156
BEEF PACKAGED:		
(Carl Buddig) smoked	1 oz.	426
(Hormel)	1 oz.	382
BEEF PEPPER ORIENTAL (La Choy):		
Canned	¾ cup	1060
Frozen	12-oz. dinner	1985
BEEF PIE:		
Home recipe (USDA) baked	4¼" pie (8 oz. before baking)	645

Food and Description	Measure or Quantity	Sodium (milligrams)
Frozen:		
(Banquet)	8-oz. pie	1292
(Stouffer's)	10-oz. pie	1600
(Swanson):		
Regular	8-oz. pie	900
Chunky	10-oz. pie	900
Hungry Man	16-oz. pie	1750
Hungry Man, steak burger	16-oz. pie	1520
BEEF ROLL (Hormel)		
Lumberjack	1 oz.	304
BEEF SHORT RIBS, frozen:		
(Armour) *Dinner Classics*, boneless	10½-oz.meal	1180
(Stouffer's) boneless, with vegetable gravy	5¾ oz.	560
BEEF SOUP (See **SOUP**, Beef)		
BEEF SPREAD, ROAST, canned (Underwood)	½ of 4¾-oz. can	515
BEEF STEW:		
Home recipe (USDA)	1 cup	91
Canned, regular pack:		
(USDA)	1 cup (8.6 oz.)	1007
Dinty Moore (Hormel):		
Regular	⅓ of 24-oz. can	980
Short Orders	7½-oz. can	939
Canned, dietetic or low calorie:		
(Dia-Mel)	8-oz. can	70
(Estee)	7½-oz. can	110
(Featherweight)	7½-oz. can	96
Frozen:		
(Banquet) *Family Entree*	2-lb. pkg.	3908
(Green Giant) Boil in Bag	9-oz. pkg.	275
(Stouffer's)	10 oz.	1675
BEEF STEW SEASONING MIX:		
*(Durkee)	1 cup	975
(French's)	1⅞-oz. pkg.	4620
BEEF STOCK BASE (French's)	1 tsp. (4 g.)	500
BEEF STROGANOFF, frozen:		
(Armour) *Dinner Classics*	11¼-oz. meal	1330

Food and Description	Measure or Quantity	Sodium (milligrams)
(Conagra) *Light & Elegant*	9-oz. entree	790
(Green Giant) twin pouch, with noodles	9-oz. entree	820
(Le Menu)	9¼-oz. dinner	930
(Stouffer's) with parsley, noodles	9¾-oz. meal	1300
*BEEF STROGANOFF SEASONING MIX (Durkee)	1 cup	870
BEER, canned:		
Regular:		
Budweiser	12 fl. oz.	5–15
Busch	12 fl. oz.	5–15
Michelob	12 fl. oz.	18
Pabst Blue Ribbon	12 fl. oz.	7
Light:		
Budweiser Light	12 fl. oz.	5–15
Gablinger's	12 fl. oz.	21
Michelob Light	12 fl. oz.	5–15
Natural Light	12 fl. oz.	5–15
BEER, NEAR, *Kingsbury* (Heileman)	12 fl. oz.	28
BEET:		
Raw (USDA):		
Whole	1 lb. (weighed with skins, without tops)	190
Diced	½ cup (2.4 oz.)	40
Boiled (USDA) drained:		
Whole	2 beets (2" dia., 3.5 oz.)	43
Diced	½ cup (3 oz.)	18
Sliced	½ cup (3.6 oz.)	44
Canned, regular pack, solids & liq.:		
(Blue Boy) harvard	½ cup	350
(Comstock):		
Regular	½ cup	100
Pickled	½ cup	500
(Del Monte):		
Pickled, sliced	½ cup (4 oz.)	375

Food and Description	Measure or Quantity	Sodium (milligrams)
Sliced, solids & liq.	½ cup (4. oz.)	290
(Larsen) *Freshlike*:		
Pickled	½ cup (4.3 oz.)	650
Sliced or whole	½ cup (4.7 oz.)	260
(Stokely-Van Camp):		
Cut	½ cup	253
Diced	½ cup	260
Harvard	½ cup (4½ oz.)	123
Pickled	½ cup (4.3 oz.)	290
Whole	½ cup (4.3 oz.)	223
Canned, dietetic pack, solids & liq.:		
(USDA)	½ cup (4.4 oz.)	57
(Comstock) water pack	½ cup	100
(Del Monte) no salt added	½ cup	100
(Featherweight) sliced	½ cup	55
(Larsen) *Fresh-Lite*, no salt added	½ cup	49
(S&W) *Nutradiet*, sliced	½ cup	40
BEET GREENS (USDA):		
Raw, whole	1 lb. (weighed untrimmed)	330
Boiled, leaves & stems, drained	½ cup (2.6 oz.)	55
BEET PUREE, canned, dietetic pack (Larsen)	1 cup	120
BERRY DRINK, canned, *Ssips* (Johanna Farms)	8.45-fl.-oz. container	15
BIG H, burger sauce (Hellmann's)	1 T.	143
BIG MAC (See McDONALD'S)		
BIG WHEEL (Hostess)	1.3-oz. cake	132
BISCUIT, home recipe (USDA) baking powder	1-oz. biscuit (2″ dia.)	175
BISCUIT DOUGH, refrigerated (Pillsbury):		
Baking Powder, *1869 Brand*	1 biscuit	293
Big Country	1 biscuit	358
Big Country, Good 'N Buttery	1 biscuit	355

Food and Description	Measure or Quantity	Sodium (milligrams)
Buttermilk:		
Regular	1 biscuit	215
Ballard Oven Ready	1 biscuit	300
1869 Brand	1 biscuit	295
Extra Lights	1 biscuit	263
Extra rich, *Hungry Jack*	1 biscuit	205
Flaky, *Hungry Jack*	1 biscuit	290
Fluffy, *Hungry Jack*	1 biscuit	303
Butter Tastin', 1869 Brand	1 biscuit	295
Butter Tastin', Hungry Jack	1 biscuit	275
Country style	1 biscuit	215
Dinner, baking powder or buttermilk tenderflake	1 biscuit	175
Flaky, *Hungry Jack*	1 biscuit	290
Heat 'N Eat, *1869 Brand*	1 biscuit	283
Oven Ready, Ballard	1 biscuit	300
Prize	1 biscuit	232
*BISCUIT MIX (USDA) baked from mix, with added milk	1-oz. biscuit	276
BITTERS (Angostura)	1 tsp. (4.6 g.)	Tr.
BLACKBERRY:		
Fresh (USDA) includes boysenberry, dewberry, youngsberry:		
With hulls	1 lb. (weighed untrimmed)	4
Hulled	½ cup (2.6 oz.)	Tr.
Canned, regular pack (USDA) solids & liq.:		
Juice pack	4-oz. serving	1
Light syrup	4-oz. serving	1
Heavy syrup	½ cup (4.6 oz.)	1
Extra heavy syrup	4-oz. serving	1
Frozen (USDA):		
Sweetened, unthawed	4-oz. serving	1
Unsweetened, unthawed	4-oz. serving	1
BLACKBERRY JELLY:		
Sweetened:		
(Home Brands)	1 T.	15
(Smucker's)	1 T.	4
Dietetic (See **BLACKBERRY SPREAD**)		

Food and Description	Measure or Quantity	Sodium (milligrams)
BLACKBERRY JUICE, canned		
(USDA) unsweetened	½ cup	1
BLACKBERRY PRESERVE or JAM:		
Sweetened (Smucker's)	1 T. (.7 oz.)	2
Dietetic or low calorie:		
(Dia-Mel)	1 T.	<3
(Diet Delight)	1 T.	19
(Louis Sherry)	1 T.	<3
BLACKBERRY SPREAD, low sugar:		
(Diet Delight)	1 T.	45
(Featherweight)	1 T.	40-50
(Slenderella)	1 T.	16
(Smucker's)	1 T.	16
BLACK-EYED PEA (See also **COWPEA**):		
Canned:		
(Allen's) regular	½ cup	370
(Goya)	½ cup	486
(Trappey's):		
With bacon, in sauce	½ cup	410
With jalapeño pepper & bacon, in sauce	½ cup	480
Frozen:		
(USDA) boiled, drained	½ cup (3 oz.)	33
(Frosty Acres)	3.3 oz.	5
(Larsen)	3.3 oz.	5
(McKenzie)	3.3 oz.	19
(Southland)	⅕ of 16-oz. pkg.	5
BLANCMANGE (See **PUDDING OR PIE FILLING,** Vanilla)		
BLINTZ, frozen:		
(Empire Kosher):		
Apple	2½-oz. piece	115
Blueberry	2½-oz. piece	116
Cherry	2½-oz. piece	105
Cheese	2½-oz. piece	126
Potato	2½-oz. piece	224
(King Kold) cheese	2½-oz. piece	250

Food and Description	Measure or Quantity	Sodium (milligrams)
BLOODY MARY MIX:		
(Bar-Tender's) dry	1 serving	510
(Holland House) liquid, *Smooth*		
& Spicy	1 oz.	329
BLUEBERRY:		
Fresh (USDA):		
Whole	1 lb. (weighed untrimmed)	4
Trimmed	½ cup (2.6 oz.)	<1
Canned solids & liq.:		
(USDA):		
Syrup pack, extra heavy	½ cup (4.4 oz.)	1
Water pack	½ cup (4.3 oz.)	1
(Thank You Brand):		
Heavy syrup	½ cup (4.3 oz.)	6
Water pack	½ cup (4.2 oz.)	<1
Frozen (USDA):		
Sweetened, solids & liq.	½ cup (4 oz.)	1
Unsweetened, solids & liq.	½ cup (2.9 oz.)	<1
BLUEBERRY PIE (See **PIE,** Blueberry)		
BLUEBERRY PRESERVE or JAM, sweetened (Smucker's)	1 T.	6
BLUEFISH (USDA):		
Raw:		
Whole	1 lb. (weighed whole)	171
Meat only	4 oz.	84
Baked or broiled, with butter or margarine	4.4-oz. piece (3½″ × 3″ × ½″)	130
Fried, prepared with egg, milk or water & bread crumbs	5.3-oz. piece (3½″ × 3″ × ½″)	219
BODY BUDDIES, cereal (General Mills):		
Brown sugar & honey	1 cup (1 oz.)	290
Natural fruit flavor	1 cup (1 oz.)	280

Food and Description	Measure or Quantity	Sodium (milligrams)
BOLOGNA:		
(Ekrich):		
Beef:		
Regular	1 slice (8-oz. pkg.)	280
Smorgas Pac	¾-oz. slice	230
Thick sliced	1.5-oz. slice	400
Thick sliced	1.8-oz. slice	510
Garlic	1-oz. slice	290
German brand:		
Chub	1 oz.	360
Sliced	1-oz. slice	350
Lunch, chub	1 oz.	290
Meat:		
Regular	1-oz. slice	290
Smorgas Pac	¾-oz. slice	230
Smorgas Pac	1-oz. slice	310
Thick sliced	1.7-oz. slice	490
Thin sliced	1 slice	160
Ring:		
Regular	1 oz.	280
Pickled	1 oz.	290
Sandwich	1-oz. slice	310
(Hormel):		
Beef:		
Regular	1 slice	296
Ring, coarse ground	1 oz.	288
Coarse ground, ring	1 oz.	289
Fine ground, ring	1 oz.	298
Meat, regular	1 slice	300
(Ohse):		
Beef	1 oz.	310
15% chicken	1 oz.	320
Chicken, beef & pork	1 oz.	280
(Oscar Mayer):		
Beef:		
Regular	.5-oz. slice	165
Regular	.8-oz. slice	253
Thick slice	1.3-oz. slice	418
Meat:		
Round	.8-oz. slice	241

Food and Description	Measure or Quantity	Sodium (milligrams)
Square	1-oz. slice	298
Thick, round	1.3-oz. slice	398
Thin, round	.5-oz. slice	157
BOLOGNA & CHEESE, packaged:		
(Eckrich)	.7-oz. slice	290
(Oscar Mayer)	.8-oz. slice	242
BOO*BERRY, cereal		
(General Mills)	1 cup (1 oz.)	210
BORSCHT, canned:		
Regular pack (Mother's) old fashioned	8-oz. serving	907
Dietetic or low calorie:		
(Manischewitz)	8 oz.	725
(Mother's):		
Artificially sweetened	8-oz. serving	943
Unsalted	8-oz. serving	51
(Rokeach) unsalted	1 cup (8 fl. oz.)	50
BOURBON WHISKEY, un-flavored (See **DISTILLED LIQUOR**)		
BOYSENBERRY:		
Fresh (See **BLACKBERRY**)		
Frozen (USDA) sweetened	10-oz. pkg.	3
BOYSENBERRY JELLY, sweetened (Smucker's)	1 T. (.7 oz.)	3
BOYSENBERRY PRESERVE or JAM:		
Sweetened:		
(Home Brands)	1 T.	15
(Smucker's)	1 T.	5
Dietetic or low calorie		
(Slenderella)	1 T. (.6 oz.)	16
BRAINS, all animals, raw (USDA)	1 oz.	35
BRAN:		
Crude (USDA)	1 oz.	3
Miller's (Elam's)	1 oz.	5
BRAN BREAKFAST CEREAL:		
(Kellogg's)		
All-Bran	⅓ cup (1 oz.)	270

Food and Description	Measure or Quantity	Sodium (milligrams)
Bran-Buds	⅓ cup (1 oz.)	150
Cracklin' Oat Bran	½ cup (1 oz.)	190
40% bran flakes	¾ cup (1 oz.)	220
Fruitful Bran	¾ cup	230
Raisin	¾ cup (1.3 oz.)	210
(Loma Linda)	1 oz.	115
(Post):		
40% bran flakes	(1 oz.)	230
With raisins	(1 oz.)	180
(Quaker) *Corn Bran*	⅔ cup (1 oz.)	245
(Ralston Purina):		
Bran Chex	⅔ cup (1 oz.)	267
40% bran flakes	⅔ cup (1 oz.)	294
Honey bran	⅞ cup (1 oz.)	157
Raisin	¾ cup (1 oz.)	286
BRANDY, unflavored (See **DISTILLED LIQUOR**		
BRAUNSCHWEIGER:		
(Eckrich) chub	1 oz.	400
(Hormel)	1 oz.	322
(Oscar Mayer) Chub	1-oz. serving	319
BRAZIL NUT:		
Whole, in shell (USDA)	1 cup (4.3 oz.)	Tr.
Shelled (USDA)	½ cup (2½ oz.)	<1
Shelled (USDA)	4 nuts (.6 oz.)	<1
Roasted (Fisher)	¼ cup (1 oz.)	57
BREAD (listed by type or brand name):		
Boston Brown (USDA)	1.7-oz. slice 3″ × ¾″)	120
Bran'nola (Arnold)	1.3-oz. slice	135
Cinnamon (Pepperidge Farm)	.9-oz. slice	100
Cracked-wheat:		
(USDA) 18 slices to 1 lb.	.8-oz. slice	122
(Pepperidge Farm) thin	.9-oz. slice	145
(Wonder)	1-oz. slice	151
Crisp Bread, *Wasa:*		
Mora	3¼-oz. slice	514
Rye:		
Golden	.4-oz. slice	43

Food and Description	Measure or Quantity	Sodium (milligrams)
Lite	.3-oz. slice	20
Sesame	.5-oz. slice	35
Sport	.4-oz. slice	66
Flatbread, *Ideal:*		
Bran	.2-oz. slice	47
Extra thin	.1-oz. slice	25
Whole grain	.2-oz. slice	47
French:		
(USDA)	.8-oz. slice	133
(Arnold) *Francisco,* regular	1/16 of loaf	110
(Wonder)	1-oz. slice	170
Garlic (Arnold)	1-oz. slice	120
Hi-fibre (Monks')	1-oz. slice	110
Hillbilly (Wonder)	1-oz. slice	170
Hollywood (Wonder):		
Dark	1-oz. slice	162
Light	1-oz. slice	170
Honey bran (Pepperidge Farm)	1.2-oz. slice	175
Honey Wheatberry:		
(Arnold)	1.1-oz. slice	140
(Pepperidge Farm)	.9-oz. slice	163
Italian:		
(USDA)	1-oz. slice	166
(Arnold) *Francisco*	1 slice	110
(Pepperidge Farm)	2-oz. serving	320
Low sodium (Wonder)	1-oz. slice	3
Multi-Grain:		
(Arnold) *Milk & Honey*	1-oz. slice	150
(Pepperidge Farm) thin	.5-oz. slice	75
Oat (Arnold):		
Bran'nola	1.3-oz. slice	170
Milk & Honey	1-oz. slice	150
Oatmeal (Pepperidge Farm)	.9-oz. slice	185
Protein (Thomas)	.7-oz. slice	94
Pumpernickel:		
(USDA) regular size	1.1-oz. slice (5″ × 4″ × ⅜″)	178
(USDA) snack size	7 g. (2½″ × 2″ × ¼″)	40
(Arnold)	1.1-oz. slice	200

Food and Description	Measure or Quantity	Sodium (milligrams)
(Levy's)	1.1-oz. slice	200
(Pepperidge Farm):		
Regular	1.1-oz. slice	305
Party	.2-oz. slice	55
Raisin:		
(USDA)	.9-oz. slice	91
(Arnold) tea	.9-oz. slice	85
(Monks') & cinnamon	1-oz. slice	85
(Pepperidge Farm) cinnamon	.9-oz. slice	95
Roman Meal	1-oz. slice	159
Rye:		
(USDA) light:		
Regular size	.9 oz. (4¾″ × 3¾″ × ⁷⁄₁₆″ slice)	142
Snack size	7 g. (2½″ × 2″ × ¼″ slice)	39
(Arnold):		
Dill, with seeds	1.1-oz. slice	190
Jewish, with or without seeds	1.1-oz. slice	170
Melba thin	.7-oz. slice	110
(Levy's)	1.1-oz. slice	170
(Pepperidge Farm):		
Family	1.1-oz. slice	245
Party, fresh or frozen	.2-oz. slice	104
(Wonder)	1-oz. slice	170
Sahara (Thomas'):		
White:		
Regular	2-oz. piece	300
Mini	1-oz. piece	150
Large	3-oz. piece	440
Whole wheat:		
Regular	2-oz. piece	320
Mini	1-oz. piece	150
Salt rising (USDA)	.9-oz. slice	66
7-Grain (Home Pride)	1-oz. slice	135
Sourdough, *DiCarlo*	1-oz. slice	156
Sunflower & bran (Monks')	1-oz. slice	80
Toaster cake (See **TOASTER CAKE or PASTRY**)		

Food and Description	Measure or Quantity	Sodium (milligrams)
Vienna (USDA)	.8-oz. slice	133
Wheat (See also Cracked Wheat, *Honey Wheatberry* and Whole Wheat):		
America's Own (Arnold):	1-oz. slice	155
Bran'nola:		
Dark	1.3-oz. slice	170
Hearty	1.3-oz. slice	200
Brick Oven	.8-oz. slice	100
Country	1.3-oz. slice	150
Less or Liteway	.8-oz. slice	120
Milk & Honey	1-oz. slice	160
Very thin	.5-oz. slice	65
Fresh Horizons	1-oz. slice	148
Fresh & Natural	1-oz. slice	135
Home Pride, butter top (Pepperidge Farm):	1-oz. slice	156
Family	.9-oz. slice	195
Sandwich	.8-oz. slice	115
(Wonder)	1-oz. slice	148
Wheatberry, *Home Pride*	1-oz. slice	151
White:		
(USDA):		
Prepared with 1–4% non-fat dry milk	.8-oz. slice	117
Prepared with 5–6% non-fat dry milk	.8-oz. slice	114
America's Own, cottage (Arnold):	1-oz. slice	180
Brick Oven:		
.8-oz. slice	.8-oz. slice	130
2-lb. loaf	1.1-oz. slice	160
Country	1.3-oz. slice	200
Less	.8-oz. slice	120
Liteway	.8-oz. slice	130
Milk & Honey	1-oz. slice	160
Very thin	.5-oz. slice	85
Fresh Horizons	1-oz. slice	142
Home Pride, butter top	1-oz. slice	149

Food and Description	Measure or Quantity	Sodium (milligrams)
(Monks')	1-oz. slice	95
(Pepperidge Farm):		
Regular	1.2-oz. slice	135
Toasting	1.1-oz. slice	230
Very thin slice	.6-oz. slice	85
(Wonder):		
Regular	1-oz. slice	153
With buttermilk	1-oz. slice	170
Whole wheat:		
(USDA):		
Prepared with 2% non-fat dry milk	.8-oz. slice	121
Prepared with 2% non-fat dry milk	.9-oz. slice	132
Prepared with water	.9-oz. slice	132
(Arnold) stone ground	.8-oz. slice	100
Home Pride	1-oz. slice	142
(Monks')	1-oz. slice	110
(Pepperidge Farm):		
Thin sliced	.9-oz. slice	125
Very thin sliced	.6-oz. slice	80
(Wonder) 100%	1-oz. slice	121
BREAD, CANNED BROWN:		
(B&M) plain or raisin	½" slice (1.6 oz.)	220
(Friend's) plain or raisin	½" slice (1.6 oz.)	220
BREAD CRUMBS:		
(USDA) dry, grated, white bread	½ cup (1¾ oz.)	366
(Contadina) seasoned	½ cup (2.1 oz.)	1491
(Pepperidge Farm):		
Regular	1 oz.	255
Herb seasoned	1 oz.	260
*BREAD DOUGH:		
Frozen:		
(Pepperidge Farm):		
Country rye	⅒ of loaf (1 oz.)	185
Stone ground wheat	⅒ of loaf (1 oz.)	127
White	⅒ of loaf (1 oz.)	165
(Rich's)		
French	⅟₂₀ of loaf	138

Food and Description	Measure or Quantity	Sodium (milligrams)
Italian	½₀ of loaf	300
Raisin	½₀ of loaf	107
Wheat	.5-oz. slice	375
White	.8-oz. slice	96
Refrigerated (Pillsbury):		
French	1″ slice	120
Wheat or white	1″ slice	170
*BREAD MIX:		
Home Pride:		
French	⅜″ slice	160
Rye	⅜″ slice	180
White	⅜″ slice	130
(Pillsbury):		
Banana, blueberry nut or date	¹⁄₁₂ of loaf	150
Cranberry	¹⁄₁₂ of loaf	160
Nut	¹⁄₁₂ of loaf	190
BREAD PUDDING, with raisins, home recipe (USDA)	1 cup (9.3 oz.)	556
BREADFRUIT, fresh (USDA):		
Whole	1 lb. (weighed untrimmed)	17
Peeled & trimmed	4 oz.	17
BREAD STICK DOUGH, refrigerated (Pillsbury) soft	1 piece	230
BREAKFAST DRINK, instant (Pillsbury):		
Chocolate or chocolate malt	1 pouch	185
Strawberry	1 pouch	180
Vanilla	1 pouch	210
BROCCOLI:		
Raw (USDA):		
Whole	1 lb. (weighed untrimmed)	42
Large leaves removed	1 lb. (weighed partially trimmed)	53
Boiled (USDA) without salt:		
½″ pieces, drained	½ cup (2.8 oz.)	8
Whole, drained	1 med. stalk (6.3 oz.)	18

Food and Description	Measure or Quantity	Sodium (milligrams)
Frozen:		
(USDA) boiled, drained	10-oz. pkg.	34
(Birds Eye):		
In cheese sauce	5 oz.	490
Chopped, spears, or baby deluxe spears	⅓ of 10-oz. pkg.	15
Cuts or deluxe florets	⅓ of 10-oz. pkg.	20
Spears:		
Regular	⅓ of 10-oz. pkg.	20
Deluxe	⅓ of 10-oz. pkg.	20
& water chestnuts with selected seasonings	⅓ of 10-oz. pkg.	215
(Frosty Acres)	3.3 oz.	20
(Green Giant):		
Regular:		
In cheese sauce	½ cup	425
Spears in butter sauce	3.3 oz.	325
Harvest Fresh:		
Cuts or spears	½ cup	160
Spears, mini	⅛ of pkg.	10
Polybag	½ cup	10
(Larsen)	3.3 oz.	30
(McKenzie):		
Chopped	3.3 oz.	23
Spears	3.3 oz.	28
(Stouffer's) in cheddar cheese sauce	½ of 9-oz. pkg.	970
BROWNIE (See **COOKIE**)		
BRUSSELS SPROUTS:		
Raw (USDA)	1 lb.	54
Boiled (USDA) drained, 1¼"- 1½" dia.	1 cup (7–8 sprouts, 5.5 oz.)	16
Frozen:		
(Birds Eye):		
Regular	⅓ of 10-oz. pkg.	15
With cheese sauce, baby	5 oz.	420
(Frosty Acres)	3.3 oz.	12
(Green Giant):		
Regular:		
In butter sauce	½ cup	275

Food and Description	Measure or Quantity	Sodium (milligrams)
In cheese sauce	½ cup	475
Polybag	½ cup	15
(Larsen)	3.3 oz.	20
(McKenzie)	3.3 oz.	19
BUC*WHEATS, cereal (General Mills)	¾ cup (1 oz.)	235
BULGUR (from hard red winter wheat) (USDA) canned:		
Unseasoned	4-oz. serving	679
Seasoned	4-oz. serving	522
BUN (See **ROLL or BUN**)		
BURGER KING:		
Apple pie	1 serving	412
Breakfast Croissan'wich:		
Bacon	1 sandwich	762
Ham	1 sandwich	987
Sausage	1 sandwich	1042
Cheeseburger:		
Regular	1 burger	439
Double:		
Plain	1 burger	615
Bacon	1 burger	728
Condiments:		
Ketchup	1 serving	121
Mustard	1 serving	31
Pickles	1 serving	60
Chicken Specialty Sandwich:		
Plain	1 sandwich	1280
Condiments:		
Lettuce	1 serving on sandwich	1
Mayonnaise	1 serving on sandwich	142
Chicken Tenders	1 piece	106
Coffee, regular	1 serving	2
Danish, great	1 piece	288
Egg platter, scrambled:		
Bacon	1 serving	167
Croissant	1 serving	298
Eggs	1 serving	317

Food and Description	Measure or Quantity	Sodium (milligrams)
Hash browns	1 serving	193
Sausage	1 serving	405
French fries	1 regular order	160
French toast sticks	1 serving	498
Hamburger:		
Plain	1 burger	297
Condiments:		
Ketchup	1 serving on burger	121
Mustard	1 serving on burger	31
Pickles	1 serving on burger	60
Ham & cheese specialty sandwich:		
Plain	1 sandwich	1461
Condiments:		
Lettuce	1 serving on sandwich	1
Mayonnaise	1 serving on sandwich	71
Tomato	1 serving on sandwich	1
Milk:		
2% lowfat	1 serving	122
Whole	1 serving	119
Onion rings	1 order	665
Orange juice	1 serving	2
Salad dressing:		
Regular:		
Bleu cheese	1 serving	309
House	1 serving	269
1000 Island	1 serving	228
Dietetic, Italian	1 serving	426
Shakes, regular:		
Chocolate	1 serving	202
Strawberry	1 serving	213
Vanilla	1 serving	205
Whaler, fish sandwich:		
Plain	1 sandwich	389

Food and Description	Measure or Quantity	Sodium (milligrams)
Condiments:		
Lettuce	1 serving on sandwich	1
Tartar sauce	1 serving on sandwich	202
Whopper:		
Regular:		
Plain	1 burger	467
With cheese	1 burger	751
Condiments:		
Ketchup	1 serving on burger	183
Lettuce	1 serving on burger	2
Mayonnaise	1 serving on burger	107
Onion	1 serving on burger	1
Pickles	1 serving on burger	119
Tomato	1 serving on burger	1
Jr.		
Plain	1 burger	297
With cheese	1 burger	439
Condiments:		
Ketchup	1 serving on burger	91
Lettuce	1 serving on burger	1
Mayonnaise	1 serving on burger	36
Pickles	1 serving on burger	60
Tomato	1 serving on burger	1
BURGUNDY WINE:		
(Gold Seal) 12% alcohol	3 fl. oz.	3
(Great Western) 12% alcohol	3 fl. oz.	36

Food and Description	Measure or Quantity	Sodium (milligrams)
BURGUNDY WINE, SPARKLING:		
(Barton & Guestier)	3 fl. oz.	2
(Gold Seal)	3 fl. oz.	3
BURRITO:		
*Canned (Del Monte)	1 burrito	616
Frozen:		
(Hormel):		
Beef	1 burrito	780
Cheese	1 burrito	792
Chicken & rice	1 burrito (4 oz.)	594
Grande	5½-oz. serving	877
Hot chili	1 burrito	619
(Swanson) bean & beef	15¼-oz. dinner	1630
(Van de Kamp's):		
Regular, crispy fried, with guacamole sauce	6 oz.	823
Sirloin, grande	11 oz.	1120
***BURRITO FILLING MIX,** canned (Del Monte)	½ cup (4.3 oz.)	900
BUTTER:		
Salted:		
(USDA)	1 pat (1″ × ⅓″)	49
(USDA)	1 T. (.5 oz.)	138
(USDA)	½ cup (4 oz.)	1119
(Breakstone)	1 T. (.5 oz.)	95
(Sealtest)	1 T. (.5 oz.)	117
Whipped:		
(USDA)	1 T. (.3 oz.)	89
(Breakstone)	1 T. (.3 oz.)	64
Unsalted:		
(USDA)	1 stick (4 oz.)	11
(USDA)	1 T. (.5 oz.)	1
(USDA)	1 pat (1″ × ⅓″)	<1
(Breakstone)	1 T.	<1
Whipped (USDA)	1 T.	<1
BUTTER BEAN (See BEAN, LIMA)		
BUTTERMILK (See MILK)		

Food and Description	Measure or Quantity	Sodium (milligrams)
BUTTERSCOTCH MORSELS		
(Nestlé) artificial	1 oz.	15
BUTTER SUBSTITUTE, *Butter*		
Buds:		
Dry	⅛ oz.	170
Liquid	1 oz.	170
Sprinkles	1 tsp.	66

C

CABBAGE:
  White (USDA):
    Raw:
      Whole — 1 lb. (weighed untrimmed) — 72

Finely shredded or chopped	1 cup (3.2 oz.)	18
Coarsely shredded or sliced	1 cup (2.5 oz.)	14
Wedge	3½″ × 4½″ (3½ oz.)	20

Boiled, without salt:
Shredded, in small amount of water, short time, drained — ½ cup (2.6 oz.) — 10
Wedges, in large amount of water, long time, drained — ½ cup (3.2 o.z) — 12
Dehydrated — 1 oz. — 54
Red:
Raw (USDA) whole — 1 lb. (weighed untrimmed) — 93
Canned, solids & liq.:
(Comstock) — ½ cup — 480
(Greenwood) — ½ cup — 475
Savory (USDA) raw, whole — 1 lb. (weighed untrimmed) — 79

Food and Description	Measure or Quantity	Sodium (milligrams)
Savory (USDA) coarsely shredded	1 cup (2.5 oz.)	15
CABBAGE, CHINESE or **CELERY,** raw (USDA):		
Whole	1 lb. (weighed untrimmed)	101
1″ pieces, leaves with stalk	½ cup (1.3 oz.)	9
CABBAGE, STUFFED, frozen (Green Giant) with beef in tomato sauce	½ of pkg.	800
CAKE:		
Not frozen:		
Plain:		
Home recipe, with butter & boiled white icing	⅑ of 9″ square	299
Home recipe, with butter & chocolate icing	⅑ of 9″ square	280
Angel food, home recipe	1/12 of 8″ cake	113
Caramel, home recipe:		
Without icing	⅑ of 9″ square	262
With caramel icing	⅑ of 9¼″ square	214
Chocolate, home recipe, with chocolate icing, 2-layer	1/12 of 9″ cake	234
Coffee, Danish, without fruit or nuts	2.3-oz. piece	238
Crumb (See also **ROLL** or **BUN**) (Hostess)	1¼-oz. piece	98
Devil's food, home recipe:		
Without icing	3″ × 2″ × 1½″ piece	162
With chocolate icing, 2-layer	1/16 of 9″ cake	176
Fruit, home recipe:		
Dark	1/30 of 8¼″ loaf	24
Light, made with butter	1/30 of 8″ loaf	29
Fruit Loaf (Hostess)	2½ oz.	263
Honey (Holland Honey Cake) low sodium:		
Fruit and raisin	½″ slice (.9 oz.)	2
Orange and premium unsalted	½″ slice (.9 oz.)	1

Food and Description	Measure or Quantity	Sodium (milligrams)
Pound, home recipe:		
Equal weights flour, sugar, butter and eggs	3½″ × 3½″ slice (1.1 oz.)	33
Traditional, made with butter	3½″ × 3½″ slice (1.1 oz.)	53
Sponge, home recipe	¹⁄₁₂ of 10″ cake	110
White, home recipe:		
Made with butter, without icing, 2-layer	⅑ of 9″ wide, 3″ high cake	303
Made with butter, with coconut icing, 2-layer	¹⁄₁₂ of 9″ wide, 3″ high cake	270
Yellow, home recipe, made with butter, without icing, 2-layer	¹⁄₁₉ of cake	249
Frozen:		
Banana (Sara Lee)	⅛ of 13¾-oz. cake	154
Banana nut layer (Sara Lee)	⅛ of 20-oz. cake	167
Black forest (Sara Lee)	⅛ of 21-oz. cake	140
Boston cream (Pepperidge Farm) Supreme	¼ of 11¾-oz. cake	190
Butterscotch pecan (Pepperidge Farm) large	¹⁄₁₀ of 17 oz. cake	110
Carrot:		
(Pepperidge Farm) with cream cheese icing	⅛ of 11¾-oz. cake	150
(Sara Lee)	⅛ of 12¼-oz. cake	124
(Weight Watchers)	3-oz. serving	340
Cheesecake:		
(Morton) *Great Little Desserts:*		
Cherry, cream or strawberry	6-oz. cake	350

Food and Description	Measure or Quantity	Sodium (milligrams)
Pineapple	6-oz. cake	355
(Rich's) Viennese	1/16 of 42-oz. cake	298
(Sara Lee):		
Blueberry, cream cheese:		
Regular	1/6 of 19-oz. cake	175
For 2	1/2 of 11.3-oz. cake	326
Cherry, cream cheese:		
Regular	1/6 of 19-oz. cake	185
For 2	1/2 of 11.3-oz. cake	262
Cream cheese:		
Large	1/6 of 17-oz. cake	175
Small	1/3 of 10-oz. cake	206
French, cream cheese	1/8 of 23½-oz. cake	136
Strawberry, cream cheese:		
Regular	1/6 of 19-oz. cake	170
For 2	1/2 of 11.3-oz. cake	268
Strawberry, French, cream cheese	1/8 of 26-oz. cake	128
(Weight Watchers):		
Regular	3.9 oz.	220
Black cherry	3.9 oz.	190
Strawberry	3.9 oz.	220
Chocolate:		
(Pepperidge Farm):		
Large:		
Fudge	1/10 of 17-oz. cake	140
German	1/10 of 17-oz. cake	170
Supreme, regular	1/4 of 11½-oz. cake	140
(Sara Lee):		
Regular	1/8 of 13¼-oz. cake	168
Bavarian	1/8 of 22½-oz. cake	78
German	1/8 of 12¼-oz. cake	134
Layer, 'n cream	1/8 of 18-oz. cake	136
Layer, double	1/8 of 18-oz. cake	138
(Weight Watchers):		
Regular	2½ oz.	290

Food and Description	Measure or Quantity	Sodium (milligrams)
German	2½ oz.	350
Coconut (Pepperidge Farm) layer	⅒ of 17-oz. cake	120
Coffee (Sara Lee):		
Almond	⅛ of 11¾-oz. cake	158
Almond ring	⅛ of 9½-oz. cake	124
Apple:		
Regular	⅛ of 15-oz. cake	208
For 2	½ of 9-oz. cake	502
Blueberry ring	⅛ of 9¾-oz. cake	135
Butter, *For 2*	½ of 6½-oz. cake	391
Maple crunch ring	⅛ of 9¾-oz. cake	131
Pecan:		
Large	⅛ of 11¼-oz. cake	159
Small	¼ of 6½-oz. cake	184
Raspberry ring	⅛ of 9¾-oz. cake	120
Streusel:		
Butter	⅛ of 11½-oz. cake	178
Cinnamon	⅛ of 10.9-oz. cake	156
Devil's Food (Pepperidge Farm) layer	⅒ of 17-oz. cake	135
Golden (Pepperidge Farm) layer	⅒ of 17-oz. cake	115
Grand Marnier (Pepperidge Farm) supreme	1½ oz.	85
Lemon Coconut (Pepperidge Farm) Supreme	¼ of 12¼-oz. cake	220
Orange (Sara Lee)	⅛ of 13¾-oz. cake	170
Pineapple cream (Pepperidge Farm) Supreme	⅟₁₂ of 24-oz. cake	130
Pound:		
(Pepperidge Farm) butter	⅒ of 10¾-oz. cake	150

Food and Description	Measure or Quantity	Sodium (milligrams)
(Sara Lee):		
Regular	⅒ of 10¾-oz. cake	104
Banana nut	⅒ of 11-oz. cake	104
Chocolate	⅒ of 10¾-oz. cake	134
Chocolate swirl	⅒ of 11.8-oz. cake	83
Family size	⅕ of 16½-oz. cake	106
Home style	⅒ of 9½-oz. cake	97
Raisin	⅒ of 12.9-oz. cake	108
Spice (Weight Watchers)	3-oz. serving	350
Strawberry cream:		
(Pepperidge Farm) Supreme	¹⁄₁₂ of 24-oz. cake	120
(Sara Lee) layer	⅛ of 20½-oz. cake	150
Strawberry shortcake (Sara Lee)	⅛ of 21-oz. cake	81
Torte (Sara Lee):		
Apples 'n cream	⅛ of 21-oz. cake	146
Fudge & nut	⅛ of 15¾-oz. cake	144
CAKE or COOKIE ICING		
(Pillsbury) all flavors	1 T.	0
CAKE ICING:		
Butter pecan (Betty Crocker) *Creamy Deluxe*	¹⁄₁₂ of can	85
Caramel, home recipe (USDA)	4-oz. serving	94
Caramel pecan (Pillsbury) *Frosting Supreme*	¹⁄₁₂ of can	70
Cherry (Betty Crocker) *Creamy Deluxe*	¹⁄₁₂ of can	95
Chocolate:		
Home recipe (USDA)	4-oz. serving	168
(Betty Crocker) *Creamy Deluxe:*		
Regular	¹⁄₁₂ of can	95

Food and Description	Measure or Quantity	Sodium (milligrams)
Chip	1/12 of can	85
Fudge, dark dutch	1/12 of can	125
Milk	1/12 of can	95
Nut	1/12 of can	95
Sour cream	1/12 of can	110
(Duncan Hines):		
Regular or milk	1/12 of can	84
Fudge, dark dutch	1/12 of can	95
(Pillsbury) *Frosting Supreme:*		
Chip	1/12 of can	70
Fudge	1/12 of can	80
Milk	1/12 of can	60
Mint	1/12 of can	80
Coconut, home recipe (USDA)	4-oz. serving	196
Coconut almond (Pillsbury) *Frosting Supreme*	1/12 of can	60
Coconut pecan (Pillsbury) *Frosting Supreme*	1/12 of can	60
Cream cheese:		
(Betty Crocker) *Creamy Deluxe*	1/12 of can	100
(Pillsbury) *Frosting Supreme*	1/12 of can	115
Double dutch (Pillsbury) *Frosting Supreme*	1/12 of can	45
Lemon:		
(Betty Crocker) *Sunkist, Creamy Deluxe*	1/12 of can	95
(Pillsbury) *Frosting Supreme*	1/12 of can	80
Orange (Betty Crocker) *Creamy Deluxe*	1/12 of can	95
Strawberry (Pillsbury) *Frosting Supreme*	1/12 of can	75
Vanilla:		
(Betty Crocker) *Creamy Deluxe*	1/12 of can	95
(Duncan Hines)	1/12 of can	86
(Pillsbury) *Frosting Supreme:*		
Regular	1/12 of can	75
Sour cream	1/12 of can	80

Food and Description	Measure or Quantity	Sodium (milligrams)
White:		
Home recipe (USDA):		
Boiled	4-oz. serving	162
Uncooked	4-oz. serving	56
(Betty Crocker) *Creamy*		
Deluxe	¹⁄₁₂ of can	95
*CAKE ICING MIX:		
Regular:		
Banana (Betty Crocker)		
Chiquita, creamy	¹⁄₁₂ of pkg.	100
Butter Brickle (Betty Crocker)		
creamy	¹⁄₁₂ of pkg.	115
Butter pecan (Betty Crocker)		
creamy, deluxe	¹⁄₁₂ of pkg.	100
Cherry (Betty Crocker)		
creamy	¹⁄₁₂ of pkg.	100
Chocolate:		
(Betty Crocker):		
Regular, creamy	¹⁄₁₂ of pkg.	75
Dark, creamy	¹⁄₁₂ of pkg.	100
Milk, creamy	¹⁄₁₂ of pkg.	80
Sour cream	¹⁄₁₂ of pkg.	75
(Pillsbury) Frost It Hot	⅛ of pkg.	50
(Pillsbury) *Rich 'n Easy:*		
Fudge	¹⁄₁₂ of pkg.	70
Milk	¹⁄₁₂ of pkg.	55
Coconut almond (Pillsbury)	¹⁄₁₂ of pkg.	95
Coconut pecan:		
(Betty Crocker) creamy	¹⁄₁₂ of pkg.	100
(Pillsbury)	¹⁄₁₂ of pkg.	105
Cream cheese & nut (Betty Crocker) creamy	¹⁄₁₂ of pkg.	100
Lemon, (Betty Crocker)		
Sunkist, creamy	¹⁄₁₂ of pkg.	100
White:		
(Betty Crocker):		
Creamy	¹⁄₁₂ of pkg.	100
Fluffy	¹⁄₁₂ of pkg.	40
Sour cream, creamy	¹⁄₁₂ of pkg.	100
(Pillsbury) fluffy	¹⁄₁₂ of pkg.	65

Food and Description	Measure or Quantity	Sodium (milligrams)
Dietetic or low calorie (Betty Crocker) *Lite:*		
Chocolate	¹⁄₁₂ of pkg.	55
Lemon or vanilla	¹⁄₁₂ of pkg.	50
CAKE MEAL (Manischewitz)	½ cup (2.6 oz.)	2
CAKE MIX:		
Regular:		
Angel food:		
*(USDA)	¹⁄₁₂ of 10″ cake (1.9 oz.)	77
(Betty Crocker):		
Chocolate	¹⁄₁₂ of pkg.	275
Confetti	¹⁄₁₂ of pkg.	275
Lemon custard	¹⁄₁₂ of pkg.	265
One-step	¹⁄₁₂ of pkg.	250
Strawberry	¹⁄₁₂ of pkg.	270
Traditional	¹⁄₁₂ of pkg.	140
(Duncan Hines)	¹⁄₁₂ of pkg.	119
*Apple cinnamon (Betty Crocker) *Supermoist*	¹⁄₁₂ of cake	275
*Applesauce raisin (Betty Crocker) *Snackin' Cake*	¹⁄₉ of cake	250
*Banana:		
(Betty Crocker) *Supermoist*	¹⁄₁₂ of cake	255
(Pillsbury), *Pillsbury Plus*	¹⁄₁₂ of cake	290
Banana walnut (Betty Crocker) *Snackin' Cake*	¹⁄₉ of pkg.	260
*Black forest cherry (Pillsbury) *Bundt*	¹⁄₁₆ of cake	310
*Boston cream (Pillsbury) *Bundt*	¹⁄₁₆ of cake	310
*Butter (Pillsbury), *Pillsbury Plus*	¹⁄₁₂ of cake	370
Butter Brickle (Betty Crocker) *Supermoist*	¹⁄₁₂ of cake	265
*Butter pecan (Betty Crocker) layer, *Supermoist*	¹⁄₁₂ of cake	250
*Butter yellow (Betty Crocker) *Supermoist*	¹⁄₁₂ of cake	295

Food and Description	Measure or Quantity	Sodium (milligrams)
*Carrot (Betty Crocker):		
Stir N' Frost, with cream		
cheese icing	⅙ of cake	200
Supermoist	¹⁄₁₂ of cake	255
*Carrot nut (Betty Crocker)		
Snackin' Cake	⅑ of cake	240
*Carrot'n spice, *Pillsbury*		
Plus	¹⁄₁₂ of cake	330
*Cheesecake:		
(Jello-O)	⅛ of 8" cake	350
(Royal) No Bake:		
Lite	⅛ of cake	380
Real	⅛ of cake	370
*Cherry chip (Betty Crocker)		
layer, *Supermoist*	¹⁄₁₂ of cake	265
Chocolate:		
(Betty Crocker):		
Almond, *Snackin' Cake*	⅑ of pkg.	215
With chocolate frosting,		
Stir 'N Frost	⅙ of pkg.	200
Fudge, *Stir 'N Frost*,		
with vanilla frosting	⅙ of pkg.	250
*Fudge, *Supermoist*	¹⁄₁₂ of cake	450
Fudge chip, *Snackin'*		
Cake	⅑ of pkg.	205
*German chocolate,		
layer, *Supermoist*	¹⁄₁₂ of cake	420
*Milk, layer, *Supermoist*	¹⁄₁₂ of cake	290
*Pudding recipe	⅙ of cake	255
*Sour cream, *Supermoist*	¹⁄₁₂ of cake	430
*(Pillsbury):		
Fudge, dark, *Pillsbury*		
Plus	¹⁄₁₂ of cake	440
Fudge marble, *Pillsbury*		
Plus	¹⁄₁₂ of cake	300
Fudge, tunnel of, *Bundt*	¹⁄₁₆ of cake	310
German chocolate, *Pillsbury Plus*	¹⁄₁₂ of cake	340
German chocolate,		
Streusel Swirl	¹⁄₁₆ of cake	290

Food and Description	Measure or Quantity	Sodium (milligrams)
Macaroon, *Bundt*	1/16 of cake	300
Microwave:		
Plain	1/8 of cake	260
With chocolate frosting	1/8 of cake	310
Supreme, double	1/8 of cake	340
Tunnel of Fudge	1/8 of cake	320
*Cinnamon (Pillsbury) *Streusel Swirl:*		
Regular	1/16 of cake	200
Microwave	1/8 of cake	180
Coconut pecan (Betty Crocker) *Snackin' Cake*	1/9 of pkg.	255
Coffee cake:		
*(Aunt Jemima)	1/8 of cake	34
*(Pillsbury), apple cinnamon	1/8 of cake	150
*Date nut (Betty Crocker) *Snackin' Cake*	1/9 of cake	265
Devil's food:		
*(Betty Crocker) layer, *Supermoist*	1/12 of cake	425
(Duncan Hines) deluxe	1/12 of pkg.	363
*(Pillsbury) *Pillsbury Plus*	1/12 of cake	370
Golden chocolate chip (Betty Crocker) *Snackin' Cake*	1/9 of pkg.	255
Lemon:		
*(Betty Crocker):		
Chiffon	1/12 of cake	190
Layer, *Supermoist*	1/12 of cake	260
& lemon frosting, *Stir 'N Frost*	1/6 of cake	210
Pudding recipe	1/6 of cake	270
*(Pillsbury):		
Bundt, tunnel of	1/16 of cake	300
Microwave:		
Plain	1/8 of cake	180
With lemon frosting	1/8 of cake	220
Supreme, deluxe	1/8 of cake	210
Pillsbury Plus	1/12 of cake	290

Food and Description	Measure or Quantity	Sodium (milligrams)
Streusel Swirl	1/16 of cake	340
*Marble (Betty Crocker) layer, *Supermoist*	1/12 of cake	255
*Orange (Betty Crocker) layer, *Supermoist*	1/12 of cake	280
*Pineapple cream (Pillsbury) *Bundt*	1/16 of cake	300
*Pound:		
(Betty Crocker) golden	1/12 of cake	155
(Dromedary)	1/2" slice	340
Spice (Betty Crocker):		
*Layer, *Supermoist*	1/12 of cake	260
Raisin, *Snackin' Cake*	1/9 of pkg.	250
*With vanilla frosting, *Stir 'N Frost*	1/6 of cake	305
*Spice (Betty Crocker) *Supermoist*	1/12 of cake	260
*Strawberry:		
(Betty Crocker) layer, *Supermoist*	1/12 of cake	260
Pillsbury Plus	1/12 of cake	300
*Upside down (Betty Crocker) pineapple	1/9 of cake	215
White:		
*(Betty Crocker):		
With milk chocolate frosting, *Stir 'N Frost*	1/6 of cake	235
Layer, *Supermoist*	1/12 of cake	275
Sour cream, *Supermoist*	1/12 of cake	260
(Duncan Hines) deluxe	1/12 of pkg.	251
Pillsbury Plus	1/12 of cake	290
Yellow:		
*(Betty Crocker):		
With chocolate frosting, *Stir 'N Frost*	1/6 of cake	210
Layer, *Supermoist*	1/12 of cake	270
(Duncan Hines) deluxe	1/12 of pkg.	271
*(Pillsbury):		
Microwave:		
Plain	1/8 of cake	170

Food and Description	Measure or Quantity	Sodium (milligrams)
With chocolate frosting	⅛ of cake	220
Pillsbury Plus	¹⁄₁₂ of cake	300
*Pillsbury Plus	¹⁄₁₂ of cake	300
*Dietetic or low calorie (Estee):		
Chocolate	¹⁄₁₀ of cake	110
Lemon pound or spice	¹⁄₁₀ of cake	75
CANADIAN WHISKY (See **DISTILLED LIQUOR**)		
CANDY, The following values of candies from the U.S. Department of Argiculture are representative of the types sold commercially. These values may be useful when individual brands or sizes are not known:		
Almond:		
Chocolate-coated	1 cup (6.3 oz.)	106
Chocolate-coated	1 oz.	17
Sugar-coated or Jordan	1 oz.	6
Butterscotch	1 oz.	19
Candy corn	1 oz.	60
Caramel:		
Plain	1 oz.	64
Plain with nuts	1 oz.	58
Chocolate	1 oz.	64
Chocolate with nuts	1 oz.	58
Chocolate-flavored roll	1 oz.	56
Chocolate:		
Bittersweet	1 oz.	<1
Milk:		
Plain	1 oz.	27
With almonds	1 oz.	23
With peanuts	1 oz.	19
Semisweet	1 oz.	<1
Sweet	1 oz.	9
Chocolate discs, sugar-coated	1 oz.	20
Coconut center, chocolate-coated	1 oz.	56

Food and Description	Measure or Quantity	Sodium (milligrams)
Fondant, plain	1 oz.	60
Fondant, chocolate-covered	1 oz.	52
Fudge:		
Chocolate fudge	1 oz.	54
Chocolate fudge, chocolate-coated	1 oz.	65
Chocolate fudge with nuts	1 oz.	48
Chocolate fudge with nuts, chocolate-coated	1 oz.	58
Vanilla fudge	1 oz.	59
Vanilla fudge with nuts	1 oz.	53
With peanuts & caramel, chocolate-coated	1 oz.	36
Gum drops	1 oz.	10
Hard	1 oz.	9
Honeycombed hard candy, with peanut butter, chocolate-covered	1 oz.	46
Jelly beans	1 oz.	3
Marshmallows	1 oz.	11
Mints, uncoated	1 oz.	60
Nougat & caramel, chocolate-covered	1 oz.	49
Peanut bar	1 oz.	3
Peanut brittle	1 oz.	9
Peanuts, chocolate-covered	1 oz.	17
Raisins, chocolate-covered	1 oz.	18
Vanilla creams, chocolate-covered	1 oz.	52
CANDY, COMMERCIAL:		
Regular:		
Almond Joy (Peter Paul Cadbury)	1.5-oz. bar	90
Baby Ruth	2-oz. serving	120
Bar None (Hershey's)	1½ oz.	50
Bonkers (Nabisco)	1 piece	0
Breath Savers (Life Savers)	1 piece	0
Bridge mix (Nabisco)	1 piece (2 grams)	1
Butterfinger	2-oz. serving	100
Butternut (Hollywood Brands)	2¼-oz. bar	120

Food and Description	Measure or Quantity	Sodium (milligrams)
Caramel Nip (Pearson's)	1 piece	17
Charleston Chew	2-oz. piece	80
Cherry, chocolate covered (Welch's) dark or milk	1 piece (.7 oz.)	10
Chocolate bar:		
Brazil nut, *Cadbury's* (Peter Paul Cadbury)	2 oz.	82
Caramello, *Cadbury's* (Peter Paul Cadbury)	2 oz.	108
Crunch (Nestlé)	1¹⁄₁₆-oz. bar	50
Fruit & nut, *Cadbury's* (Peter Paul Cadbury)	2 oz.	77
Hazelnut, *Cadbury's* (Peter Paul Cadbury)	2 oz.	88
Milk:		
Cadbury's (Peter Paul Cadbury)	2 oz.	94
(Hershey's)	.35-oz. miniature	9
(Hershey's)	1.65-oz. bar	45
(Hershey's)	4-oz. bar	109
(Nestlé)	.35-oz. miniature	7
(Nestlé)	1¹⁄₁₆-oz. bar	21
Special Dark (Hershey's)	1.45-oz. bar	5
Special Dark (Hershey's)	4-oz. bar	14
Chocolate bar with almonds:		
Cadbury's (Peter Paul Cadbury)	2 oz.	82
(Hershey's) milk	.35-oz. miniature	8
(Hershey's) milk	1.55-oz. bar	60
(Nestlé)	1-oz. serving	15
Chocolate Parfait (Pearson's)	1 piece (.2 oz.)	17
Chocolate, Petite (Andes)	1 piece (.15 oz.)	4
Chuckles, any flavor	1 oz.	10
Coffee Nips (Pearson's)	1 piece (.2 oz.)	17
Coffioca (Pearson's)	1 piece (6.5 g.)	17
Creme De Menthe (Andes)	1 piece (.2 oz.)	3
Eggs (Nabisco) *Chuckles*	½ oz.	5
5th Avenue Bar (Hershey's)	1.93-oz. serving	110
Fudge (Nabisco) bar	1 piece (.7 oz.)	20
Good Stuff (Nab)	1.8-oz. piece	90

Food and Description	Measure or Quantity	Sodium (milligrams)
Halvah (Sahadi)	1 oz.	45
Hard (Jolly Rancher):		
Apple; fire; grape; lemon; lemonade, pink; fruit punch; raspberry & watermelon	1 piece	5
Butterscotch	1 piece	37
Cherry; peppermint; strawberry	1 piece	3
Orange	1 piece	4
Holidays (M&M/Mars):		
Plain	1 oz.	40
Peanut	1 oz.	35
Jelly, *Chuckles*:		
Bar	1 oz.	10
Bean	½ oz.	15
Rings	1 oz.	10
Ju-Jubes (Nabisco) *Chuckles*	½ oz.	7
Kisses (Hershey) milk chocolate	1 piece (5 g.)	4
Kit Kat (Hershey's)	.6-oz. bar	16
Kit Kat (Hershey's)	1.62-oz. bar	60
Krackel Bar (Hershey's)	1.65-oz. bar	85
Licorice Nip (Pearson's)	1 piece (6.5 g.)	17
Lollipop (Life Savers)	1 piece	10
Mars Bar (M&M/Mars)	1.7-oz. serving	82
Marshmallow eggs (Nabisco) *Chuckles*	1 oz.	0
Mary Jane	.25-oz. piece	4
Mary Jane	1½-oz. piece	23
Milky Way (M&M/Mars)	2.24-oz. bar	150
Mint Parfait (Andes)	.2-oz. piece	3
Mint Pattie (Nabisco):		
Junior pattie	.1-oz. piece	<1
Peppermint	.5-oz. piece	5
M&M's (M&M/Mars):		
Peanut	1.83-oz. serving	60
Plain	1.69-oz. serving	65
Mounds (Peter Paul Cadbury)	1.65-oz. bar	87
Mr. Goodbar (Hershey's)	.35-oz. miniature	6

Food and Description	Measure or Quantity	Sodium (milligrams)
Mr. Goodbar (Hershey's)	1.85-oz. serving	20
Munch bar (M&M/Mars)	1 oz.	77
My Buddy (Tom's)	1.8-oz. serving	60
Naturally Nut & Fruit Bar (Planters):		
Almond/apricot	1 oz.	75
Almond/pineapple	1 oz.	80
Peanut/raisin	1 oz.	70
Walnut/apple	1 oz.	90
Nougat center (Nabisco) *Chuckles*	1 oz.	10
$100,000 Bar (Nestlé)	1¼-oz. bar	50
Orange slice (Nabisco) *Chuckles*	1 oz.	10
Park Avenue (Tom's)	1.8-oz. serving	120
Peanut bar (Planters)	1.6-oz. piece	110
Peanut butter cup (Reese's)	1 cup	90
Peanut Butter Pals (Tom's)	1.3-oz. serving	100
Peanut butter parfait (Pearson)	1 piece	17
Peanut, chocolate covered (Nabisco)	1 piece	1
Peanut crunch (Saladi)	¾-oz. bar	10
Peanut parfait (Andes)	1 piece	11
Peanut Plank (Tom's)	1.7-oz. serving	30
Peanut roll (Tom's)	1¾-oz. serving	120
Pom Poms (Nabisco)	1 oz.	70
Powerhouse (Peter Paul Cadbury)	2 oz.	193
Raisin, chocolate covered (Nabisco)	1 piece	<1
Reese's Pieces (Hershey's)	1.95-oz. pkg.	95
Rolo (Hershey's)	1 piece (6 g.)	12
Rolo (Hershey's)	1¾-oz. roll	109
Royals (M&M/Mars)	1½-oz. serving	34
Sesame crunch bar (Sahadi)	¾-oz. bar	55
Sesame Tahini (Sahadi)	1 oz.	75
Skittles (M&M/Mars)	1 oz.	13
Skor (Hershey's) toffee bar	1.4-oz. bar	125
Snickers (M&M/Mars)	2.16-oz. bar	170

Food and Description	Measure or Quantity	Sodium (milligrams)
Spearmint leaves (Nabisco) *Chuckles*	1 oz.	15
Spice flavored sticks & drops (Nabisco) *Chuckles*	1 oz.	10
Spice flavored strings (Nabisco) *Chuckles*	1 oz.	10
Starburst (M&M/Mars)	1-oz. serving	15
Stars, chocolate (Nabisco)	1 piece	3
Sugar Babies (Nabisco)	1⅝-oz. pkg.	85
Sugar Daddy (Nabisco)	1⅜-oz. pop	85
Sugar Mama (Nabisco)	¾-oz. piece	30
3 Musketeers Bar (M&M/ Mars)	2.13-oz. serving	120
Ting-A-Ling (Andes)	.2-oz. bar	7
Tootsie Roll:		
Regular:		
Chocolate	.23-oz. midgee	1
Chocolate	.63-oz. bar	4
Chocolate	¾-oz. bar	5
Chocolate	1-oz. bar	6
Chocolate	1¼-oz. bar	8
Flavored	.16-oz. square	1
Flavored	.23-oz. midgee	2
Pop:		
Caramel	.49-oz. pop	4
Chocolate	.49-oz. pop	4
Flavored	.49-oz. pop	Tr.
Pop drop:		
Caramel	.17-oz. piece	1
Chocolate	.17-oz. piece	Tr.
Flavored	.17-oz. piece	Tr.
Twix, cookie bar (M&M/ Mars)	.85-oz. serving	48
Twix, cookie bar, peanut butter (M&M/Mars)	.8-oz. serving	69
Whatchamacallit (Hershey's)	1.8-oz. bar	90
Wispa (Peter Paul Cadbury)	1 oz.	47
Y&S Bites (Hershey's)	1 oz.	85
Zagnut Bar (Clark)	1.5-oz. bar	43

Food and Description	Measure or Quantity	Sodium (milligrams)
Dietetic or low calorie:		
Carob bar, *Joan's Natural:*		
Coconut	1 section of 3-oz. bar (¼ oz.)	10
Coconut	3-oz. bar	117
Fruit & nut	1 section of 3-oz. bar (¼ oz.)	10
Fruit & nut	3-oz. bar	115
Honey bran	1 section of 3-oz. bar (¼ oz.)	9
Honey bran	3-oz. bar	114
Peanut	1 section of 3-oz. bar (¼ oz.)	9
Peanut	3-oz. bar	109
Chocolate or chocolate flavored bar:		
Coconut (Estee)	1 section of 2½-oz. bar	5
Coconut (Estee)	2½-oz. bar	61
Crunch (Estee)	1 section of 2½-oz. bar	5
Crunch (Estee)	2½-oz. bar	65
Fruit & nut (Estee)	1 section of 2½-oz. bar	5
Fruit & nut (Estee)	2½-oz. bar	59
Milk (Estee)	1 section of 2½-oz. bar	6
Milk (Estee)	2½-oz. bar	68
Estee-Ets, peanut	1.4-g. piece	2
Gum drops (Estee) fruit and licorice	1 piece (2 g.)	1
Hard (Louis Sherry)	1 piece	2
Lollipop (Estee)	1 pop	5
Mint (Estee)	1 piece	0
Peanut butter cup (Estee)	1 piece (.3 oz.)	10
Raisin, chocolate covered (Estee)	1 piece (1 g.)	2
TV mix (Estee)	1 piece (2 g.)	2
CANNELONI, frozen:		
(Blue Star) *Dining Lite:*		
Cheese	9-oz. meal	940

Food and Description	Measure or Quantity	Sodium (milligrams)
Veal & vegetable	9-oz. meal	790
(Calentano) florentine	12-oz. pkg.	540
(Stouffer's):		
Beef & pork with mornay		
sauce	9⅝-oz. meal	940
Cheese, with tomato sauce	9⅛-oz. meal	885
(Weight Watchers) Florentine,		
one-compartment meal	13-oz. meal	894
CANTALOUPE, fresh (USDA):		
Whole, medium	1 lb. (weighed with skin & cavity contents)	27
Cubed	½ cup (2.9 oz.)	10
CAP'N CRUNCH, cereal (Quaker):		
Regular	¾ cup (1 oz.)	185
Crunchberries	¾ cup (1 oz.)	166
Peanut butter	¾ cup (1 oz.)	210
CARAMBOLA, raw (USDA):		
Whole	1 lb. (weighed whole)	9
Flesh only	4 oz.	2
CARAWAY SEED (French's)	1 tsp.	Tr.
CARDAMOM SEED (French's)	1 tsp.	Tr.
CARL'S JR. RESTAURANT:		
Bacon	2 strips	200
Cake, chocolate	3.2-oz. piece	335
California Roast Beef 'n Swiss		
sandwich	1 sandwich	1070
Cheese:		
American	.6-oz. piece	290
Swiss	.6-oz. piece	221
Chicken sandwich:		
Charbroiler BBQ	6.3-oz. sandwich	955
Charbroiler Club	8.2-oz. sandwich	1165
Danish	3.5-oz. piece	550
Egg, scrambled	2.4-oz. serving	105
Fish filet sandwich	7.9-oz. sandwich	945
French toast dips, without syrup	4.7-oz. serving	576

Food and Description	Measure or Quantity	Sodium (milligrams)
Hamburger:		
Plain:		
Famous Star	8.1-oz. burger	890
Happy Star	3-oz. burger	445
Old Time Star	5.9-oz. burger	760
Super Star	10.6-oz. burger	990
Cheeseburger, *Western Bacon:*		
Regular	7.5-oz. burger	1415
Double	10.4-oz. burger	1620
Hot cakes, with margarine, excluding syrup	1 serving	1190
Milk, 2% lowfat	10 fl. oz.	550
Muffins:		
Blueberry	3½-oz. muffin	360
Bran	4-oz. muffin	300
English, with margarine	2-oz. serving	275
Onion rings	3.2-oz. serving	105
Orange juice	1 small serving	2
Potato:		
Baked:		
Bacon & cheese	1 potato	1820
Broccoli & cheese	1 potato	690
Cheese	1 potato	785
Fiesta	1 potato	1230
Lite	1 potato	35
Sour cream & chive	1 potato	140
French fries	1 regular order	626
Hash brown nuggets	3-oz. serving	350
Salad dressing:		
Regular:		
Bleu cheese	2-oz. serving	278
House	2-oz. serving	329
1000 Island	2-oz. serving	435
Dietetic, Italian	2-oz. serving	360
Sausage	1.5-oz. patty	275
Shake	1 regular size	255
Soft drink:		
Regular	1 regular drink	37
Dietetic	1 regular drink	13

Food and Description	Measure or Quantity	Sodium (milligrams)
Soup:		
Broccoli, cream of	6 fl. oz.	845
Chicken & noodle	6 fl. oz.	605
Chowder, Boston Clam	6 fl. oz.	861
Vegetable	6 fl. oz.	807
Steak sandwich, country fried	7.2-oz. sandwich	1290
Sunrise Sandwich:		
Bacon	4.5-oz. sandwich	750
Sausage	6.1-oz. sandwich	990
Tea, iced	1 regular drink	0
Zucchini	4.3-oz. serving	480
CARNATION-DO-IT-YOURSELF DIET PLAN	2 scoops	110
CARNATION INSTANT BREAKFAST:		
Bar:		
Chocolate chip	1 bar	180
Chocolate crunch	1 bar	145
Peanut butter with chocolate chips or peanut butter crunch	1 bar	170
Dry:		
Chocolate or vanilla	1 packet	135
Chocolate malt	1 packet	160
Coffee	1 packet	130
Eggnog	1 packet	185
Strawberry	1 packet	195
CARP, raw (USDA):		
Whole	1 lb. (weighed whole)	68
Meat only	4 oz.	57
CARROT:		
Raw (USDA):		
Whole	1 lb. (weighed with full tops)	126
Partially trimmed	1 lb. (weighed without tops, with skins)	175
Trimmed	5½″ × 1″ carrot (1.8 oz.)	24

Food and Description	Measure or Quantity	Sodium (milligrams)
Trimmed	25 thin strips (1.8 oz.)	24
Chunks	½ cup (2.4 oz.)	32
Diced	½ cup (1½ oz.)	34
Grated or shredded	½ cup (1.9 oz.)	26
Slices	½ cup (2.2. oz.)	30
Strips	½ cup (2 oz.)	27
Boiled without salt, drained (USDA):		
Chunks	½ cup (2.9 oz.)	27
Diced	½ cup (2½ oz.)	23
Slices	½ cup (2.7 oz.)	25
Canned, regular pack, solids & liq.:		
(Comstock)	½ cup	320
(Del Monte), Diced	½ cup (4 oz.)	265
(Stokely-Van Camp):		
Diced, solids & liq.	½ cup (4.3 oz.)	290
Sliced, solids & liq.	½ cup (4.3 oz.)	263
Canned, dietetic or low calorie, solids & liq.:		
(Blue Boy) sliced	½ of 8¼-oz. can	43
(Featherweight) sliced	½ cup	30
(Larsen) *Fresh-Lite*	½ cup (4.4 oz.)	40
(S&W) *Nutridiet*, sliced	½ cup	50
Dehydrated (USDA)	1 oz.	76
Frozen:		
(Birds Eye) baby, whole deluxe	⅓ of 10-oz. pkg.	45
(Frosty Acres):		
Crinkle cut	3.3 oz.	130
Whole, baby	3.3 oz.	45
(Green Giant) crinkle cuts in butter sauce	½ cup	315
(Larsen)	3.3 oz.	40
(McKenzie)	3.3-oz.	56
CASABA MELON, fresh (USDA):		
Whole	1 lb. (weighed whole)	27

Food and Description	Measure or Quantity	Sodium (milligrams)
Flesh	4 oz.	14
CASHEW NUT:		
(USDA) salted	1 oz.	57
(USDA) salted	½ cup (2.5 oz.)	140
(USDA) salted	5 large or 8 med.	21
All America Nut (Adams)	1 oz.	85
(Eagle Snacks) *Honey Roast*	1 oz.	170
(Fisher) salted:		
Dry	1 oz.	140
Honey roasted	1 oz.	70
Oil:		
Whole or pieces	1 oz.	110
Halves	1 oz.	160
Lightly salted	1 oz.	40
(Guy's) whole, salted	1 oz.	140
(Planters):		
Dry:		
Salted	1 oz.	230
Unsalted	1 oz.	0
Honey roasted, with or without peanuts	1 oz.	170
Oil, salted, halves or fancy	1 oz.	135
(Tom's)	1 oz.	122
CATAWBA WINE (Great Western) pink, 12% alcohol	3 fl. oz.	36
CATFISH:		
Raw, fillet (USDA)	4 oz.	68
Frozen (Mrs. Paul's) breaded & fried:		
Fillet	3.6-oz. fillet	243
Finger	½ of 8-oz. pkg.	260
CATSUP:		
Regular pack:		
(USDA)	1 T. (.6 oz.)	188
(USDA)	½ cup (4.8 oz.)	735
(Del Monte)	1 T. (.7 oz.)	181
(Hunt's)	1 T. (.5 oz.)	160
(Smucker's)	1 T. (.6 oz.)	135

Food and Description	Measure or Quantity	Sodium (milligrams)
Dietetic or low calorie:		
(Del Monte) no salt added	1 T.	6
(Dia-Mel)	1 T.	20
(Featherweight)	1 T. (.6 oz.)	5
(Hunt's)	1 T.	0
(Tillie Lewis) *Tasti Diet*	1 T. (.5 oz.)	6
CAULIFLOWER:		
Raw (USDA):		
Whole	1 lb. (weighed untrimmed)	23
Flowerbuds	½ cup (1.8 oz.)	6
Slices	½ cup (1.5 oz.)	5
Boiled (USDA) flowerbuds, without salt, drained	½ cup (2.2 oz.)	5
Frozen:		
(Birds Eye):		
Regular	⅓ of 10-oz. pkg.	20
With cheese sauce	5 oz.	480
(Frosty Acres)	3.3 oz.	15
(Green Giant):		
In cheese sauce	½ cup (3.3 oz.)	450
Polybag, cuts	½ cup	30
In white cheddar cheese sauce	½ cup (3.3 oz.)	415
(Larsen)	3.3 oz.	45
(McKenzie)	3.3 oz.	28
CAVATELLI, frozen (Celentano)	⅕ of 16-oz. pkg.	100
CAVIAR, STURGEON (USDA) whole eggs	1 T. (.6 oz.)	352
CELERIAC ROOT, raw (USDA):		
Whole	1 lb. (weighed unpared)	390
Pared	4 oz.	113
CELERY, all varieties (USDA):		
Fresh:		
Whole	1 lb. (weighed untrimmed)	429

Food and Description	Measure or Quantity	Sodium (milligrams)
1 large outer stalk	8" × 1½" at root end (1.4 oz.)	50
Diced, chopped or cut in chunks	½ cup (2.1 oz.)	67
Slices	½ cup (1.9 oz.)	63
Boiled, drained solids:		
Diced or cut in chunks	½ cup (2.7 oz.)	67
Slices	½ cup (3 oz.)	74
Frozen (Larsen)	3½ oz.	90
CELERY CABBAGE (See **CABBAGE, CHINESE**)		
CELERY SALT (French's)	1 tsp. (4.6 g.)	1505
CELERY SEED (French's)	1 tsp. (2.4 g.)	4
CEREAL (See kind of cereal, such as **CORN FLAKES** or brand names such as **KIX, CHEX,** etc.)		
CERVELAT (Hormel) Viking, chub	1 oz.	325
CHABLIS WINE:		
(Great Western) 12% alcohol	3 fl. oz.	31
(Great Western) Diamond, 12% alcohol	3 fl. oz.	<1
CHAMPAGNE: (Great Western):	3 fl. oz.	31
CHARD, Swiss (USDA):		
Raw, whole	1 lb. (weighed untrimmed)	613
Raw, trimmed	4 oz.	167
Boiled, without salt, drained solids	½ cup (3.4 oz.)	83
CHARLOTTE RUSSE, with ladyfingers, whipped cream filling, home recipe (USDA)	4 oz.	49
CHAYOTE, raw (USDA):		
Whole	1 lb. (weighed unpared)	19
Pared	4 oz.	6
CHEERIOS, cereal (General Mills):		
Regular	1¼ cups (1 oz.)	290

Food and Description	Measure or Quantity	Sodium (milligrams)
Honey-nut	¾ cups (1 oz.)	250
CHEESE:		
American or cheddar:		
(USDA):		
Natural	1″ cube (.6 oz.)	119
Natural, diced	1 cup (4.6 oz.)	917
Natural, grated or shredded	1 cup (3.9 oz.)	777
Natural, grated or shredded	1 T. (.7 g.)	48
Process	1″ cube (.6 oz.)	204
(Dorman's) *Chedda-De Lite*	1 oz.	100
(Featherweight) low sodium	1 oz.	6
(Kraft):		
Regular:		
American singles	1 oz.	310
Cheddar	1 oz.	180
Old English, cheddar, sharp	1 oz.	440
(Laughing Cow)	1 oz.	227
(Polly-O) cheddar, shredded	1 oz.	180
(Sargento):		
Crock, sharp	1 oz.	274
Midget, midget Longhorn or shredded, regular or sharp	1 oz.	176
Shredded, non-dairy	1 oz.	269
Sliced or stick, sharp	1 oz.	176
Bleu or blue:		
(Frigo)	1 oz.	511
(Sargento) cold pack or crumbled	1 oz.	396
Bonbino (Laughing Cow)	1 oz.	227
Brick (Sargento) sliced	1 oz.	159
Brie (Sargento) *Danish Danko*	1 oz.	282
Burgercheese (Sargento)	1 oz.	406
Camembert (Sargento) *Danish Danko*	1 oz.	233
Cheddar (See American)		
Colby:		
(Featherweight) low sodium	1 oz.	4
(Kraft)	1 oz.	180
(Pauly) low sodium	1 oz.	5

Food and Description	Measure or Quantity	Sodium (milligrams)
(Sargento) midget Longhorn, shredded or sliced	1 oz.	171
Cottage:		
Unflavored:		
(USDA)	1 oz.	65
(USDA)	1 T.	34
(Borden):		
Regular, 4% milkfat:		
Salted	½ cup	400
Unsalted	½ cup	40
Dry curd, 0.5% milkfat	½ cup	20
Lite-Line, 1.5% milkfat	½ cup	400
(Breakstone's):		
Low fat	4 oz.	470
Smooth & creamy	4 oz.	370
Tangy	4 oz.	420
(Friendship) low fat or no salt added	1 oz.	7
(Johanna):		
Large or small curd	½ cup	450
Low fat	½ cup	430
No salt	½ cup	70
(Sealtest) large or small curd	4 oz.	460
Cream cheese:		
Plain, unwhipped:		
(USDA)	1 oz.	71
(Kraft) *Philadelphia Brand:*		
Regular	1 oz.	85
Lite	1 oz.	160
Flavored, unwhipped (Kraft)		
Philadelphia Brand:		
With chives & onion	1 oz.	100
With olives & pimiento	1 oz.	150
Edam:		
(House of Gold)	1 oz.	204
(Kaukauna)	1 oz.	275

Food and Description	Measure or Quantity	Sodium (milligrams)
(Laughing Cow)	1 oz.	227
(Sargento)	1 oz.	274
Farmer:		
(Friendship) no salt added	1 oz.	2
(Sargento)	1 oz.	132
Feta (Sargento) Danish, cups	1 oz.	316
Gjetost (Sargento) Norwegian	1 oz.	170
Gouda:		
(Kaukauna) any flavor	1 oz.	230
(Laughing Cow)	1 oz.	227
(Sargento) baby, caraway or smoked	1 oz.	232
Wispride	1 oz.	298
Grated:		
(Kraft) Italian blend	1 oz.	435
(Polly-O)	1 oz.	530
Gruyère, *Swiss Knight*	1 oz.	362
Havarti (Sargento): Creamy	1 oz.	198
Hoop (Friendship)	1 oz.	3
Hot pepper (Sargento) sliced	1 oz.	171
Jarlsberg (Sargento) Norwegian, sliced	1 oz.	130
Kettle Moraine (Sargento) sliced	1 oz.	17
Limburger (Sargento) natural	1 oz.	227
Monterey Jack:		
(Kaukauna) natural	1 oz.	150
(Kraft)	1 oz.	190
(Sargento) shredded or sliced	1 oz.	152
Mozzarella:		
(Dorman's) shredded, low sodium, light	1 oz.	90
(Kraft) 100% natural	1 oz.	190
(Polly-O):		
Fior di Latte	1 oz.	20
Lite	1 oz.	120
Part skim milk, regular or shredded	1 oz.	280
Smoked	1 oz.	240
Whole milk:		
Regular	1 oz.	280

Food and Description	Measure or Quantity	Sodium (milligrams)
Old fashioned:		
Regular	1 oz.	200
Shredded	1 oz.	220
Shredded or slices	1 oz.	220
Muenster:		
(Dorman's) sliced, low sodium	1 oz.	95
(Kaukauna) natural	1 oz.	180
(Sargento) red rind	1 oz.	178
Wispride	1 oz.	129
Nibblin' curds (Sargento)	1 oz.	176
Parmesan:		
(Frigo):		
Regular	1 oz.	341
Grated	1 T. (6 g.)	88
(Polly-O) grated	1 oz.	530
(Sargento):		
Grated, non-dairy	1 T. (7 g.)	105
Wedge	1 oz.	454
Pizza (Sargento) shredded or sliced, non-dairy	1 oz.	306
Provolone:		
(Frigo)	1 oz.	284
(Sargento) sliced	1 oz.	248
Ricotta (Polly-O):		
Lite	1 oz.	32
Old fashioned	1 oz.	25
Part skim milk:		
Regular	1 oz.	22
No salt	1 oz.	10
Whole milk:		
Regular	1 oz.	22
No salt	1 oz.	10
Romano (Sargento) wedge	1 oz.	340
Roquefort, natural (USDA)	1 oz.	465
Samsoe (Sargento) Danish	1 oz.	198
Semi-soft:		
Bill Paese	1 oz.	196
Laughing Cow:		
Babybel	1 oz.	227

Food and Description	Measure or Quantity	Sodium (milligrams)
Bombel	1 oz.	227
Slim Jack (Dorman's)	1 oz.	90
String (Sargento)	1 oz.	150
Swiss:		
(Dorman's) light, no salt added	1 oz.	8
(Sargento) sliced:		
Domestic	1 oz.	74
Imported, Finland	1 oz.	74
Taco (Sargento) shredded	1 oz.	47
CHEESE DIP (See **DIP**)		
CHEESE FONDUE:		
Home recipe (USDA)	4 oz.	615
Swiss Knight	1-oz. serving	186
CHEESE FOOD, process:		
American or cheddar:		
(Borden) *Lite-Line:*		
American	1 oz.	410
Cheddar, sharp	1 oz.	440
(Pauly)	.8-oz. slice	431
(Sargento) logs with almonds & with port wine & almonds; with port wine and sharp, cold pack	1 oz.	274
Wispride, cheddar:		
Regular	1 oz.	180
& port wine	1 oz.	190
Cheez'n Crackers, process (Kraft)	1.1-oz. piece	466
Cheez-ola (Fisher) process	1 oz.	454
Colby (Pauly) low sodium	1 oz.	5
Cracker snack (Sargento)	1 oz.	406
Garlic & herb, *Wispride*	1 oz.	180
Jalapeño (Borden) *Lite-Line*	1 oz.	430
Low sodium (Borden) *Lite-Line*	1 oz.	200
Monterey Jack (Borden) *Lite-Line*	1 oz.	450
Muenster (Borden) *Lite-Line*	1 oz.	450
Mun-chee (Pauly) chunk	1 oz.	485
Pimiento (Pauly)	.8-oz. slice	426

Food and Description	Measure or Quantity	Sodium (milligrams)
Swiss:		
(Borden) *Lite-Line*	1 oz.	330
(Kraft) reduced fat, light natural	1 oz.	55
CHEESE SPREAD:		
American, process:		
(USDA)	1 T. (.5 oz.)	228
(Nabisco) Easy Cheese	1 tsp. (6 g.)	70
Wispride	1 oz.	304
Blue (Laughing Cow)	1 oz.	312
Cheddar:		
(Laughing Cow)	1 oz.	312
(Nabisco) *Easy Cheese:*		
Regular	1 tsp.	74
Chive	1 tsp.	68
Sharp	1 tsp.	64
Wispride, sharp	1 oz.	304
Cheese & bacon (Nabisco) Easy Cheese	1 tsp. (6 g.)	70
Count Down (Fisher)	1 oz.	435
Gruyère (Laughing Cow) *La Vache Qui Rit*	1 oz.	312
Imitation (Fisher) *Chef's Delight*	1 oz.	380
Nacho (Nabisco) *Easy Cheese*	1 tsp.	68
Pimiento:		
(Pauly)	¾-oz. serving	386
(Price's)	1 oz.	335
Provolone (Laughing Cow)	1 oz.	312
Sharp (Pauly)	.8-oz. serving	437
Swiss (Pauly) process	.8-oz. serving	391
Velveeta (Kraft):		
Regular	1 oz.	430
Mexican, with jalapeño pepper	1 oz.	440
CHEESE STRAW (USDA)	5″ × ⅜″ piece (6 g.)	43
CHELOIS WINE (Great Western)		
12% alcohol	3 fl. oz.	37

Food and Description	Measure or Quantity	Sodium (milligrams)
CHERRY:		
Sour (USDA):		
Fresh:		
Whole	1 lb. (weighed with stems)	7
Whole	1 lb. (weighed without stems)	8
Pitted	½ cup (2.7 oz.)	2
Canned, syrup pack, pitted:		
Light syrup	4 oz. (with liq.)	1
Heavy syrup	½ cup (with liq.)	1
Extra heavy syrup	4 oz. (with liq.)	1
Canned, water pack, pitted, solids & liq.	½ cup (4.3 oz.)	2
Frozen, pitted:		
Sweetened	½ cup (4.6 oz.)	3
Unsweetened	4 oz.	2
Sweet:		
Fresh (USDA):		
Whole	1 lb. (weighed with stems)	8
Whole, with stems	½ cup (2.3 oz.)	1
Pitted	½ cup (2.9 oz.)	2
Canned, syrup pack:		
(USDA):		
Light syrup, pitted	4 oz. (with liq.)	1
Heavy syrup, pitted	½ cup (with liq., 4.2 oz.)	1
Extra heavy syrup, pitted	4 oz. (with liq.)	1
(Del Monte) solids & liq.:		
Dark	½ cup (4.3 oz.)	<10
Light	½ cup (4.3 oz.)	<10
(Stokely-Van Camp) pitted, solids & liq.	½ cup (4.2 oz.)	18
Canned, dietetic or water pack, solids & liq.:		
(Diet Delight)	½ cup (4.4 oz.)	5
(Featherweight):		
Dark	½ cup	<10
Light	½ cup	<10

Food and Description	Measure or Quantity	Sodium (milligrams)
CHERRY DRINK:		
Canned:		
(Hi-C)	6 fl. oz.	4
Ssips (Johanna Farms)	8.45-fl.-oz. container	20
*Mix (Hi-C)	6 fl. oz.	23
CHERRY JELLY:		
Sweetened:		
(Home Brands)	1 T.	15
(Smucker's)	1 T.	3
Dietetic or low calorie		
(Featherweight)	1 T.	40–50
CHERRY PIE (See **PIE,** Cherry)		
CHERRY PIE FILLING (See **PIE FILLING,** Cherry)		
CHERRY PRESERVE or JAM:		
Sweetened (Home Brands)	1 T. (.7 oz.)	15
Dietetic (Louis Sherry)	1 T.	<3
CHERVIL (Spice Island)	1 tsp.	Tr.
CHESTNUT (USDA):		
Fresh:		
In shell	1 lb. (weighed in shell)	22
Shelled	4 oz.	7
Dried:		
In shell	1 lb. (weighed in shell)	45
Shelled	4 oz.	14
CHEWING GUM, sweetened or unsweetened:		
Beechies	1 tablet	0
Beech-Nut	1 stick	Tr.
Beemans	1 stick	
Big Red	1 stick	Tr.
Doublemint (Wrigley's)	1 stick	Tr.
Freedent (Wrigley's)	1 stick	Tr.
Juicy Fruit (Wrigley's)	1 stick	Tr.
Orbit, regular or bubble	1 stick	Tr.
Spearmint (Wrigley's)	1 stick (3 g.)	Tr.

Food and Description	Measure or Quantity	Sodium (milligrams)
CHEX, cereal (Ralston Purina):		
Bran (See **BRAN BREAKFAST CEREAL**)		
Corn	1 cup (1 oz.)	295
Rice	1⅛ cups (1 oz.)	243
Wheat	⅔ cup (1 oz.)	192
Wheat & raisin	¾ cup (1⅓ oz.)	216
CHICKEN (See also **CHICKEN, CANNED**): (USDA):		
Broiler, cooked, meat only	4 oz.	75
Fryer:		
Raw, ready-to-cook	1 lb. (weighed ready-to-cook)	0
Hen and cock:		
Stewed:		
Meat only	4 oz.	62
Chopped	½ cup (2.5 oz.)	40
Diced	½ cup (2.4 oz.)	37
Ground	½ cup (2 oz.)	31
Roaster:		
Roasted:		
Dark meat without skin	4 oz.	100
Light meat without skin	4 oz.	75
CHICKEN À LA KING:		
Home recipe (USDA)	1 cup (8.6 oz.)	760
Canned (Swanson)	½ of 10½-oz. can	690
Frozen:		
(Banquet)	4-oz. pkg.	555
(Blue Star) *Dining Lite*, with rice	9½-oz. meal	910
(Green Giant) twin pouch	9-oz. entree	1545
(Le Menu)	10¼-oz. dinner	1050
(Morton) Light	8-oz. dinner	600
(Stouffer's) with rice	9½-oz. meal	900
(Weight Watchers) boil-in-bag	9-oz. pkg.	1060
CHICKEN BOUILLON/ BROTH, cube or powder (See also **SOUP**, Chicken):		
(Borden) *Lite-Line*	1 tsp.	5

Food and Description	Measure or Quantity	Sodium (milligrams)
(Featherweight) low sodium	1 tsp.	5
(Herb-Ox):		
Cube	4-g. cube	950
Powder	5-g. packet	960
(Maggi)	1 cube	746
MBT	1 packet (.2 oz.)	575
(Wyler's):		
Cube	1 cube	900
Instant	1 tsp.	900
CHICKEN, CANNED, BONED:		
(Featherweight) low sodium	5 oz.	99
(Hormel):		
Breast	6¾-oz. can	855
Dark	6¾-oz. can	933
White & dark:		
Regular	6¾-oz. can	857
Low sodium	6¾-oz. can	75
(Swanson):		
Regular	½ of 5-oz. can	240
Mixin' style	½ of 5-oz. can	225
White	½ of 5-oz. can	230
CHICKEN DINNER or		
ENTREE:		
Canned:		
(Hunt's) *Minute Gourmet Microwave Entree Maker:*		
Barbecued:		
Without chicken	3.1 oz.	1040
With chicken	6.8 oz.	1110
Cacciatore:		
Without chicken	4.6 oz.	780
With chicken	8.3 oz.	840
Sweet & sour:		
Without chicken	4.1 oz.	360
With chicken	7.8 oz.	420
(Swanson) & dumplings	7½ oz.	960
Frozen:		
(Armour):		
Classic Lites:		
Breast medallions marsala	11-oz. meal	970

Food and Description	Measure or Quantity	Sodium (milligrams)
Burgundy	11¼-oz. meal	1220
Oriental	10-oz. meal	880
Sweet & sour	11-oz. meal	640
Dinner Classics:		
Fricassee	11¾-oz. meal	1210
Hawaiian	11½-oz. meal	700
Milan	11½-oz. meal	1360
Sweet & sour	11-oz. meal	1240
(Banquet):		
Dinner:		
American Favorites, fried	11-oz. dinner	1831
Family Favorites & dumplings	9-oz. dinner	944
Entree:		
Family Entree & dumpling	32-oz. pkg.	3712
Gourmet Entree:		
Cacciatore	10-oz. pkg.	510
French	10-oz. pkg.	850
(Blue Star) *Dining Lite*:		
Glazed, with vegetables & rice	8½-oz. meal	880
With vegetables & vermicelli	12¾-oz. meal	960
(Celentano):		
Parmigiana, cutlets	9-oz. pkg.	750
Primavera	11½-oz. pkg.	650
(Conagra) *Light & Elegant*:		
Glazed	8-oz. entree	660
Parmigiano	8-oz. entree	680
(Green Giant):		
Baked:		
In BBQ sauce with corn on cob	1 meal	885
In herb butter with stuffed potato	1 meal	965
Stir fry, & cashews	10-oz. entree	965
Stir fry, & vegetables	10-oz. entree	705
Stir fry, sweet & sour	10-oz. entree	585

Food and Description	Measure or Quantity	Sodium (milligrams)
Twin pouch:		
& broccoli with rice in cheese sauce	9½-oz. entree	915
& pea pods in sauce with rice & vegetables	10-oz. entree	995
(La Choy) *Fresh and Lite*, almond	9¾-oz. entree	820
(Le Menu):		
Parmigiana, breast of	11½-oz. dinner	890
Sweet & sour	11½-oz. dinner	980
(Morton):		
Regular; boneless	11-oz. dinner	500
Fried	11-oz. dinner	1400
(Stouffer's):		
Regular:		
Creamed	6½-oz. pkg.	680
Divan	8½-oz. meal	830
Lean Cuisine:		
Glazed, with vegetable rice	8½-oz. meal	830
& vegetables, with vermicelli	12¾-oz. meal	1220
(Swanson):		
Regular:		
& dumplings	7½-oz. meal	965
Fried, 4-compartment:		
Barbecue flavor	9¼-oz. meal	960
Breast portion	10¾-oz. meal	1580
Dark meat	10¼-oz. meal	1390
Hungry Man:		
Boneless	17½-oz. dinner	1640
Fried:		
Breast	14-oz. dinner	2120
Dark portion	14-oz. dinner	1680
Parmigiana	20-oz. dinner	2080
(Weight Watchers):		
Cacciatori, boil-in-bag	10-oz. pkg.	1110
Parmigiana, 2-compartment	8-oz. meal	960

Food and Description	Measure or Quantity	Sodium (milligrams)
Southern fried patty, 2-compartment	6½-oz. serving	787
Sweet & sour, with oriental style vegetables	9-oz. pkg.	800
CHICKEN & DUMPLINGS (See **CHICKEN DINNER or ENTREE**)		
CHICKEN FRICASSEE, home recipe (USDA)	1 cup (8½ oz.)	370
CHICKEN, FRIED, frozen:		
(Banquet):		
Assorted or hot & spicy	32-oz. pkg.	6005
Breast portion	22-oz. pkg.	3860
Drum snackers	12-oz. pkg.	2128
Thigh & drumstick	25-oz. pkg.	4460
Wings	12-oz. pkg.	2128
(Swanson) Plump & Juicy:		
Assorted, regular	3¼ oz. serving	600
Breast portion	4½-oz. serving	830
Cutlet	3½-oz. serving	440
Dipsters	3-oz. serving	400
Drumlets	3-oz. serving	390
Nibbles (wings)	3¼-oz. serving	640
Take-out style	3¼-oz. serving	660
Thighs & drumsticks	3¼-oz. serving	550
CHICKEN GIZZARD (USDA):		
Raw	2-oz. serving	37
Simmered	2-oz. serving	32
***CHICKEN HELPER** (General Mills):		
Crispy:		
& biscuits	⅕ of pkg.	1240
& seasoned rice	⅕ of pkg.	1490
& dumplings	⅕ of pkg.	1320
& mushroom	⅕ of pkg.	900
Potato & gravy	⅕ of pkg.	1000
Stuffing	⅕ of pkg.	1600
Teriyaki	⅕ of pkg.	1010
Tetrazzini	⅕ of pkg.	870

Food and Description	Measure or Quantity	Sodium (milligrams)
CHICKEN LIVER (See **LIVER**)		
CHICKEN & NOODLES:		
Home recipe (USDA)	1 cup (8½ oz.)	600
Frozen:		
(Green Giant)	9-oz. pkg.	940
(Stouffer's):		
Escalloped	11½-oz. meal	1440
Paprikash	10½-oz. meal	1325
CHICKEN NUGGETS, frozen		
(Banquet) breaded & fried,		
regular	12-oz. pkg.	2292
CHICKEN, PACKAGED:		
(Carl Buddig) smoked	1 oz.	340
(Eckrich) breast, sliced	1 slice	210
CHICKEN PATTIE, frozen		
(Banquet) breaded & fried	12-oz. pkg.	2052
CHICKEN PIE:		
Home recipe (USDA) baked	8-oz. pie (4¼" dia.)	581
Frozen:		
(Banquet)	8-oz. pie	966
(Stouffer's)	10-oz. pie	1530
(Swanson):		
Regular	8-oz. pie	840
Chunky	10-oz. pie	850
Hungry Man	16-oz. pie	1670
CHICKEN SALAD, canned		
(Carnation) *Spreadable*	¼ of 7½-oz. can	230
CHICKEN SOUP (See **SOUP,**		
Chicken)		
CHICKEN SPREAD, canned:		
(Hormel):		
Lunche Loaf	1 oz.	304
Sandwich Makins	1 oz.	252
(Swanson)	1-oz. serving	140
(Underwood) chunky	½ of 4¾-oz. can	575
CHICKEN STEW:		
Canned, regular pack:		
(Libby's) with dumplings	⅓ of 24-oz. can	976
(Swanson)	7⅝-oz. serving	960

Food and Description	Measure or Quantity	Sodium (milligrams)
Canned, dietetic or low calorie:		
(Dia-Mel)	8-oz. can	65
(Featherweight)	7½-oz. can	53
CHICKEN STICKS, frozen		
(Banquet) breaded-fried	12-oz. pkg.	2264
CHICKEN STOCK BASE		
(French's)	1 tsp. (3 g.)	475
CHICK-FIL-A:		
Brownie, fudge, with nuts	2.8-oz. piece	213
Carrot-raisin salad:		
Small	1 cup (2.7 oz.)	8
Large	1 pint (13.1 oz.)	37
Chargrill:		
Without bun	3.6 oz.	770
With bun	5¾ oz.	1027
Chicken Salad:		
Cup	3.4-oz. serving	543
Plate	11.8-oz. serving	1839
Sandwich	5.7-oz. sandwich	888
Chicken soup, hearty	8.5-oz. serving	530
Chick-fil-A:		
Regular:		
Without bun	3.6 oz.	552
With bun	5.7 oz.	1174
Nuggets:		
8-pack	4 oz.	1326
12-pack	6 oz.	1989
Coleslaw:		
Cup	3.7 oz.	158
Pint	15¼ oz.	648
Icedream	4½ oz.	51
Pie, lemon	4.1 oz. slice	300
Potato Salad:		
Cup	3.8 oz.	337
Pint	16½ oz.	1448
Potato fries, waffle	1 regular order (3 oz.)	45
CHICK PEAS or GARBANZOS:		
Dry (USDA)	1 cup (7.1 oz.)	52

Food and Description	Measure or Quantity	Sodium (milligrams)
Canned, regular pack, solids & liq:		
(Allen's)	½ cup	330
(Furman's)	⅓ cup (2.6 oz.)	275
CHICORY, WITLOOF, Belgian or French endive, raw, bleached head (USDA):		
Untrimmed	½ lb.	14
Trimmed, cut	½ cup (1.6 oz.)	1
CHILI or CHILI CON CARNE:		
Canned, beans only:		
(Comstock)	½ cup	540
(Hormel) in sauce	5 oz.	453
(Hunt's)	½ cup (3½ oz.)	430
Canned, regular pack, with beans:		
(USDA)	1 cup (8.8 oz.)	1328
(Gebhardt) Hot	½ of 15-oz. can	1000
(Hormel):		
Regular:		
Hot	½ of 15-oz. can	1121
Mild	½ of 15-oz. can	1127
Short Orders:		
Hot	7½-oz. can	1086
Mild	7½-oz. can	1134
(Libby's)	½ of 15-oz. can	810
(Old El Paso)	1 cup	907
Canned, regular pack, without beans:		
(Gebhardt)	½ of 15-oz. can	1040
(Hormel):		
Regular:		
Hot	½ of 15-oz. can	985
Mild	½ of 15-oz. can	1012
Short Orders	7½-oz. can	961
(Libby's)	½ of 15-oz. can	1182
Frozen, with beans (Stouffer's)	8¾-oz. meal	1265
CHILI MAC (Hormel) *Short Orders*	7½-oz. can	1418

Food and Description	Measure or Quantity	Sodium (milligrams)
CHILI SAUCE:		
Regular:		
(USDA)	1 T. (.5 oz.)	201
(Del Monte)	1 oz.	417
(El Molino) green, mild	1 T.	105
(Ortega) hot	1-oz. serving	181
Dietetic:		
(USDA) low sodium	1 T. (.5 oz.)	Tr.
(Featherweight)	1 T. (.5 oz.)	10
CHILI SEASONING MIX:		
*(Durkee)	1 cup	979
(French's) *Chili-O*, plain	1¾-oz. pkg.	3780
CHINESE DINNER, frozen (See individual listings such as **CHOP SUEY, CHOW MEIN,** etc.)		
CHIPS (See **POTATO CHIPS** or **CRACKERS, PUFFS and CHIPS**)		
CHOCO-DILES (Hostess)	2-oz. piece	284
CHOCOLATE, BAKING:		
(Baker's):		
Bitter or unsweetened	1-oz. square	1
Semi-sweet:		
Regular	1-oz. square	<1
Chips	¼ cup (1½ oz.)	<9
Sweetened, German	1-oz. square	<1
(Hershey's):		
Bitter or unsweetened	1-oz. square	5
Semi-sweet, chips	1 oz.	3
Sweetened, chips:		
Dark, regular or mini	1 oz.	65
Milk	1 oz.	35
(Nestlé):		
Bitter or unsweetened, *Choco-Bake*	1-oz. packet	5
Semi-sweet, morsels	1 oz.	0
Sweetened, milk, morsels	1 oz.	20
CHOCOLATE CAKE (See **CAKE,** Chocolate)		

Food and Description	Measure or Quantity	Sodium (milligrams)
CHOCOLATE CANDY (See **CANDY**)		
CHOCOLATE, HOT, home recipe (USDA)	1 cup (8.8 oz.)	120
CHOCOLATE ICE CREAM (See **ICE CREAM,** Chocolate)		
CHOCOLATE PIE (See **PIE,** Chocolate)		
CHOCOLATE PUDDING or PIE FILLING (See **PUDDING or PIE FILLING,** Chocolate)		
CHOCOLATE SYRUP (See **SYRUP,** Chocolate)		
CHOP SUEY:		
Home recipe (USDA) with meat	1 cup (8.8 oz.)	1052
Canned (USDA) with meat	1 cup (8.8 oz.)	1378
Frozen (Banquet) beef:		
Buffet Supper	2-lb. pkg.	5336
Cookin' Bag	7-oz. pkg.	1140
Dinner	12-oz. dinner	1802
*Mix (Durkee)	1¾ cups	5582
CHOW CHOW (USDA):		
Sour	1 oz.	379
Sweet	1 oz.	149
CHOW MEIN:		
Home recipe (USDA) chicken, without noodles	8-oz. serving	652
Canned, regular pack:		
(Chun King) chicken, *Divider-Pak*	¼ of pkg.	821
(La Choy):		
Beef	¾ cup	890
*Beef, bi-pack	¾ cup	840
Chicken	¾ cup	800
*Chicken, bi-pack	¾ cup	970
Meatless	¾ cup	780
*Pepper oriental, bi-pack	¾ cup	950
*Pork, bi-pack	¾ cup	950
Shrimp	¾ cup	820
*Shrimp, bi-pack	¾ cup	860

Food and Description	Measure or Quantity	Sodium (milligrams)
Frozen:		
(Armour) *Chicken Lites*	10½-oz. meal	1180
(Blue Star) *Dining Lite*,		
chicken & rice	11¼-oz. meal	1450
(Green Giant):		
Beef, twin pouch with rice		
& vegetables	10-oz. entree	1050
Chicken, twin pouch, with		
rice & vegetables	9-oz. entree	1075
(La Choy):		
Regular:		
Chicken:		
Dinner	12-oz. dinner	1740
Entree	⅔ cup	720
Shrimp:		
Dinner	12-oz. dinner	1740
Entree	⅔ cup	820
Fresh & Lite, imperial		
chicken	11-oz. entree	950
(Morton) light, chicken:		
Dinner	11-oz. dinner	700
Entree	8-oz. entree	500
(Stouffer's) *Lean Cuisine*,		
chicken with rice	11¼-oz. meal	1155
(Van de Kamp's) Mandarin:		
Beef	11-oz. meal	1700
Chicken	11-oz. meal	1180
CHOW MEIN NOODLES (See **NOODLES, CHOW MEIN**)		
CHOW MEIN SEASONING MIX (Kikkoman)	1⅛-oz. pkg.	3
CHURCH'S FRIED CHICKEN:		
Chicken, fried:		
Breast	4.3-oz. serving	560
Leg	2.9-oz. serving	286
Thigh	4.2-oz. serving	448
Wing-breast	4.8-oz. serving	583
Corn, with butter oil	1 serving	20
French fries	1 regular order (3 oz.)	126

Food and Description	Measure or Quantity	Sodium (milligrams)
CIDER (See **APPLE CIDER**)		
CINNAMON, GROUND:		
(USDA)	1 tsp. (2.3 g.)	1
(French's)	1 tsp. (1.7 g.)	Tr.
CINNAMON SUGAR (French's)	1 tsp.	0
CITRON, CANDIED (USDA)	1 oz.	82
*CITRUS BERRY BLEND, mix, dietetic (Sunkist)	8 fl. oz.	20
CITRUS COOLER DRINK, canned (Hi-C)	6 fl. oz.	4
CLAM:		
Raw (USDA):		
Hard or round, meat only	1 cup (8 oz.)	465
Soft, meat only	1 cup (8 oz.)	82
Canned (Gorton's) minced, drained solids	1 can	1280
Frozen:		
(Gorton's) fried strips, crunchy	1 pkg.	920
(Mrs. Paul's) batter fried, light	½ of 5-oz. pkg.	385
CLAMATO COCKTAIL, canned (Mott's)	6 fl. oz.	815
CLARET WINE (Gold Seal)	3 fl. oz.	3
CLOVE, GROUND (French's)	1 tsp. (1.7 g.)	4
CLUB SODA (See SOFT DRINK)		
COCOA:		
Dry:		
(USDA):		
Low fat	1 T. (5 g.)	<1
Medium-low fat	1 T. (5 g.)	<1
Medium-high fat	1 T. (5 g.)	<1
High fat	1 T.	<1
(Hershey's) unsweetened, American process	⅓ cup (1 oz.)	10
Home recipe (USDA)	1 cup (8.8 oz.)	128

Food and Description	Measure or Quantity	Sodium (milligrams)
Mix, regular pack:		
(Alba '66) instant, low fat, regular and chocolate with marshmallow flavor	6 fl. oz.	89
(Carnation) instant	1-oz. pkg.	120
(Hershey's) instant	3 T. (¾ oz.)	45
(Nestlé)	1.5-oz. pkg.	110
(Ovaltine) hot'n rich	1-oz. packet	183
Swiss Miss:		
Regular:		
Double rich	1 envelope	160
Milk chocolate	1 envelope	170
With mini marshmallows	1 envelope	150
European creme:		
Amaretto	1 envelope	120
Chocolate	1 envelope	180
Creme de menthe or mocha	1 envelope	120
Mix, dietetic or low calorie:		
(Carnation) *70 Calorie*	.73-oz. pkg.	125
(Estee)	1 packet	75
(Ovaltine) reduced calorie	.45-oz. packet	88
Swiss Miss:		
Lite	1 envelope	210
Milk chocolate or with sugar-free marshmallows	1 envelope	190
COCOA KRISPIES, cereal (Kellogg's)	¾ cup (1 oz.)	195
COCOA PUFFS, cereal (General Mills)	1 cup (1 oz.)	200
COCONUT:		
Fresh (USDA):		
Whole	1 lb. (weighed in shell)	54
Meat only	4 oz.	26
Meat only	2″ × 2″ × ½″ piece (1.6 oz.)	10
Grated or shredded, loosely packed	½ cup (1.4 oz.)	15

Food and Description	Measure or Quantity	Sodium (milligrams)
Dried, canned or packaged:		
(Baker's):		
Angel flake, bag	⅓ cup	73
Cookie	⅓ cup	109
Premium shred	⅓ cup	84
(Durkee) shredded	¼ cup	5
COCONUT, CREAM OF,		
canned:		
(Coco Lopez)	1 T.	5
(Holland House)	1 oz.	21
COCO WHEATS, cereal	1 T. (.42 oz.)	3
COD(USDA):		
Raw:		
Whole	1 lb.	98
Meat only	4 oz.	79
Broiled	4 oz.	124
Dehydrated, lightly salted	4 oz.	9185
Frozen:		
(Frionor) *Norway Gourmet*	4-oz. fillet	106
(Gorton's) *Fishmarket Fresh*	4 oz.	70
(Van de Kamp's) *Today's*		
Catch	4 oz.	150
COD DINNER OR ENTREE,		
frozen:		
(Armour) *Dinner Classics,*		
almondine	12-oz.meal	1440
(Blue Star) *Dining Lite*	10-oz. meal	570
(Frionor) *Norway Gourmet:*		
With dill sauce	4.5-oz. fillet	169
With toasted bread crumbs	4.5-oz. fillet	359
COFFEE:		
Ground:		
(Chase & Sanborn) drip or		
electric perk; *Max-Pax;*		
(Maxwell House) regular or		
Electra-Perk; (Yuban)		
regular, drip or *Electra*		
Matic	6 fl. oz.	Tr.
Mellow Roast	6 fl. oz.	1

Food and Description	Measure or Quantity	Sodium (milligrams)
Decaffeinated:		
Brim, regular, drip or electric perk	6 fl. oz.	5
Decaf, Nescafé	6 fl. oz.	<10
Sanka	6 fl. oz.	1
Freeze-dried, *Taster's Choice*	6 fl. oz.	0
Instant:		
(Chase & Sanborn)	5 fl. oz.	1
(General Foods) *International Coffee:*		
Café Amaretto	6 fl. oz.	25
Café Francais	6 fl. oz.	24
Café Irish Crème	6 fl. oz.	19
Café Vienna	6 fl. oz.	93
Irish Mocha Mint	6 fl. oz.	24
Orange Cappuccino	6 fl. oz.	98
Suisse Mocha	6 fl. oz.	24
Mellow Roast	6 fl. oz.	2
Sunrise	6 fl. oz.	<10
COFFEE CAKE (See **CAKE,** Coffee)		
COFFEE SOUTHERN, liqueur	1 fl. oz.	Tr.
COGNAC (See **DISTILLED LIQUOR**)		
COLA SOFT DRINK (See **SOFT DRINK,** Cola)		
COLD DUCK WINE (Great Western) pink, 12% alcohol	3 fl. oz.	31
COLESLAW, solids & liq. (USDA):		
Prepared with commercial French dressing	4-oz. serving	304
Prepared with homemade French dressing	4-oz. serving	149
Prepared with mayonnaise	4-oz. serving	136
Prepared with mayonnaise type salad dressing	1 cup (4.2 oz.)	149
COLLARDS:		
Raw (USDA) leaves, including stems	1 lb.	195

Food and Description	Measure or Quantity	Sodium (milligrams)
Canned (Sunshine) chopped, solids & liq.	½ cup (4.1 oz.)	378
Frozen:		
(USDA):		
Not thawed	10-oz. pkg.	51
Boiled, chopped, drained	½ cup (3 oz.)	14
(Frosty Acres)	3.3 oz.	45
(McKenzie) chopped	3.3 oz.	56
(Southland) chopped	⅓ of 16-oz. pkg.	45
COLLINS MIXER (See **SOFT DRINK,** Tom Collins)		
COMPLETE CEREAL (Elam's)	1-oz. serving	5
CONCORD WINE:		
(Gold seal) 13-14% alcohol	3 fl. oz.	3
(Pleasant Valley) red, 12½% alcohol	3 fl. oz.	23
COOKIE (Listed by type or brand name. See also **COOKIE, DIETETIC; COOKIE DOUGH; COOKIE, HOME RECIPE** and **COOKIE MIX**)		
Almond supreme (Pepperidge Farm)	1 piece	21
Animal:	1 piece (3 g.)	9
(USDA)	1 oz.	86
(Dixie Belle)	1 piece	7
(Nabisco) *Barnum's*	1 piece	11
(Ralston)	1 piece	7
(Sunshine)	1 piece	13
(Tom's)	1.7 oz.	200
Apple Newtons (Nabisco)	1 piece	30
Apricot-raspberry (Pepperidge Farm)	1 cookie	26
Assortment:		
(Nabisco) *Famous Assortment:*		
Baronet creme sandwich	1 piece	25
Biscos sugar wafer	1 piece	6
Butter flavored	1 piece	23
Cameo creme sandwich	1 piece	28

Food and Description	Measure or Quantity	Sodium (milligrams)
Kettle cookie	1 piece	29
Lorna Doone	1 piece	34
Oreo, chocolate	1 piece	57
(Pepperidge Farm):		
Butter	1 piece	27
Champagne, Original		
Pirouettes	1 piece	18
Seville	1 piece	25
Southport	1 piece	35
Blueberry (Pepperidge Farm)	1 piece	23
Blueberry Newtons (Nabisco)	1 piece	53
Bordeaux (Pepperidge Farm)	1 cookie	23
Brown edge wafer (Nabisco)	1 piece	16
Brownie:		
(Hostess):		
Large	2-oz. piece	122
Small	1¼-oz. piece	76
(Nabisco) *Almost Home*	1 piece	75
(Pepperidge Farm):		
Chocolate nut	1 piece (.4 oz.)	27
Nut, large	1 piece (.9 oz.)	65
(Sara Lee) frozen	⅛ of 13-oz. pkg.	108
Brussels (Pepperidge Farm):		
Regular	1 cookie	32
Mint	1 cookie	40
Butter flavored:		
(Nabisco)	1 piece	23
(Sunshine)	1 piece	37
Buttercup (Keebler)	1 piece	30
Cappucino (Pepperidge Farm)	1 cookie	20
Capri (Pepperidge Farm)	1 cookie	45
Cherry Newton (Nabisco)	1 piece	53
Chessman (Pepperidge Farm)	1 cookie	26
Chocolate & chocolate covered:		
(USDA)	1 oz.	39
(Keebler) fudge stripes	1 piece	50
(Nabisco):		
Famous Wafer	1 cookie	40
Pinwheels, cake	1.1-oz. piece	35
Snaps	1 piece	20

Food and Description	Measure or Quantity	Sodium (milligrams)
(Sunshine) nugget	1 cookie	18
Chocolate chip:		
(USDA)	1 oz.	114
(Keebler) *Rich 'n Chips*	1 piece	70
(Nabisco):		
Almost Home:		
Fudge	1 cookie	65
Real	1 cookie	50
Chips Ahoy!:		
Regular	1 cookie	32
Chewy	1 cookie	55
Chips 'n More:		
Coconut	1 cookie	47
Fudge	1 cookie	30
Original	1 cookie	35
Snaps	1 cookie	17
(Pepperidge Farm):		
Old fashioned	1 cookie	30
Chocolate	1 cookie	25
(Sunshine):		
Chip-A-Roos:		
Regular	1 cookie	50
Chocolate	1 cookie	80
Chippy Chews, any flavor	1 cookie	35
(Tom's)	1½ g.	110
Chocolate peanut bar (Nabisco)	1 cookie	65
Cinnamon raisin (Nabisco)		
Almost Home	1 cookie	47
Creme stick (Dutch Twin)	1 piece	3
Danish (Nabisco) imported	1 cookie	14
Date nut granola (Pepperidge Farm) Kitchen Hearth	1 cookie	32
Date pecan (Pepperidge Farm)	1 cookie	20
Devil's food cake (Nabisco)	1⅓-oz. piece	90
Fig bar:		
(Nabisco) *Fig Newtons*	1 piece (.6 oz.)	50
(Sunshine) Chewies	1 cookie	30
(Tom's)	1.8-oz. serving	130
Fruit Stick (Nabisco) *Almost Home*:		
Apple	1 cookie	30

Food and Description	Measure or Quantity	Sodium (milligrams)
Blueberry	1 cookie	90
Cherry	1 cookie	100
Iced dutch apple	1 cookie	40
Geneva (Pepperidge Farm)	1 piece	21
Gingerman (Pepperidge Farm)	1 piece	25
Gingersnap:		
(Archway)	1 cookie	20
(Nabisco) old fashioned	1 cookie	50
(Sunshine)	1 cookie	23
Golden fruit raisin (Sunshine)	1 piece (smallest portion after breaking on score line)	40
Hazelnut (Pepperidge Farm)	1 piece	37
Heyday (Nabisco)	1 cookie	45
Ladyfinger (USDA)	3¼″ × 1¾″ × 1⅛″	8
Lemon cooler (Sunshine) cooler	1 cookie	22
Lemon nut crunch (Pepperidge Farm)	1 piece	25
Lido (Pepperidge Farm)	1 piece	42
Macaroon (Nabisco) soft	1 piece	65
Mallo Puffs (Sunshine)	1 cookie	60
Marshmallow (Nabisco):		
Mallomars	1 piece	17
Puffs, cocoa covered	1 piece	55
Sandwich	1 piece	20
Twirls	1 cookie	55
Milano (Pepperidge Farm)	1 piece	26
Molasses:		
(Archway)	1 cookie	155
(Nabisco) *Pantry*	1 cookie	65
Molasses crisp (Pepperidge Farm)	1 piece	25
Nassau (Pepperidge Farm)	1 piece	45
Nilla wafer (Nabisco)	1 piece	14
Oatmeal:		
(Archway):		
Regular	1 cookie	90
Apple filled	1 cookie	115
Date filled	1 cookie	105

Food and Description	Measure or Quantity	Sodium (milligrams)
(Keebler) old fashioned:	1 piece	115
(Nabisco) *Bakers Bonus*	1 cookie	45
(Pepperidge Farm):		
Irish	1 piece	40
Raisin	1 piece	57
(Sunshine):		
Country style	1 cookie	60
Peanut sandwich	1 cookie	65
Orange Milano (Pepperidge Farm)	1 piece	35
Orbits (Sunshine):		
Butter flavored	1 cookie	19
Chocolate	1 cookie	21
Orleans (Pepperidge Farm)	1 piece	10
Peanut or peanut butter:		
(Nabisco):		
Almost Home:		
Regular	1 cookie	47
Fudge	1 cookie	45
Creme pattie	1 piece	25
Nutter Butter, sandwich	1 piece	50
(Sunshine) wafer	1 cookie	17
Pecan Sandies (Keebler)	1 piece	52
Raisin (Nabisco) *Almost Home*:		
Fudge chocolate chip	1 cookie	42
Iced applesauce	1 cookie	35
Iced oatmeal	1 cookie	40
Oatmeal	1 cookie	50
Sandwich:		
(Keebler):		
Fudge creme	1 cookie	30
Oatmeal creme	1 cookie	60
Pitter Patter	1 cookie	120
(Nabisco):		
Almost Home: (See "A")		
Baronet	1 cookie	25
Cameo	1 cookie	28
Gaity, fudge chocolate	1 cookie	
Giggles:		
Chocolate	1 cookie	35

Food and Description	Measure or Quantity	Sodium (milligrams)
Vanilla	1 cookie	25
I Screame	1 cookie	35
Mystic Mint	1 cookie	47
Oreo:		
Regular	1 cookie	57
Double Stuf	1 cookie	60
Mint	1 cookie	80
"A":		
Fudge & chocolate creme	1 cookie	120
Fudge & vanilla creme	1 cookie	110
Oatmeal creme	1 cookie	150
Peanut butter creme	1 cookie	120
(Sunshine):		
Regular:		
Chocolate fudge	1 cookie	55
Cup custard	1 cookie	75
Hydrox	1 cookie	45
Vienna Fingers	1 cookie	60
Chips 'n Middles:		
Fudge	1 cookie	65
Peanut butter	1 cookie	70
Tru Blu	1 cookie	75
Shortbread:		
(Nabisco):		
Lorna Doone	1 piece	33
Pecan	1 piece	40
Striped	1 piece	37
(Pepperidge Farm)	1 piece	43
Social Tea (Nabisco)	1 piece	18
Sprinkles (Sunshine)	1 piece	65
Strawberry (Pepperidge Farm)	1 piece	23
Sugar:		
(Nabisco) rings	1 piece	50
(Pepperidge Farm)	1 piece	38
Sugar wafer:		
(Keebler) *Krisp Kreem*	1 piece	14
(Nabisco) *Biscos*	1 piece	4
(Sunshine) wafer	1 piece	12
Sugar Heroes (Nabisco)	1 piece	11

Food and Description	Measure or Quantity	Sodium (milligrams)
Tahiti (Pepperidge Farm)	1 piece	25
Toy (Sunshine)	1 piece	18
Vanilla wafer (Tom's)	1.7-oz. serving	160
Waffle creme (Nabisco) *Biscos*	1 piece	10
COOKIE, DIETETIC:		
Chocolate chip:		
(Estee)	1 piece	5
(Featherweight)	1 piece	6
Coconut (Estee)	1 piece	<5
Lemon:		
(Estee) thin	1 piece	<5
(Featherweight)	1 piece	3
Oatmeal raisin (Estee)	1 piece	<5
Sandwich:		
(Estee) duplex	1 piece	5
(Featherweight)	1 piece	3
Vanilla:		
(Estee) thins	1 piece	<5
(Featherweight)	1 piece	6
Wafer:		
(Estee):		
Chocolate covered	1 piece	10
Vanilla creme	1 piece	<5
(Featherweight) creme, chocolate, pecan or vanilla	1 piece	14
COOKIE CRISP, cereal (Ralston-Purina):		
Chocolate chip	1 cup (1 oz.)	188
Vanilla	1 cup (1 oz.)	200
COOKIE DOUGH:		
Refrigerated:		
(USDA):		
Unbaked, plain	1 oz.	141
Baked, plain	1 oz.	155
*(Pillsbury):		
Brownie, fudge:		
Regular	1/24 of pkg.	115
Microwave, with chocolate-flavored chips	1/9 of pkg.	110

Food and Description	Measure or Quantity	Sodium (milligrams)
Chocolate chip	1 piece	55
Chocolate chocolate chip	1 cookie	35
Oatmeal raisin	1 cookie	60
Peanut butter	1 piece	70
Sugar	1 piece	70
*Frozen (Rich's):		
Chocolate chip	1 piece	120
Oatmeal	1 piece	90
Oatmeal with raisin	1 piece	73
Oatmeal, super jumbo	1 piece	226
Peanut butter	1 piece	185
Ranger	1 piece	90
Sugar	1 piece	111

COOKIE, HOME RECIPE
(USDA):

Brownie with nuts	1¾″ × 1¾″ × ⅞″	50
Chocolate chip	1 oz.	99
Sugar, soft, thick	1 oz.	90

COOKIE MIX:
Regular:
Brownie:
*(Betty Crocker):
Fudge:

Regular size	¹⁄₁₆ of pkg.	100
Family size	¹⁄₂₄ of pkg.	95
Supreme	¹⁄₂₄ of pkg.	85
Walnut, Regular size	¹⁄₁₆ of pkg.	80
(Duncan Hines)	¹⁄₂₄ of pkg.	98

*(Pillsbury) fudge:
Deluxe:

Plain	¹⁄₁₆ of pkg.	100
Family size	¹⁄₂₄ of pkg.	95
Walnut	¹⁄₁₆ of pkg.	90
Microwave	⅑ of pkg.	105

Ultimate:

Caramel fudge chunk, chunky triple fudge or double fudge	¹⁄₁₆ of pkg.	105
Rocky road	¹⁄₁₆ of pkg.	95

Food and Description	Measure or Quantity	Sodium (milligrams)
Chocolate (Duncan Hines) double	⅟₃₆ of pkg.	38
Chocolate chip:		
*(Betty Crocker) *Big Batch*	1 cookie	100
(Duncan Hines)	⅟₃₆ of pkg.	42
*(Quaker)	1 cookie	70
Date bar (Betty Crocker)	⅟₃₂ of pkg.	35
Macaroon, coconut (Betty Crocker)	⅟₂₄ of pkg.	15
Oatmeal:		
(Duncan Hines) raisin	⅟₃₆ of pkg.	31
*(Nestlé) raisin	1 cookie	43
*(Quaker)	1 cookie	71
Peanut Butter:		
(Duncan Hines)	⅟₃₆ of pkg.	57
*(Nestlé)	1 cookie	90
Sugar:		
*(Betty Crocker) *Big Batch*	1 cookie	95
(Duncan Hines) golden	⅟₃₆ of pkg.	33
*(Nestlé)	1 cookie	65
**Vienna Dream Bar* (Betty Crocker)	⅟₂₄ of pkg.	65
*Dietetic (Estee) brownie	2″ × 2″ piece	15
COOKING FATS (See **FAT**)		
CORIANDER (HEW/FAO)		
Raw:		
Untrimmed	1 lb.	333
Leaves only	4 oz.	107
CORIANDER SEED (French's)	1 tsp. (1.4 grams)	Tr.
CORN:		
Fresh, white or yellow (USDA):		
Raw:		
Untrimmed, on the cob	1 lb. (weighed in husk)	Tr.
Trimmed, on cob	1 lb. (husk removed)	Tr.
Boiled:		
Kernels, cut from cob, drained	1 cup (5.8 oz.)	Tr.

Food and Description	Measure or Quantity	Sodium (milligrams)
Whole	4.9-oz. ear (5″ × 1¾″)	Tr.
Canned, regular pack: (USDA):		
Golden or yellow, whole kernel, solids & liq., vacuum pack	½ cup (3.7 oz.)	250
Golden or yellow, whole kernel,wet pack	½ cup (4.5 oz.)	302
Golden or yellow, whole kernel, drained solids, wet pack	½ cup (3 oz.)	203
White kernel, solids & liq.	½ cup (4.5 oz.)	302
White kernel, drained solids	½ cup (2.8 oz.)	189
White, whole kernel, drained liq., wet pack	4 oz.	268
Cream style	½ cup (4.4 oz.)	295
(Comstock) solids & liq.:		
Cream style	½ cup	350
Whole kernel	½ cup	440
(Del Monte):		
Cream style, golden or white	½ cup	355
Whole kernel, solids & liq.	½ cup	355
(Festal):		
Cream style:		
Golden, wet pack	½ cup (4¼ oz.)	411
White, wet pack	½ cup (4¼ oz.)	281
Whole kernel:		
Golden white, solids & liq.	½ cup (4¼ oz.)	316
Golden or white, drained solids	½ cup (4 oz.)	285
Golden or yellow, vacuum pack, solids & liq.	½ cup (4. oz.)	233
White, drained solids	½ cup (4 oz.)	319
(Green Giant) solids & liq.:		
Cream style, golden kernel	½ of 8½-oz. can	380
Whole kernel:		
Golden or yellow	¼ of 17-oz. can	270

Food and Description	Measure or Quantity	Sodium (milligrams)
Golden or yellow, vacuum pack	½ of 7-oz. can	230
Golden, *Mexicorn*	½ of 7-oz. can	335
White, vacuum pack	½ of 7½-oz. can	315
(Kounty Kist):		
Cream style	½ of 8½-oz. can	437
Whole kernel:		
Golden, liquid pack, solids & liq.	½ of 7-oz. can	259
Golden, vacuum pack	⅓ of 12-oz. can	295
(Larsen) *Freshlike:*		
Cream style, golden	½ cup	290
Whole kernel:		
Regular, solids & liq.	½ cup	320
Vacuum pack:		
Plain	½ cup	260
With pepper	½ cup	300
(Le Sueur) golden, whole kernel, solids & liq.	¼ of 17-oz. can	376
(Libby's):		
Cream style	½ cup (4.3 oz.)	295
Whole kernel, solids & liq.	½ cup (4.4 oz.)	264
(Lindy)		
Cream style	½ of 8½-oz. can	437
Whole kernel:		
Golden, liquid pack, solids & liq.	½ of 7-oz. can	259
Golden, vacuum pack	½ cup	295
(Stokely-Van Camp):		
Cream style:		
Golden	½ cup (4½ oz.)	383
White	½ cup (4.6 oz.)	360
Whole kernel:		
Golden or yellow, solids & liq.	½ cup (4.5 oz.)	290
Golden, vacuum pack	½ cup (4.4 oz.)	418
White, solids & liq.	½ cup (4.5 oz.)	248
Canned, dietetic pack:		
(USDA):		
Whole kernel:		
Solids & liq.	4 oz.	2

Food and Description	Measure or Quantity	Sodium (milligrams)
Drained solids	4 oz.	2
Liquid only	4 oz.	2
Cream style	4 oz.	2
(Del Monte) no salt added, solids & liq.	½ cup	<10
(Diet Delight) whole kernel, solids & liq.	½ cup (4.4 oz.)	5
(Featherweight) whole kernel, solids & liq.	4 oz.	<10
(Larsen) *Fresh-Lite*, solids & liq.	½ cup	5
(S & W) *Nutradiet:*		
Cream style	½ cup	<10
Whole kernel, solids & liquid	½ cup	<10
Frozen:		
(USDA):		
On the cob, boiled, drained	5″ ear (4 oz.)	1
Whole kernel, boiled, drained	½ cup (3.2 oz.)	<1
(Birds Eye):		
On the cob:		
Farmside	1 ear (4.4 oz.)	4
Little Ears	1 ear (2.3 oz.)	2
Natural Ear	1 ear	5
Whole kernel:		
Regular	⅓ of 10-oz. pkg.	3
In butter sauce	⅓ of 10-oz. pkg.	178
Tendertreat	⅓ of 10-oz. pkg.	3
(Frosty Acres):		
On the cob:		
Whole	1 ear	0
Piece	1 piece	0
Cut	3.3 oz.	0
(Green Giant):		
On the cob:		
Niblets	1 ear (2.7 oz.)	10
Niblet Ears	1 ear (4.9 oz.)	20
Cream style	½ cup	315

Food and Description	Measure or Quantity	Sodium (milligrams)
Whole kernel:		
Niblets:		
In butter sauce	½ cup	280
In cream sauce	½ cup	295
Harvest Fresh	½ cup	280
Polybag	½ cup	5
Shoe peg, white, in butter sauce	½ cup	290
(Larsen):		
On the cob	1 piece	5
Cut	3.3 oz.	5
(McKenzie):		
On the cob	5″ ear (4.4 oz.)	25
Whole kernel	3.3 oz.	19
CORNBREAD, HOME RECIPE (USDA):		
Corn pone, prepared with white, whole-ground cornmeal	4 oz.	449
Johnnycake, prepared with yellow, degermed cornmeal	4 oz.	782
Southern style, prepared with degermed cornmeal	2½″ × 2½″ × 1⅝″ piece (2.9 oz.)	491
Southern-style, prepared with whole-ground cornmeal	4 oz.	712
Spoon bread, prepared with white, whole-ground cornmeal	4 oz.	547
CORNBREAD MIX:		
(USDA):		
Dry	1 oz.	328
*Prepared with egg and milk	2⅜″ muffin (1.4 oz.)	298
*(Aunt Jemima)	⅙ of pkg.	600
*(Pillsbury) *Ballard*	⅛ of pkg.	570
*CORN DOG, frozen (Hormel)	1 wiener	656
CORNED BEEF:		
Uncooked (USDA) boneless, medium fat	1 lb.	5897

Food and Description	Measure or Quantity	Sodium (milligrams)
Cooked (USDA) medium fat, boneless	4 oz.	1973
Canned:		
(Libby's)	⅓ of 7-oz. can	720
Dietetic (Featherweight) loaf	2½ oz.	53
Packaged:		
(Carl Buddig) smoked	1 oz.	380
(Eckrich)	1 oz.	340
(Oscar Mayer)	.7 oz.	248
CORNED BEEF HASH:		
Canned:		
(USDA) with potato	1 cup (7.8 oz.)	1197
(Libby's)	1 cup (8 oz.)	1330
Mary Kitchen (Hormel):		
Regular	7½-oz. serving	1386
Short Orders	7½-oz. can	1368
Frozen (Banquet)	10-oz. dinner	1752
CORNED BEEF SPREAD		
(Underwood)	½ of 4½-oz. can	605
CORN FLAKE CRUMBS		
(Kellogg's)	¼ cup (1 oz.)	285
CORN FLAKES, cereal:		
Regular:		
(USDA):		
Regular	1 cup (.9 oz.)	291
Crushed	1 cup (3 oz.)	704
Frosted	1 cup (1.4 oz.)	310
(General Mills) *Country*	1 cup (1 oz.)	310
(Kellogg's):		
Regular	1 cup (1 oz.)	280
Honey & Nut	¾ cup (1 oz.)	190
Sugar frosted	¾ cup (1 oz.)	190
(Post) *Post Toasties*	1¼ cups (1 oz.)	299
(Ralston Purina):		
Regular	1 cup (1 oz.)	267
Sugar frosted	¾ cup (1 oz.)	179
Low sodium (Featherweight)	1¼ cups (1 oz.)	10
CORN FRITTER (See **FRITTER,** corn)		

Food and Description	Measure or Quantity	Sodium (milligrams)
CORN GRITS (See **HOMINY**)		
CORNMEAL, WHITE or YELLOW:		
Dry:		
Bolted:		
(USDA)	1 cup (4.3 oz.)	1
(Aunt Jemima/Quaker)	1 cup (4 oz.)	1
Degermed (USDA)	1 cup (4.9 oz.)	Tr.
Self-rising, degermed:		
(USDA)	1 cup (5 oz.)	1946
(Aunt Jemima)	1 cup (6 oz.)	2292
CORN POPS, cereal (Kellogg's)	1 cup (1 oz.)	95
CORN PUDDING, home recipe (USDA)	1 cup (8.6 oz.)	1068
CORN PUREE, canned (Larsen)	½ cup	6
CORNSTARCH:		
(USDA)	1 cup (4.5 oz.)	Tr.
(Argo; Duryea's or Kingsford's)	1 T. (9.5 g.)	Tr.
CORN STICK (See **CORNBREAD**)		
COTTAGE PUDDING, home recipe (USDA):		
Without sauce	2 oz.	170
With chocolate sauce	2 oz.	132
With strawberry sauce	2 oz.	132
COUGH DROP:		
(Beech-Nut)	1 drop (2 g.)	<1
(Pine Bros.)	1 drop (3 g.)	0
COUNT CHOCULA, cereal (General Mills)	1 cup (1 oz.)	205
COUNTRY CRISP, cereal (Post)	¾ cup (1 oz.)	197
COWPEA (USDA):		
Immature seeds:		
Raw, whole	1 lb. (weighed in pods)	5
Raw, shelled	½ cup (2.5 oz.)	1
Boiled, without salt, drained solids	½ cup (2.9 oz.)	<1
Canned, solids & liq.	4 oz.	268

Food and Description	Measure or Quantity	Sodium (milligrams)
Frozen (See **BLACK-EYED PEAS**, frozen)		
Young pods, with seeds:		
Raw, whole	1 lb. (weighed untrimmed)	17
Boiled, drained solids	4 oz.	3
Mature seeds, dry:		
Raw	1 lb.	159
Raw	½ cup (3 oz.)	29
Boiled	½ cup (4.4 oz.)	10
CRAB, all species:		
Canned (USDA) drained solids	4 oz.	1134
Frozen (Wakefield's) Alaska		
King, thawed & drained	4 oz.	Tr.
CRAB APPLE, fresh (USDA):		
Whole	1 lb. (weighed whole)	4
Flesh only	4 oz.	1
CRABAPPLE JELLY, sweetened:		
(Home Brands)	1 T.	15
(Smucker's)	1 T.	3
CRABAPPLE PRESERVE or JAM, sweetened (Smucker's)	1 T.	3
CRAB AU GRATIN, frozen (Gorton's) *Light Recipe*	1 pkg.	810
CRAB, DEVILED:		
Home recipe (USDA)	1 cup (8.5 oz.)	2081
Frozen (Mrs. Paul's):		
Breaded & French-fried	3-oz. piece	385
Breaded & fried, miniatures	½ of 7-oz. pkg.	195
CRAB, IMITATION (See **SURIMI**)		
CRAB IMPERIAL:		
Home recipe (USDA)	1 cup (7.8 oz.)	1602
Frozen (Gorton's) *Light Recipe*, stuffed	1 pkg.	950
CRAB SOUP (Crosse & Blackwell)	½ of 13-oz. can	933
CRACKED WHEAT CEREAL (See **WHEAT CEREAL, CRACKED**)		

Food and Description	Measure or Quantity	Sodium (milligrams)
CRACKER, PUFFS, and CHIPS		
(See also individual listings such as **POTATO CHIPS,** etc.)		
Arrowroot biscuit (Nabisco)		
National	1 piece (5 g.)	13
Bacon flavored thins (Nabisco)	1 piece (2 g.)	30
Bran wafer (Featherweight)		
unsalted	1 piece	<1
Bugles (Tom's)	15 pieces (1 oz.)	300
Butter (Pepperidge Farms)	1 piece	33
Cafe (Sunshine)	1 piece (smallest portion after breaking on scoreline)	45
Cheese-flavored (See also individual brand names in this grouping):		
(USDA)	1 oz.	295
American Heritage (Sunshine):		
Cheddar	1 piece	30
Parmesan	1 piece	45
Better Blue Cheese (Nabisco)	1 piece	26
Better Cheddar (Nabisco)	1 piece	20
Better Nacho (Nabisco)	1 piece	24
Better Swiss (Nabisco)	1 piece	23
Cheddar Sticks (Flavor Tree)	1 oz.	445
Cheese Bites (Tom's)	1½ oz.	540
Chee•Tos:		
Crunchy:		
Regular	1 oz.	280
Light	1 oz.	360
Puffed balls	1 oz.	360
Puffs	1 oz.	330
Cheez Balls (Planters)	1 oz.	270
Cheez Curls (Planters)	1 oz.	290
Cheez-It (Sunshine)	1 piece	11
Corn cheese (Tom's):		
Crunchy	1⅝ oz.	270
Puffed, baked	1⅛ oz.	300

Food and Description	Measure or Quantity	Sodium (milligrams)
Dip In A Chip (Nabisco)	1 piece	16
(Dixie Bell)	1 piece	10
Nachips (Old El Paso)	1 oz.	193
Nips (Nabisco)	1 piece	10
(Ralston)	1 piece	10
Tid-Bit (Nabisco)	1 piece (<1 g.)	12
Cheese & peanut butter sandwich (USDA)	1 oz.	281
Chicken in a Biskit (Nabisco)	1 piece (2 g.)	16
Cinnamon Treats (Nabisco)	1 piece	16
Club cracker (Keebler)	1 piece	39
Corn chips:		
(Featherweight) low sodium	1 oz.	3
(Flavor Tree)	1 oz.	260
Fritos:		
Regular	1 oz.	230
Bar-B-Q	1 oz.	320
Chili cheese	1 oz.	310
Crisp 'N Thin or king size	1 oz.	210
(Laura Scudder's)	1 oz.	125
(Planters)	1 oz.	224
(Tom's):		
Regular	1 oz.	200
BBQ	1 oz.	220
Corn Stick (Flavor Tree)	1 oz.	220
Country Cheddar (Nabisco)	1 piece	24
Crown Pilot (Nabisco)	1 piece (.6 oz.)	65
English Water Biscuit (Pepperidge Farm)	1 piece	22
Escort (Nabisco)	1 piece	37
Goldfish (Pepperidge Farm):		
Thins:		
Cheese	1 piece (3.5 g.)	15
Lightly salted or wheat	1 piece (3.5 g.)	16
Tiny:		
Cheddar cheese, lightly salted, pizza or pretzel	1 piece	4
Parmesan	1 piece	6
Graham:		
(USDA)	2½" sq. (7 g.)	47

Food and Description	Measure or Quantity	Sodium (milligrams)
(Dixie Belle) sugar-honey coated	1 piece	26
(Keebler) cinnamon crisp or honey	1 piece	21
(Nabisco):		
Regular	1 piece	57
Sugar-honey coated, *Honey Maid*	1 piece	45
(Ralston) sugar-honey coated	1 piece	26
(Sunshine):		
Cinnamon	1 piece (after breaking on scoreline)	24
Honey	1 piece (after breaking on scoreline)	22
Great Crisps (Nabisco):		
French onion	1 piece	13
Nacho	1 piece	31
Real bacon	1 piece	26
Savory garlic	1 piece	24
Sesame	1 piece	21
Tomato & celery	1 piece	18
Hi-Ho (Sunshine)	1 piece	31
Meal Mates (Nabisco)	1 piece	47
Nacho Rings (Tom's)	1 oz.	330
Oyster:		
(USDA)	10 pieces (.4 oz.)	110
(USDA)	1 cup (1 oz.)	312
(Dixie Belle)	1 piece	11
(Nabisco):		
Dandy	1 piece	11
Oysterettes	1 piece	7
(Ralston)	1 piece	11
(Sunshine)	1 piece	12
Party Mix (Flavor Tree):		
Regular	1 oz.	400
No salt added	1 oz.	10
Rich & Crisp (Dixie Belle)	1 piece	18

Food and Description	Measure or Quantity	Sodium (milligrams)
Ritz (Nabisco):		
Regular	1 piece	30
Low salt	1 piece	15
Roman Meal Wafer boxed	1 piece (2.2 g.)	20
Royal Lunch (Nabisco)	1 piece (1.7 g.)	80
Rusk (Nabisco) Holland	1 piece	35
Rye toast (Keebler)	1 piece	29
RyKrisp:		
Regular	1 triple cracker	48
Seasoned	1 triple cracker	65
Sesame	1 triple cracker	75
Saltine:		
(Dixie Belle)		
Regular	1 piece	36
Unsalted top	1 piece	21
(Keebler) *Zesta*	1 piece	41
(Nabisco) *Premium*:		
Regular	1 piece	36
Unsalted Top	1 piece	23
(Ralston):		
Regular	1 piece	36
Unsalted Top	1 piece	21
(Sunshine) *Krispy*:		
Regular	1 piece	42
Unsalted	1 piece	24
Sea Rounds (Nabisco)	1 piece	140
Sesame Chip (Flavor Tree)	1 oz.	410
Sesame Crunch (Flavor Tree)	1 oz.	70
Sesame Stick (Flavor Tree):		
Plain	1 oz.	405
With bran	1 oz.	370
No salt added	1 oz.	10
Sesame Toast (Keebler)	1 piece	20
Snackers (Dixie Belle)	1 piece	23
Snackin' Crisp (Durkee) *O&C*	1 oz.	257
Snack Sticks (Pepperidge Farm):		
Cheese	1 piece	43
Pumpernickel	1 piece	48

Food and Description	Measure or Quantity	Sodium (milligrams)
Sesame or cheese	1 piece	43
Sociables (Nabisco)	1 piece (2 g.)	22
Soda:		
(USDA)	1 oz.	312
(USDA)	2½″ sq. (6 g.)	60
Sour cream & onion stick (Flavor Tree)	1 oz.	415
Taco chip (Laura Scudder's) mini	1 oz.	200
Tortilla chip:		
Doritos:		
Regular	1 oz.	230
Cool Ranch:		
Regular	1 oz.	190
Light	1 oz.	240
Nacho cheese:		
Regular	1 oz.	240
Light	1 oz.	290
Salsa Rio	1 oz.	170
Taco flavored	1 oz.	220
(La Famous):		
Regular	1 oz.	180
No salt added	1 oz.	5
(Laura Scudder's)	1 oz.	90
Santitas:		
Regular	1 oz.	75
Strips	1 oz.	65
(Tom's)	1 oz.	173
Tostitos:		
Jalapeño & cheese	1 oz.	160
Sharp nacho	1 oz.	200
Traditional	1 oz.	170
Tortilla Strip (Laura Scudder's)	1 oz.	140
Town House (Keebler)	1 piece	29
Triscuit (Nabisco):		
Regular	1 piece	30
Low salt	1 piece	12
Tuc (Keebler)	1 piece	28
Twigs (Nabisco)	1 piece	40
Uneeda Biscuit (Nabisco)	1 piece	33

Food and Description	Measure or Quantity	Sodium (milligrams)
Unsalted (Estee)	1 piece	<5
Vegetable thins (Nabisco)	1 piece	14
Waverly (Nabisco)	1 piece (4 g.)	40
Wheat (Pepperidge Farm):		
Cracked	1 piece	50
Hearty	1 piece	45
Wheat Nuts (Flavor Tree)	1 oz.	185
Wheat Snack (Dixie Belle)	1 piece	12
Wheat Thins (Nabisco):		
Regular	1 piece	15
Cheese	1 piece	24
Low salt	1 piece	4
Nutty	1 piece	36
Wheat Toast (Keebler)	1 piece	30
Wheat Wafer (Estee) *6 Calorie*	1 piece	<5
CRACKER CRUMBS, GRAHAM:		
(USDA)	1 cup (3 oz.)	576
(Nabisco)	⅛ of 9" pie shell or 2T. (.5 oz.)	90
(Nabisco)	1 cup (3 oz.)	540
(Sunshine)	½ cup (2¼ oz.)	495
CRACKER MEAL:		
(USDA)	1 T. (.4 oz.)	110
(Nabisco) unsalted	½ cup (1.5 oz.)	0
CRANAPPLE juice drink (Ocean Spray) canned:		
Regular pack	6 fl. oz.	4
Low calorie or dietetic	6 fl. oz.	8
CRANBERRY:		
Fresh:		
(USDA)		
Untrimmed	1 lb. (weighed with stems)	9
Trimmed, stems removed	1 cup (4 oz.)	2
(Ocean Spray)	½ cup (2 oz.)	<1
Dehydrated (USDA)	1 oz.	5
CRANBERRY JUICE COCKTAIL, canned (Ocean Spray):		
Regular	6 fl. oz.	3

Food and Description	Measure or Quantity	Sodium (milligrams)
Low calorie	6 fl. oz.	6
CRANBERRY-ORANGE RELISH (Ocean Spray)	2 oz.	18
CRANBERRY-RASPBERRY SAUCE, canned (Ocean Spray) jellied	2-oz. serving	14
CRANBERRY SAUCE:		
Home recipe (USDA) sweetened, unstrained	4 oz.	1
Canned:		
(USDA) sweetened, strained	½ cup (4.8 oz.)	1
(Ocean Spray):		
Jellied	2-oz. serving	17
Whole berry	2-oz. serving	16
CRANGRAPE, drink (Ocean Spray)	6 fl. oz.	5
CRANICOT, drink (Ocean spray)	6 fl. oz.	<10
CRANPRUNE **JUICE DRINK** (Ocean Spray)	6 fl. oz.	3
CRAN-RASPBERRY SAUCE, canned (Ocean Spray) jellied	2-oz. serving	14
CRAZY COW, cereal (General Mills) chocolate	1 cup (1 oz.)	185
CREAM (See also **CREAM SUBSTITUTE**):		
Half & Half:		
(USDA)	1 T.	7
(USDA)	½ cup (4.3 oz.)	56
(Johanna)	1 T. (.5 oz.)	6
Light, table or coffee:		
(USDA)	1 T. (.5 oz.)	6
(Johanna) 18% butterfat	1 T.	6
(Sealtest)	1 T. (.5 oz.)	6
Light whipping:		
(USDA)	1 cup (8.4 oz.)	86
(USDA)	1 T. (.5 oz.)	5
(Sealtest) 30% fat	1 T. (.5 oz.)	5
Heavy whipping (unwhipped):		
(USDA)	1 cup (8.4 oz.)	76
(Dean)	1 T. (.5 oz.)	5

Food and Description	Measure or Quantity	Sodium (milligrams)
(Johanna) 36% butterfat	1 T.	6
Sour:		
(USDA)	1 cup (8.1 oz.)	99
(Dean)	1 T. (.5 oz.)	6
(Johanna)	1 T.	8
Sour, imitation (Pet)	1 T. (.5 oz.)	25
CREAM PUFF:		
Home recipe (USDA) with custard filling	3½″ × 2″ piece (4.6 oz.)	108
Frozen (Rich's):		
Bavarian	1⅓-oz. piece	83
Chocolate	1⅓-oz. piece	83
CREAM SUBSTITUTE:		
(Carnation) *Coffee-mate*	1 tsp. (1.9 g.)	4
Coffee Rich, frozen, liquid	½ oz.	7
Cremora (Borden)	1 tsp.	5
N-Rich (Sanna)	1½ tsp. (3-g. packet)	17
CREME DE MENTHE LIQUEUR, green or white (Leroux)	1 fl. oz.	<1
CREPE, frozen (Mrs. Paul's):		
Crab	½ of 5½-oz. pkg.	578
Shrimp	½ of 5½-oz. pkg.	523
CRESS, Garden (USDA):		
Raw, whole	1 lb. (weighed untrimmed)	45
Boiled, without salt, drained	1 cup (4.8 oz.)	14
CRISPIX, cereal (Kellogg's)	¾ cup (1 oz.)	230
CRISP RICE cereal:		
Regular (Ralston Purina)	1 cup (1 oz.)	208
Low Sodium (Van Brode)	1 cup (1 oz.)	2
CRISPY WHEAT 'N RAISINS cereal (General Mills)	¾ cup (1 oz.)	185
CROAKER (USDA):		
Atlantic:		
Raw, whole	1 lb. (weighed whole)	134

Food and Description	Measure or Quantity	Sodium (milligrams)
Raw, meat only	4 oz.	99
Baked	4 oz.	136
CROUTON (Kellogg's) *Croutettes*	⅔ cup (.7 oz.)	260
CRULLER (See **DOUGHNUT**)		
CUCUMBER, fresh (USDA):		
Eaten with skin	½ lb. (weighed whole)	13
Eaten without skin	½ lb. (weighed with skin)	10
Unpared, 10-oz. cucumber	7½″ × 2″ pared cucumber (7.3 oz.)	12
Pared	6 slices (2″ × ⅛″)	Tr.
Pared and diced	½ cup (2.5 oz.)	4
CUMIN SEED (French's)	1 tsp. (1.6 oz.)	3
CUPCAKE:		
Home recipe (USDA):		
Without icing	1.4-oz. cupcake	120
With chocolate icing	1.8-oz. cupcake	114
With boiled white icing	1.8-oz. cupcake	131
With uncooked white icing	1.8-oz. cupcake	114
Commercial type (Hostess):		
Chocolate	1¾-oz. cupcake	249
Orange	1½-oz. cupcake	170
Frozen (Sara Lee) yellow	1¾-oz. cupcake	161
*CUPCAKE MIX (Flako)	¹⁄₁₂ of pkg.	195
CURRANT:		
Fresh (USDA):		
Black European:		
Whole	1 lb. (weighed with stems)	13
Stems removed	4 oz.	3
Red and white:		
Whole	1 lb. (weighed with stems)	9
Stems removed	1 cup (3.9 oz.)	2
Dried:		
(Del Monte) Zante	½ cup (2.4 oz.)	<10
(Sun-Maid) Zante	½ cup (2.5 oz.)	18

Food and Description	Measure or Quantity	Sodium (milligrams)
CURRANT JELLY, sweetened:		
(Home Brands)	1 T.	15
(Smucker's)	1 T. (.7 oz.)	7
CUSTARD:		
Home recipe (USDA) baked	½ cup (4.7 oz.)	104
Canned (Thank You Brand) egg	½ cup (4.6 oz.)	195
Chilled, *Swiss Miss:*		
Chocolate flavor	4 oz.	149
Egg flavor	4 oz.	180
*Mix, dietetic (Featherweight)	½ cup	105
C.W. POST, cereal:		
Family style	¼ cup (1 oz.)	49
Family style, with raisins	¼ cup (1 oz.)	44

D

DAIRY CRISP, cereal (Pet)		
high calcium	¼ cup (1 oz.)	140
DAIRY QUEEN/**BRAZIER:**		
Banana split	13.5-oz. serving	150
Brownie Delight, hot fudge	9.4-oz. serving	225
Buster Bar	5¼-oz. piece	175
Chicken sandwich	7.8-oz. sandwich	870
Cone:		
Plain, any flavor:		
Small	3-oz. cone	47
Regular	5-oz. cone	80
Large	7½-oz. cone	115
Dipped, chocolate:		
Small	3¼-oz. cone	55
Regular	5½-oz. cone	100
Large	8¼-oz. cone	145
Dilly Bar	3-oz. piece	50
Double Delight	9-oz. serving	150

Food and Description	Measure or Quantity	Sodium (milligrams)
DQ Sandwich	2.1-oz. sandwich	40
Fish sandwich:		
Plain	6-oz. sandwich	875
With cheese	6¼-oz. sandwich	1035
Float	14-oz. serving	85
Freeze, vanilla	14-oz. serving	180
French fries:		
Regular	2½-oz. serving	115
Large	4-oz. serving	185
Hamburger:		
Plain:		
Single	5.2-oz. burger	630
Double	7.5-oz. burger	660
Triple	9.6-oz. burger	690
With cheese:		
Single	5.7-oz. burger	790
Double	8.4-oz. burger	980
Triple	10.62-oz. burger	1010
Hot dog:		
Regular:		
Plain	3.5-oz. serving	830
With cheese	4-oz. serving	990
With chili	4½-oz. serving	985
Super:		
Plain	6.2-oz. serving	1365
With cheese	6.9-oz. serving	1605
With chili	7.7-oz. serving	1595
Lettuce	½ oz.	<10
Malt, chocolate:		
Small	10¼-oz. serving	180
Regular	14¾-oz. serving	260
Large	20¾-oz. serving	360
Mr. Misty:		
Plain:		
Small	8¼-oz. serving	<10
Regular	11.64-oz. serving	<10
Large	15½-oz. serving	<10
Kiss	3.14-oz. serving	<10
Float	14.5-oz. serving	95
Freeze	14.5-oz. serving	140

Food and Description	Measure or Quantity	Sodium (milligrams)
Onion rings	3-oz. serving	140
Parfait	10-oz. serving	140
Peanut Butter Parfait	10¾-oz. serving	250
Shake, chocolate:		
Small	10¼-oz. serving	180
Regular	14¾-oz. serving	260
Large	20¾-oz. serving	360
Strawberry shortcake	11-oz. serving	215
Sundae, chocolate:		
Small	3¾-oz. serving	75
Regular	6¼-oz. serving	120
Large	8¾-oz. serving	165
Tomato	½ oz.	<10
DAIQUIRI COCKTAIL:		
Canned (Mr. Boston):		
Regular	3 fl. oz.	51
Strawberry	3 fl. oz.	64
Mix (Holland House):		
Instant	.56-oz. packet	21
Liquid:		
Regular	1 oz.	111
Raspberry	1 oz.	4
Strawberry	1 oz.	3
DANDELION GREENS, raw (USDA):		
Trimmed	1 lb.	345
Boiled, without salt, drained	½ cup (3.2 oz.)	40
DATE, dry:		
Domestic:		
(USDA):		
With pits	1 lb. (weighed with pits)	4
Without pits	4 oz.	1
Without pits, chopped	1 cup (6.1 oz.)	2
Imported (Bordo) Iraq	2 oz.	5
DELI'S, frozen (Pepperidge Farm):		
Beef with barbecue sauce	4-oz. piece	685
Mexican style	4-oz. piece	645
Pizza style	4-oz. piece	790

Food and Description	Measure or Quantity	Sodium (milligrams)
Reuben in rye pastry	4-oz. piece	650
Savory chicken salad	4-oz. piece	625
Scrambled eggs, Canadian bacon & cheese	3½-oz. piece	665
Sliced beef with brown sauce	4-oz. piece	560
Turkey, ham & cheese	4-oz. piece	740
Western style omelet	4-oz. piece	555
DESSERT CUPS (Hostess)	¾-oz. piece	120
DEWBERRY, fresh (See **BLACKBERRY,** fresh)		
DILL SEED (French's)	1 tsp. (2.1 g.)	Tr.
DING DONG (Hostess)	1.3-oz. cake	132
DIP:		
Acapulco (Ortega):		
Plain	1 oz.	1
With American cheese	1 oz.	172
With cheddar cheese	1 oz.	106
With Monterey Jack cheese	1 oz.	124
Bleu cheese (Dean) tang	1 oz.	14
Enchilada, *Fritos*	1 oz.	97
Garlic (Dean)	1 oz.	16
Jalapeno (Wise)	1 T.	50
Onion (Thank You Brand)	1 T. (.8 oz.)	191
Picante sauce (Wise)	1 T.	65
Taco:		
(Thank You Brand)	1 T.	129
(Wise)	1 T.	57
DISTILLED LIQUOR. The values below would apply to unflavored bourbon whiskey, brandy, Canadian whiskey, gin, Irish whiskey, rum, rye whiskey, Scotch whiskey, tequila and vodka. The caloric content of distilled liquors depends on the percentage of alcohol. The proof is twice the alcohol percent and the following values apply to all rands (USDA):		
80 proof	1 fl. oz.	<1

Food and Description	Measure or Quantity	Sodium (milligrams)
86 proof	1 fl. oz.	<1
90 proof	1 fl. oz.	<1
94 proof	1 fl. oz.	<1
100 proof	1 fl.oz.	<1
DOCK, including **SHEEP SORREL** (USDA):		
Raw, whole	1 lb. (weighed untrimmed)	16
Boiled, without salt, drained	4 oz.	3
DOUGHNUT:		
(USDA):		
Cake type	1.1-oz. piece	160
Yeast-leavened	.6-oz. piece	40
Commercial type (Hostess):		
Regular:		
Chocolate coated	1-oz. piece	151
Cinnamon	1-oz. piece	111
Krunch	1-oz.piece	134
Old fashioned:		
Regular	1½-oz. piece	217
Glazed	2-oz. piece	217
Plain	1-oz. piece	135
Powdered sugar	1-oz. piece	153
Donettes:		
Frosted	1 piece	50
Powdered	1 piece	51
Frozen (Morton):		
Regular:		
Bavarian creme	2-oz. piece	75
Boston creme	2⅓-oz. piece	90
Chocolate iced	1½-oz. piece	75
Glazed	1½-oz. piece	75
Jelly	1.8-oz. piece	75
Mini	1.1-oz. piece	200
Donut Holes:		
Devil's food	⅕ of 7¾-oz. pkg.	105
Honey wheat	⅕ of 7¾-oz. pkg.	140
Vanilla	⅕ of 7¾-oz. pkg.	123
Morning Light:		
Chocolate	2-oz. serving	177

Food and Description	Measure or Quantity	Sodium (milligrams)
Glazed	2-oz. serving	176
Jelly	2-oz. serving	193
DRUM, raw (USDA):		
Freshwater:		
Whole	1 lb. (weighed whole)	83
Meat only	4 oz.	79
Red:		
Whole	1 lb. (weighed whole)	102
Meat only	4 oz.	62
DRUMSTICK, frozen, in a cone:		
Ice cream:		
Topped with peanuts	1 piece	82
Topped with peanuts & cone bisque	1 piece	72
Ice milk:		
Topped with peanuts	1 piece	87
Topped with peanuts & cone bisque	1 piece	77
DUCK, raw (USDA) domesticated meat only	4 oz.	84
DULCITO, frozen (Hormel):		
Apple	4 oz.	350
Cherry	4 oz.	345
DUMPLING stuffed, canned, dietetic:		
(Dia-Mel)	8-oz. serving	70
(Featherweight)	7½-oz. serving	117

E

ECLAIR:
Home recipe (USDA) with custard filling & chocolate icing 4-oz. piece 93

Food and Description	Measure or Quantity	Sodium (milligrams)
Frozen (Rich's) chocolate	2.6-oz. piece	194
EGG (USDA) (See also **EGG SUBSTITUTE**):		
Chicken:		
Raw:		
White only	1 large egg (1.2 oz.)	48
White only	1 cup (9 oz.)	372
Yolk only	1 large egg (.6 oz.)	9
Yolk only	1 cup (8.5 oz.)	125
Whole, small	1 egg (1.3 oz.)	45
Whole, medium	1 egg (1.5 oz.)	53
Whole, large	1 egg (1.8 oz.)	61
Whole	1 cup (8.8 oz.)	306
Whole, extra large	1 egg (2 oz.)	70
Whole, jumbo	1 egg (2.3 oz.)	79
Cooked:		
Boiled, without salt	1 large egg (1.8 oz.)	61
Fried in butter	1 large egg	155
Omelet, mixed with milk & cooked in fat	1 large egg	159
Poached	1 large egg	130
Scrambled, mixed with milk & cooked in fat	1 large egg	164
Scrambled, mixed with milk & cooked in fat	1 cup (7.8 oz.)	565
Dried:		
Whole	1 cup (3.8 oz.)	461
White, powder	1 oz.	313
Yolk	1 cup (3.4 oz.)	96
Duck, raw, whole	1 egg (2.8 oz.)	98
EGG DINNER OR ENTREE,		
frozen (Swanson):		
Omelet:		
With cheese sauce & ham	7-oz. meal	1160
Spanish style	8-oz. meal	840
Scrambled with sausage & potatoes	6¼-oz. meal	790

Food and Description	Measure or Quantity	Sodium (milligrams)
*EGG FOO YOUNG, canned:		
(Chun King) stir fry	5-oz. serving	517
(La Choy)	1 patty plus ¼ cup sauce	760
EGG MIX (Durkee):		
*Omelet:		
With bacon	½ of pkg.	276
Puffy	½ of pkg.	333
Western	½ of pkg.	823
Scrambled:		
With bacon	1.3-oz. pkg.	476
Plain	.8-oz. pkg.	320
EGG NOG, dairy:		
(Borden)	½ cup	80
(Johanna)	½ cup	69
EGG NOG COCKTAIL (Mr. Boston)	3 fl. oz.	71
EGGPLANT:		
Raw (USDA) whole	1 lb. (weighed untrimmed)	7
Boiled (USDA) without salt, drained, diced	1 cup (7.1 oz.)	2
Frozen:		
(Buitoni) Parmigiana	5-oz. serving	684
(Celentano):		
Parmigiana	½ of 16-oz. pkg.	405
Rollettes	11-oz. pkg.	510
(Mrs. Paul's):		
Parmigiana	½ of 11-oz. pkg.	905
Sticks, breaded and fried	½ of 7-oz. pkg.	610
(Weight Watchers) parmigiana, 1-compartment meal	13-oz. meal	1073
EGG ROLL, frozen:		
(Chun King):		
Chicken	.65-oz. piece	110
Chicken	.8-oz. piece	139
Meat & shrimp	.65-oz. piece	104
Meat & shrimp	.8-oz. piece	133
Meat & shrimp	2.6-oz. piece	427

Food and Description	Measure or Quantity	Sodium (milligrams)
Shrimp	.65-oz. piece	105
Shrimp	.8-oz. piece	134
(La Choy):		
Chicken	.5-oz. piece	62
Lobster	.5-oz. piece	70
Lobster	3-oz. piece	485
Meat & shrimp	.24-oz. piece	42
Meat & shrimp	.5-oz. piece	73
Shrimp	.5-oz. piece	70
Shrimp	3-oz. piece	575
EGG ROLL DINNER OR		
ENTREE, frozen:		
(La Choy) entrees:		
Almond chicken	2 egg rolls	1020
Beef & broccoli	2 egg rolls	1060
Spicy oriental chicken	2 egg rolls	690
Sweet & sour pork	2 egg rolls	720
(Van de Kamp's) Cantonese	10½-oz. meal	1100
EGG SUBSTITUTE:		
Egg Beaters (Fleischmann) plain	¼ cup (2.1 oz.)	80
Egg Magic (Featherweight)	½ envelope	123
*Scramblers (Morningstar Farms)	1 egg equivalent	75
Second Nature (Avoset)	3 T.	68
ELDERBERRY JELLY, sweetened (Smucker's)	1 T.	Tr.
ELDERBERRY PRESERVE or		
JAM, sweetened (Smucker's)	1 T.	Tr.
ENCHILADA:		
Canned (Old El Paso) beef	1 enchilada	215
Frozen:		
Beef:		
(Banquet):		
Dinner	12-oz. dinner	1805
Entree, family	2-lb. pkg.	5908
(Green Giant) baked, Sonora style	12-oz. entree	1245

Food and Description	Measure or Quantity	Sodium (milligrams)
(Hormel)	1 enchilada	573
(Morton)	11-oz. dinner	1216
(Swanson):		
Regular:		
Dinner	15-oz. dinner	1400
Entree	11¼-oz. entree	1190
Hungry Man	16-oz. entree	2010
(Van de Kamp's):		
Dinner, regular	12-oz. dinner	2177
Entree:		
Regular	7½-oz. entree	1201
Shredded	5½-oz. serving	930
Cheese:		
(Banquet) dinner		
International Favorites	12-oz. dinner	2166
Man-Pleaser	21¼-oz. dinner	2510
(Hormel)	1 enchilada	676
(Van de Kamp's):		
Dinner	12-oz. dinner	1664
Entree:		
Regular	7½-oz. meal	963
Ranchero	5½-oz. serving	540
Chicken (Van de Kamp's):		
Regular	7½-oz. pkg.	1108
Suiza with rice & beans	14¾-oz. serving	590
ENCHILADA SAUCE:		
Canned:		
(Del Monte):		
Hot	½ cup	1151
Mild	½ cup	1072
(El Molino) hot	1 T.	50
(Old El Paso):		
Green chili	¼ cup	400
Hot	¼ cup	248
Mild	¼ cup	250
*Mix (Durkee)	1 cup	96

Food and Description	Measure or Quantity	Sodium (milligrams)
ENCHILADA SEASONING MIX (French's)	¼ of 1⅜-oz. pkg.	1130
ENDIVE, BELGIAN, or FRENCH (See **CHICORY, WITLOOF**)		
ENDIVE, CURLY, raw (USDA):		
Untrimmed	1 lb.	56
Trimmed	½ lb.	32
Cut up or shredded	1 cup (2.5 oz.)	10

F

FARINA (See also **CREAM OF WHEAT**):		
Regular:		
Dry:		
(USDA)	1 cup (6 oz.)	3
(H-O) cream, enriched	1 cup (6.1 oz.)	8
(H-O) cream, enriched	1 T.	<1
Malt-O-Meal	1 oz.	3
(3-Minute Bran)	2½ T.	<5
Cooked:		
*(USDA)	1 cup (8.4 oz.)	343
*(USDA)	4 oz.	163
*(Pillsbury) made with water and salt	⅔ cup	270
Quick-cooking:		
Dry:		
(USDA)	1 oz.	71
Malt-O-Meal	1 oz.	2

Food and Description	Measure or Quantity	Sodium (milligrams)
Cooked (USDA)	1 cup (8.6 oz.)	466
Instant-cooking (USDA):		
Dry	1 oz.	2
Cooked	4 oz.	213
FENNEL SEED (French's)	1 tsp. (2.1 grams)	2
FETTUCINI ALFREDO, frozen (Stouffer's)	5 oz.	1195
FIG:		
Fresh (USDA):		
Regular size	1 lb.	9
Small	1.3-oz. fig (1½″ dia.)	<1
Candied (Bama)	1 T. (.7 oz.)	<1
Canned, regular pack, solids & liq.:		
(USDA):		
Light syrup	4 oz.	2
Heavy syrup	3 figs & 2 T. syrup (4 oz.)	2
Heavy syrup	½ cup (4.4 oz.)	3
Extra heavy syrup	½ cup	<10
Canned, unsweetened or dietetic:		
(USDA) water pack, solids & liq.	4 oz.	2
(Diet Delight) Kadota, solids & liq.	½ cup (4.4 oz.)	4
(Featherweight) Kadota, water pack, solids & liq.	½ cup	<10
Dried (USDA):		
Chopped	1 cup (6 oz.)	58
Whole	.7-oz. fig (2″ × 1″)	7
FIG JUICE, canned (Sunsweet)	6 fl. oz.	24
FIGURINES (Pillsbury):		
Chocolate, chocolate peanut butter or vanilla	1 bar	45
Chocolate caramel	1 bar	55
Chocolate mint	1 bar	118
Chocolate peanut butter	1 bar	120

Food and Description	Measure or Quantity	Sodium (milligrams)
Double chocolate	1 bar	130
Vanilla	1 bar	103
FILBERT or HAZELNUT:		
(USDA):		
Whole	1 lb.	4
Shelled	1 oz.	<1
(Fisher) oil dipped, salted	½ cup (2 oz.)	114
FISH (See individual listings)		
FISH CAKE, frozen (Mrs. Paul's) thins, breaded and fried	½ of 10-oz. pkg.	1020
FISH & CHIPS, frozen:		
(Gorton's)	1 pkg.	1380
(Swanson):		
Dinner:		
Regular	10½-oz. dinner	970
Hungry Man	14¾-oz. dinner	1350
Entree	5½-oz. entree	585
(Van de Kamp's) batter dipped, French-fried	7-oz. pkg.	640
FISH DINNER, frozen:		
(Banquet) American Favorites	8¾-oz. dinner	927
(Morton)	10-oz. dinner	1400
(Mrs. Paul's):		
Regular, Parmesan	5 oz.	540
Light:		
Dijon	8½ oz.	650
Florentine	9 oz.	1025
Mornay	10 oz.	665
(Stouffer's) *Lean Cuisine:*		
Divan	12⅜-oz.	785
Florentine	9 oz.	815
(Van de Kamp's) fillet, regular	12-oz. dinner	1820
(Weight Watchers) fillet:		
Au gratin	9¼-oz. meal	910
Oven fried	6¾-oz. serving	470
FISH FILLET, frozen:		
(Frionor) *Norway Gourmet,* breaded	1.5-oz. piece	150

Food and Description	Measure or Quantity	Sodium (milligrams)
(Gorton's):		
Regular:		
Batter dipped, crispy	1 piece	440
Crunchy	1 piece	220
Potato crisp	1 piece	230
Light Recipe:		
Lightly breaded	1 piece	380
Tempura batter	1 piece	400
(Mrs. Paul's):		
Batter fried, light:		
Regular	3-oz. piece	415
Crunchy	2¼-oz. piece	417
Supreme	3.6-oz. piece	505
Breaded & fried:		
Crispy crunchy	2.1-oz. piece	325
Light & natural	6-oz. piece	770
Buttered	2½-oz. piece	390
(Van de Kamp's):		
Batter dipped, french-fried	3-oz. piece	230
Country seasoned	2-oz. piece	335
Light & crispy	2-oz. piece	175
FISH KABOBS, frozen		
(Van de Kamp's) batter dipped, French fried	4-oz.	430
FISH NUGGET, frozen		
(Frionor) *Bunch O' Crunch,* breaded	.5-oz. piece	37
FISH SANDWICH, frozen		
(Frionor) *Bunch O' Crunch,* microwave	5-oz. sandwich	635
FISH SEASONING, dietetic		
(Featherweight)	¼ tsp	<1
FISH STICK, frozen:		
(Frionor) *Bunch O'Crunch,* breaded	.7-oz. piece	70
(Gorton's):		
Batter dipped, crispy	1 piece	140
Breaded	1 piece	120
Crunchy	1 piece	92
Potato crisp	1 piece	100

Food and Description	Measure or Quantity	Sodium (milligrams)
Value pack (Mrs. Paul's):	1 piece	105
Batter fried, light & crunchy	1 stick (.8 oz.)	199
Breaded and fried	1 stick (¾ oz.)	114
(Van de Kamp's) batter dipped, French-fried:		
Regular	1-oz. piece	83
Light & crispy	.9-oz. piece	75
FIT'N FROSTY (Alba '77), instant milk shake mix:		
Chocolate	¾-oz. envelope	93
Chocolate and marshmallow	1 envelope	93
Strawberry	1 envelope	115
Vanilla	1 envelope	108
FIVE ALIVE, juice drink, chilled or frozen (Snow Crop)	6 fl. oz.	1
FLOUNDER:		
Raw (USDA):		
Whole	1 lb.	117
Meat only	4 oz.	88
Baked (USDA)	4 oz.	269
Frozen:		
(Frionor) *Norway Gourmet*	4-oz. fillet	350
(Gorton's):		
Fishmarket Fresh	4 oz.	140
Light Recipe:		
Fillet, entree	1 piece	710
Stuffed	1 pkg.	880
(Mrs. Paul's) fillets:		
Batter fried, crunchy, light	2¼-oz. piece	555
Breaded & fried:		
Crispy, crunchy	2-oz. piece	400
Light & natural	3-oz. piece	487
(Van de Kamp's) *Today's Catch*	4 oz.	130
FLOUR:		
(USDA):		
Chestnut	1 oz.	3
Corn	1 cup (3.9)	1

Food and Description	Measure or Quantity	Sodium (milligrams)
Fish, from whole fish	1 oz.	48
Potato	1 oz.	10
Rice, stirred, spooned	1 cup (5.6 oz.)	8
Rye:		
Light:		
Unsifted, spooned	1 cup (3.6 oz.)	1
Sifted, spooned	1 cup (3.1 oz.)	4
Medium:	1 oz.	<1
Dark:		
Unstirred	1 cup (4.5 oz.)	1
Stirred	1 cup (4.5 oz.)	1
Sunflower seed, partially defatted	1 oz.	16
Wheat:		
All-purpose:		
Unsifted, dipped	1 cup (5 oz.)	3
Unsifted, spooned	1 cup (4.4 oz.)	3
Sifted, spooned	1 cup (4.1 oz.)	2
Bread:		
Unsifted, dipped	1 cup (4.8 oz.)	3
Unsifted, spooned	1 cup (4.3 oz.)	2
Sifted, spooned	1 cup (4.1 oz.)	2
Cake:		
Unsifted, dipped	1 cup (4.2 oz.)	2
Unsifted, spooned	1 cup (3.9 oz.)	2
Sifted, spooned	1 cup (3.5 oz.)	2
Gluten:		
Unsifted, dipped	1 cup (5 oz.)	3
Unsifted, spooned	1 cup (4.8 oz.)	3
Sifted, spooned	1 cup (4.8 oz.)	3
Self-rising:		
Unsifted, dipped	1 cup (4.6 oz.)	1403
Unsifted, spooned	1 cup (4.5 oz.)	1370
Sifted, spooned	1 cup (3.7 oz.)	1144
(Aunt Jemima) self-rising	¼ cup (1 oz.)	368
Ballard:		
All-purpose	¼ cup	<2
Self-rising	¼ cup	323
Bisquick (Betty Crocker)	¼ cup	350
Drifted Snow	¼ cup	<2

Food and Description	Measure or Quantity	Sodium (milligrams)
Elam's:		
Brown rice, stone ground, whole grain	¼ cup	2
Buckwheat, pure	¼ cup	2
Pastry	1 oz.	2
Rye, stone ground, whole grain	¼ cup	3
Soy	1 oz.	5
Whole wheat, stone ground, whole grain	1 oz.	5
Gold Medal (Betty Crocker):		
All-purpose or unbleached	¼ cup	<2
High protein	¼ cup	<2
Self-rising	¼ cup	380
La Pina	¼ cup	Tr.
(Pillsbury):		
All purpose	¼ cup	0
All purpose, unbleached	¼ cup	1
Bread	¼ cup	0
Rye, medium	¼ cup	1
Sauce & gravy	1 T.	<5
Self-rising	¼ cup	322
Whole wheat	¼ cup	3
Presto, self-rising	¼ cup (1 oz.)	322
Purasnow:		
Regular	¼ cup (1 oz.)	1
Self-rising	¼ cup (1 oz.)	380
Red Band:		
Regular or unbleached	¼ cup (1 oz.)	1
Self-rising	¼ cup (1 oz.)	380
Red Star, self-rising	¼ (1 oz.)	380
Softasilk	¼ cup (1 oz.)	<5
Swans Down, cake:		
Regular	¼ cup	0
Self-rising	¼ cup	188
White Deer	¼ cup (1 oz.)	1
Wondra	¼ cup (1 oz.)	<3
FOOD STICKS (Pillsbury)		
chocolate	1 stick	25

Food and Description	Measure or Quantity	Sodium (milligrams)
FOUR FRUIT PRESERVE, sweetened (Smucker's)	1 T.	3
FRANKEN*BERRY, cereal (General Mills)	1 cup (1 oz.)	205
FRANKFURTER, raw or cooked:		
(USDA):		
Raw, All kinds	1 frankfurter (10 per lb.)	499
(Eckrich):		
Beef	1.2-oz. frankfurter	380
Beef	1.6-oz. frankfurter	480
Beef	2-oz. frankfurter	620
Cheese	2-oz. frankfurter	650
Meat	1.2-oz. frankfurter	360
Meat	1.6-oz. frankfurter	470
Meat	2-oz. frankfurter	630
(Empire Kosher):		
Chicken	2 oz.	634
Turkey	2 oz.	746
(Hormel):		
Beef	1 frankfurter (12-oz. pkg.)	362
Beef	1 frankfurter (1-lb. pkg.)	463
Chili, *Frank 'N Stuff*	1 frankfurter	517
Meat	1 frankfurter (12-oz. pkg.)	378
Meat	1 frankfurter (1-lb. pkg.)	486
Wrangler's, smoked:		
Beef	1 frankfurter	619
Cheese	1 frankfurter	546
Range Brand	1 frankfurter	600
(Ohse):		
Beef	1 oz.	280
Wiener:		
Regular	1 oz.	300
Chicken, beef & pork	1 oz.	260
(Oscar Mayer):		
Beef	1.6-oz. frankfurter	466

Food and Description	Measure or Quantity	Sodium (milligrams)
Beef	2-oz. frankfurter	588
Beef, *Big One*	4-oz. frankfurter	1177
Little wiener	.3-oz. frankfurter	91
Wiener	1.2-oz. frankfurter	347
Wiener	1.6-oz. wiener	459
Wiener, jumbo	2-oz. frankfurter	581
FRANKS AND BEANS (See BEANS & FRANKFURTERS)		
FRENCH TOAST, frozen (Aunt Jemima):		
Regular	1½-oz. slice	216
Cinnamon swirl	1½-oz. slice	179
FRENCH TOAST & SAUSAGE, frozen (Swanson) plain	6½-oz. meal	770
FRITTER:		
Home recipe, corn (USDA)	2″ × 1½″ fritter (1.2 oz.)	541
Frozen (Mrs. Paul's):		
Apple	2-oz. fritter	385
Corn	2-oz. fritter	363
FROOT LOOPS, cereal (Kellogg's)	1 cup (1 oz.)	135
FROSTED RICE, cereal (Ralston Purina)	1 cup	151
FROSTEE (Borden):		
Chocolate	1 cup	160
Strawberry	1 cup	150
FROSTING (See CAKE ICING)		
FROZEN DESSERT (See also TOFUTTI):		
(Baskin-Robbins):		
Low, Lite 'n Luscious	½ cup (4 fl. oz.)	60–70
Special Diet	1 scoop (½ cup)	60
Eskimo bar, chocolate covered	2½-fl. oz. bar	40
FRUIT N'APPLE JUICE, canned or *frozen (Tree Top)	6 fl. oz.	10
FRUIT N'BERRY JUICE, canned or *frozen (Tree Top)	6 fl. oz.	10
FRUIT BITS, dried (Sun-Maid)	1-oz. serving	24
FRUIT N'CHERRY JUICE, canned or *frozen (Tree Top)	6 fl. oz.	10

Food and Description	Measure or Quantity	Sodium (milligrams)
FRUIT N'CITRUS JUICE,		
canned (Tree Top)	6 fl. oz.	10
FRUIT COCKTAIL:		
Canned, regular pack, solids & liq.:		
(USDA):		
Light syrup	4 oz.	6
Heavy syrup	½ cup (4.5 oz.)	6
Extra heavy syrup	4 oz.	6
(Del Monte) heavy syrup, regular or chunky fruit	½ cup (4½ oz.)	5
(Libby's) heavy syrup	½ cup (4.5 oz.)	8
(Stokely-Van Camp)	½ cup (4.5 oz.)	15
Canned, dietetic or unsweetened, solids & liq.:		
(USDA) water pack	4 oz.	6
(Del Monte) *Lite*	½ cup (4¼ oz.)	5
(Diet Delight)	½ cup (4.4 oz.)	5
(Featherweight):		
Juice pack	½ cup	<10
Water pack	½ cup	<10
(Libby's) water pack	½ cup (4.3 oz.)	10
FRUIT COMPOTE, canned (Rokeach)	½ cup (4 oz.)	4
FRUIT CUP (Del Monte):		
Mixed, solids & liq.	5-oz. container	6
Peaches, cling, diced, solids & liq.	5-oz. container	9
FRUIT & FIBER, cereal (Post):		
Apple & cinnamon	½ cup (1 oz.)	195
Dates, walnuts & raisins	½ cup (1 oz.)	170
FRUIT & JUICE BAR (Dole):		
Orange or strawberry	2½-fl.-oz. bar	6
Pineapple	2½-fl.-oz. bar	4
FRUIT, MIXED:		
Canned, regular (Hunt's) *Snack pack*	5-oz. container	5
Canned, dietetic or low calorie (Del Monte) *Lite*, solids & liq.	½ cup	5

Food and Description	Measure or Quantity	Sodium (milligrams)
Dried:		
(Del Monte)	2 oz.	10
(Sun-Maid/Sunsweet)	2 oz.	11
FRUIT & NUT MIX (Carnation)	.9-oz. pkg.	10
FRUIT PUNCH:		
Canned:		
Bama (Borden)	8.45-fl.-oz. container	15
Capri Sun	6¾ oz.	1
(Hi-C)	6 fl. oz.	<1
(Lincoln) party	6 fl. oz.	30
Ssips (Johanna Farms)	8.45-fl. oz. container	<10
Chilled:		
Five Alive (Snow Crop)	6 fl. oz.	1
(Minute Maid)	6 fl. oz.	<1
(Sunkist)	8.45 fl. oz.	0
*Frozen, *Five Alive* (Snow Crop)	6 fl. oz.	1
*Mix:		
Regular (Hi-C)	6 fl. oz.	1
Dietetic:		
Crystal Light	6 fl. oz.	<1
(Sunkist)	6 fl. oz.	15
FRUIT ROLL:		
(Betty Crocker)	½-oz. roll	5
(Flavor Tree)	¾-oz. roll	15
(Sunkist)	½-oz. roll	10
FRUIT SALAD:		
Canned, regular pack, solids & liq.:		
(USDA):		
Light syrup	4 oz.	1
Heavy syrup	½ cup (4.3 oz.)	1
Extra heavy syrup	4 oz.	1
(Del Monte):		
Fruit for salad	½ cup (4.3 oz.)	<10
Tropical	½ cup (4. oz.)	<10
(Libby's) heavy syrup	½ cup (4.4 oz.)	8

Food and Description	Measure or Quantity	Sodium (milligrams)
(Stokely-Van Camp)	½ cup (4.5 oz.)	15
Canned, unsweetened or dietetic pack, solids & liq.:		
(USDA) water pack	4 oz.	1
(Diet Delight) juice pack	½ cup (4.4 oz.)	
FRUIT SQUARES, frozen (Pepperidge Farm):		
Apple	2½-oz. piece	175
Blueberry	2½-oz. piece	190
Cherry	2½-oz. piece	185
***FUDGE JUMBLES** (Pillsbury):		
Brown sugar oatmeal, chocolate chip oatmeal & coconut oatmeal	1 bar	60
Peanut butter oatmeal	1 bar	55

G

GARLIC, raw (USDA):		
Whole	2 oz. (weighed with skin)	10
Peeled	1 oz.	5
GARLIC FLAKES (Gilroy)	1 tsp. (1.5 grams)	<1
GARLIC POWDER (Gilroy)	1 tsp.	<1
GARLIC SALT (French's)	1 tsp. (5.7 grams)	1850
GAZPACHO SOUP, canned (Crosse & Blackwell)	½ of 13-oz. can	1653
GELATIN, unflavored, dry (Knox)	1 envelope	10
GELATIN DESSERT:		
Canned, dietetic (Dia-Mel; Louis Sherry)	4 oz.	5

Food and Description	Measure or Quantity	Sodium (milligrams)
Powder:		
*Regular:		
(Jello):		
Apricot, black cherry, mixed fruit, orange, peach, raspberry, strawberry or strawberry-banana	½ cup	55
Blackberry	½ cup	54
Cherry	½ cup	77
Grape, concord	½ cup	40
Lemon or wild strawberry	½ cup	81
Lime	½ cup	62
Orange-pineapple	½ cup	70
Raspberry, black	½ cup	39
(Royal) all fruit flavors	½ cup (4.9 oz.)	90–100
*Dietetic or low calorie:		
Carmel Kosher, all flavors	½ cup	<10
(Dia-Mel) *Gel-A-Thin*	½ cup	10
(D-Zerta)	½ cup	5
(Estee)	½ cup	10
(Featherweight) all flavors, artificially sweetened	½ cup	2
(Jell-O):		
Cherry	½ cup	80
Lime	½ cup	60
Orange	½ cup	56
Raspberry or strawberry	½ cup	56
(Louis Sherry) *Shimmer*	½ cup	10
(Royal)	½ cup	70
GELATIN DRINKING (Knox) orange	1 envelope	20
GIN, unflavored (see **DISTILLED LIQUOR**)		
GINGERBREAD:		
Home recipe (USDA)	1.9-oz piece (2″ × 2″ × 2″)	130
*Mix:		
(USDA)	⅑ of 8″ sq. (2.2 oz.)	192

Food and Description	Measure or Quantity	Sodium (milligrams)
(Betty Crocker)	⅑ of pkg.	325
(Pillsbury)	3″ sq. (⅑ of pkg.)	310
GINGER ROOT, fresh (USDA):		
With skin	1 oz.	2
Without skin	1 oz.	2
GOLDEN GRAHAMS, cereal		
(General Mills)	¾ cup (1 oz.)	285
GOOSE, domesticated (USDA)		
roasted, meat only	4 oz.	141
GOOSEBERRY (USDA):		
Fresh	1 lb.	5
Fresh	1 cup (5.3 oz.)	2
Canned, water pack, solids & liq.	4 oz.	1
GRAHAM CRACKER (See **CRACKER**)		
GRAHAM CRAKOS, cereal		
(Kellogg's)	¾ cup (1 oz.)	145
GRANOLA BAR, *Nature Valley:*		
Regular:		
Almond or peanut	1 bar	80
Cinnamon, coconut or oats 'n honey	1 bar	65
Peanut butter	1 bar	90
Chewy:		
Apple or raisin	1 bar	65
Chocolate chip	1 bar	85
Peanut butter	1 bar	80
*GRANOLA BAR MIX,		
Nature Valley, Bake-A-Bar:		
Chocolate chip, oats 'n honey or raisins & spice	1 bar	40
Peanut butter	1 bar	60
GRANOLA CEREAL:		
Nature Valley	⅓ cup (1 oz.)	35
Sun Country (Kretschmer)	¼ cup (1 oz.)	10
GRANOLA CLUSTERS, *Nature Valley:*		
Almond	1.2-oz. roll	140
Apple-cinnamon	1.2-oz. roll	125

Food and Description	Measure or Quantity	Sodium (milligrams)
Caramel	1.2-oz. roll	95
Chocolate chip	1.2-oz. roll	100
Raisin	1.2-oz. roll	110
GRANOLA & FRUIT BAR,		
Nature Valley:		
Apple or raspberry	1 bar	150
Date	1 bar	135
GRANOLA SNACK		
Nature Valley, Light & Crunchy:		
Cinnamon or peanut butter	1 pouch	175
Honeynut	1 pouch	160
Oats 'n Honey	1 pouch	170
Peanut Butter	1 pouch	165
GRAPE:		
Fresh:		
American type (slip skin), Concord, Delaware, Niagara, Catawba and Scuppernong:		
(USDA)	½ lb. (weighed with stem, skin & seeds)	4
(USDA)	½ cup (2.7 oz.)	1
(USDA)	3½″ × 3″ bunch (3.5 oz.)	2
European type (adherent skin), Malaga, Muscat, Thompson seedless, Emperor & Flame Tokay:		
(USDA)	½ lb. (weighed with stem & seeds)	6
(USDA) whole	20 grapes (¾″ dia.)	2
(USDA) whole	½ cup (.3 oz.)	3
Canned, solids & liq.:		
(USDA) Thompson, seedless, heavy syrup	4 oz.	5
(USDA) Thompson, seedless, water pack	4 oz.	5

Food and Description	Measure or Quantity	Sodium (milligrams)
(Featherweight) water pack, seedless	½ cup	<10
(Thank You Brand) in heavy syrup	½ cup (4.1 oz.)	6
GRAPE DRINK:		
Canned:		
Bama (Borden)	8.45-fl.-oz. container	25
(Capri Sun)	6¾ fl. oz.	19
(Hi-C)	6 fl. oz.	<1
(Lincoln)	6 fl. oz.	30
Ssips (Johanna Farms)	8.45-fl.-oz. container	20
(Sunkist)	8.45 fl. oz.	0
*Mix:		
Regular (Hi-C)	6 fl. oz.	42
Dietetic (Sunkist)	6 fl. oz.	19
GRAPEFRUIT:		
Fresh (USDA):		
White:		
Seeded type	1 lb. (weighed with seeds & skin)	2
Seedless type	1 lb. (weighed with skin)	2
Seeded type	½ med. grapefruit (3¾" dia., 8.5 oz.)	1
Pink and red:		
Seeded type	1 lb. (weighed with seeds & skin)	2
Seedless type	1 lb. (weighed with skin)	2
Seeded type	½ med. grapefruit (3¾" dia., 8.5 oz.)	1
Canned, syrup pack (Del Monte) solids & liq.	½ cup	2

Food and Description	Measure or Quantity	Sodium (milligrams)
Canned, unsweetened or dietetic pack, solids & liq.:		
(USDA) water pack	½ cup (4.2 oz.)	5
Del Monte) sections	½ cup	2
(Diet Delight) sections, juice pack	½ cup (4.3 oz.)	5
(Featherweight) sections, juice pack	½ of 8-oz. can	<10
GRAPEFRUIT JUICE:		
Fresh (USDA) pink, red or white, all varieites	½ cup (4.3 oz.)	1
Canned:		
Sweetened:		
(USDA)	½ cup (4.4 oz.)	1
(Del Monte)	6 fl. oz.	2
(Johanna Farms)	6 fl. oz.	4
(Minute Maid)	6 fl. oz.	2
Unsweetened:		
(USDA)	½ cup (4.4 oz.)	1
(Del Monte)	6 fl. oz.	<10
(Libby's)	6 fl. oz.	5
(Ocean Spray)	6 fl. oz. (6.5 oz.)	7
(Texsun) pink	6 fl. oz.	2
Chilled (Minute Maid)	6 fl. oz.	2
*Frozen:		
Sweetened (USDA) diluted with 3 parts water	½ cup (4.4 oz.)	1
Unsweetened:		
(USDA) diluted with 3 parts water	½ cup (4.4 oz.)	1
(Minute Maid)	6 fl. oz.	<1
*Dehydrated crystals (USDA) reconstituted	½ cup (4.4 oz.)	1
GRAPEFRUIT JUICE COCKTAIL, canned (Ocean Spray) pink	6 fl. oz.	15
GRAPEFRUIT-ORANGE JUICE COCKTAIL, canned (Ocean Spray) pink	6 fl. oz.	15

Food and Description	Measure or Quantity	Sodium (milligrams)
GRAPE JAM, sweetened		
(Smucker's)	1 T.	5
GRAPE JELLY:		
Sweetened:		
(Bama)	1 T.	7
(Home Brands)	1 T.	15
Dietetic (See **GRAPE SPREAD**)		
GRAPE JUICE:		
Canned:		
(USDA)	½ cup (4.4 oz.)	3
(Seneca Foods)	6 fl. oz.	4
Sippin' Pak (Borden)	8.45-fl. oz. container	25
(Tree Ripe)	8.45-fl.-oz. container	7
(Welch's):		
Regular	6 fl. oz.	5
Red or white	6 fl. oz.	15
Sparkling red or white	6 fl. oz.	30
*Frozen, sweetened:		
(USDA)	½ cup (4.4 oz.)	1
(Minute Maid)	6 fl. oz.	2
GRAPE JUICE DRINK, canned		
(Sunkist)	8.45 fl. oz.	30
GRAPE NUT FLAKES, cereal		
(Post):		
Regular	¼ cup (1 oz.)	197
Flakes	⅞ cup (1 oz.)	218
Raisin	¼ cup (1 oz.)	160
GRAPE SPREAD, low sugar:		
(Diet Delight)	1 T. (.6 oz.)	15
(Estee)	1 T. (.6 oz.)	Tr.
(Featherweight)	1 T.	40–50
(Louis Sherry)	1 T.	<3
(Smucker's) regular	1 T.	34
GRAVY:		
Canned:		
Au jus (Franco-American)	2-oz. serving	290
Beef (Franco-American)	2-oz. serving	310

Food and Description	Measure or Quantity	Sodium (milligrams)
Brown:		
(Dawn Fresh) with mushroom broth	2-oz. serving	297
(Franco-American) with onion	2-oz. serving	340
(La Choy)	½ of 5-oz. can	555
Ready Gravy	½ cup	<1
Chicken (Franco-American)		
Regular or giblet	2-oz. serving	320
Mushroom (Franco-American)	2-oz. serving	320
Pork (Franco-American)	2-oz. serving	350
Turkey (Franco-American)	2-oz. serving	300
Mix, regular:		
Au Jus:		
(Durkee):		
*Regular	1 cup	913
Roastin' Bag	1-oz. pkg.	2628
*French's) *Gravy Makins*	1 cup	1040
*Brown:		
(Durkee):		
Regular	1 cup	1036
With mushrooms	1 cup	1402
With onions	1 cup	1356
(French's) *Gravy Makins*	1 cup	1000
(Pillsbury)	1 cup	1200
(Spatini)	1-oz. serving	205
Chicken:		
(Durkee):		
*Regular	1 cup	1710
*Creamy	1 cup	1528
Roastin' Bag:		
Regular	1.5-oz. pkg.	3597
Creamy	2-oz. pkg.	2528
Italian style	1.5-oz. pkg.	3614
*(French's) *Gravy Makins*	1 cup	1080
*(Pillsbury)	1 cup	920
*Homestyle:		
(Durkee)	1 cup	830
(French's) *Gravy Makins*	1 cup	1000

Food and Description	Measure or Quantity	Sodium (milligrams)
(Pillsbury)	1 cup	1200
Meatloaf (Durkee) *Roastin' Bag*	1.5-oz. pkg.	3472
*Mushroom:		
(Durkee)	1 cup	1170
(French's) *Gravy Makins*	1 cup	1000
*Onion:		
(Durkee)	1 cup	952
(French's) *Gravy Makins*	1 cup	1080
Pork:		
(Durkee):		
Regular	1 cup	2174
Roastin' Bag	1.5-oz. pkg.	2579
*(French's) *Gravy Makins*	1 cup	1000
Pot roast (Durkee) *Roastin' Bag:*		
Regular	1.5-oz. pkg.	2965
& onion	1.5-oz. pkg.	2864
*Swiss steak (Durkee)	¾ cup	1482
*Turkey:		
(Durkee)	1 cup	1326
(French's) *Gravy Makins*	1 cup	1160
Mix, dietetic (Weight Watchers):		
Brown:		
Regular	1 pkg.	1339
With mushroom	1 pkg.	1495
With onion	1 pkg.	1479
Chicken	1 pkg.	2087
GRAVY MASTER	1 tsp. (.2 oz.)	127
GRAVY WITH MEAT OR TURKEY:		
Canned (Morton House):		
Sliced beef	½ of 12½-oz. can	1076
Sliced pork	½ of 12½-oz. can	975
Sliced turkey	½ of 12½-oz. can	995
Frozen:		
(Banquet):		
Entree for One, & beef	4 oz.	426
Family Entree, & turkey	2-lb. pkg.	4040

Food and Description	Measure or Quantity	Sodium (milligrams)
(Morton)		
Gravy & beef sliced	8 oz.	490
Gravy & salisbury steak	8 oz.	670
Gravy & turkey, sliced	8 oz.	1310
(Swanson) with sliced beef	8-oz. entree	760
GREAT BEGINNINGS (Hormel):		
With chunky beef	5 oz.	904
With chunky chicken or pork	5 oz.	567
With chunky turkey	5 oz.	585
GREENS, MIXED, canned (Sunshine) solids & liq.	½ cup (4.1 oz.)	468
GREEN PEA (See PEA, GREEN)		
GRITS (See HOMINY GRITS)		
GUAVA, COMMON, fresh (USDA):		
Whole	1 lb. (weighed untrimmed)	18
Whole	1 guava (2.8 oz.)	3
Flesh only	4 oz.	5
GUAVA JELLY (Smucker's)	1 T.	3
GUAVA NECTAR, canned (Libby's)	6 fl. oz.	5
GUAVA, STRAWBERRY, fresh (USDA):		
Whole	1 lb. (weighed untrimmed)	18
Flesh only	4 oz.	<5

H

HADDOCK:		
Raw (USDA):		
Whole	1 lb.	133
Meat only	4 oz.	69

Food and Description	Measure or Quantity	Sodium (milligrams)
Fried, breaded (USDA)	4″ × 3″ × ½″ fillet (3.5 oz.)	176
Frozen:		
(Frionor) *Norway Gourmet*	4-oz. fillet	149
(Gorton's):		
Fishmarket Fresh	4 oz.	100
Light Recipe, fillet, entree	1 piece	570
(Mrs. Paul's):		
Batter fried, crunchy & light	2 oz.	400
Breaded & fried:		
Crispy, crunchy	6 oz.	960
Light & natural	2¼ oz.	468
(Van de Kamp's) batter dipped, french-fried	2-oz. piece	215
(Weight Watchers) with stuffing, 2-compartment meal	7-oz. meal	549
HAKE, raw (USDA):		
Whole	1 lb.	144
Meat only	4 oz.	84
HALF & HALF (milk & cream) (see **CREAM**)¾		
HALIBUT:		
Atlantic & Pacific (USDA):		
Raw:		
Whole	1 lb. (weighed whole)	145
Meat only	4 oz.	61
Broiled	4.4 oz. (4″ × 3″ × ½″ steak)	168
Frozen (Van de Kamp's) batter dipped, French-fried	½ of 8-oz. pkg.	440
HAM (See also **PORK**):		
Canned:		
(Hormel):		
Black Label	4 oz. (1½-lb. ham)	1324
Black Label	4 oz. (5-lb. ham)	1245
Chunk	6¾-oz. serving	2241

Food and Description	Measure or Quantity	Sodium (milligrams)
Chopped	3 oz. (8-lb. ham)	1062
Curemaster	4 oz.	1361
EXL	4 oz.	1382
Patties	1 patty	456
(Oscar Mayer) *Jubilee*, extra lean, cooked	¹⁄₁₂ of 3-lb. ham (4 oz.)	1384
(Swift):		
Hostess	¼″ slice (3.5 oz.)	1231
Premium	1¾-oz. slice (5″ × 2″ × ¼″)	535
Canned, deviled:		
(Hormel)	1 T.	108
(Underwood)	1 T. (.5 oz.)	142
Packaged, cooked:		
(Carl Buddig) smoked	1 oz.	400
(Eckrich):		
Chopped:		
Regular	1-oz. slice	330
Smorgas Pac	¾-oz. slice	250
Cooked	1.2-oz. slice	470
Danish	1.3-oz. slice	487
Loaf	1-oz. slice	330
Smoked, cured:		
Regular	¾-oz. slice	270
Slender-Sliced	1 oz.	360
(Hormel) chopped	1 slice	347
(Ohse):		
Chopped or cooked	1 oz.	260
Smoked:		
Regular	1 oz.	320
95% fat free	1 oz.	310
Turkey ham	1 oz.	370
(Oscar Mayer):		
Chopped	1 oz.	378
Cooked, smoked	1 oz.	382
Sliced, *Jubilee*	1-oz. slice	349
Steak, *Jubilee*	2-oz. steak	711

HAMBURGER (See **BEEF**, Ground; *McDONALD'S, BURGER KING,* etc.)

Food and Description	Measure or Quantity	Sodium (milligrams)
*HAMBURGER MIX		
Hamburger Helper (General Mills):		
Beef noodle	⅕ of pkg.	970
Beef Romanoff	⅕ of pkg.	1095
Cheeseburger macaroni	⅕ of pkg.	1025
Chili tomato	⅕ of pkg.	1230
Hash	⅕ of pkg.	920
Lasagna	⅕ of pkg.	1000
Pizza dish	⅕ of pkg.	960
Potato au gratin	⅕ of pkg.	890
Potato stroganoff	⅕ of pkg.	965
Rice oriental	⅕ of pkg.	1085
Spaghetti	⅕ of pkg.	1045
Stew	⅕ of pkg.	945
Tamale pie	⅕ of pkg.	910
HAMBURGER SEASONING MIX:		
*(Durkee)	1 cup	1012
(French's)	1-oz. pkg.	1800
HAM & CHEESE:		
Canned (Hormel):		
Loaf	3 oz.	1135
Patties	1 patty	468
Packaged:		
(Eckrich)	1-oz. slice	350
(Hormel) loaf	1 slice	334
HAM DINNER, frozen:		
(Banquet) American Favorite	10-oz. dinner	1148
(Morton)	10-oz. dinner	700
HAM SALAD SPREAD:		
(Carnation) spreadable	1½-oz. serving	264
(Oscar Mayer)	1-oz. serving	259
HAWAIIAN PUNCH, canned:		
Regular:		
Apple or grape	6 fl. oz.	13
Cherry or fruit juicy red	6 fl. oz.	17
Island fruit cocktail, orange or wild fruit	6 fl. oz.	19
Tropical fruit	6 fl. oz.	8

Food and Description	Measure or Quantity	Sodium (milligrams)
Very berry	6 fl. oz.	22
Dietetic, punch	6 fl. oz.	20
HAZELNUT (see FILBERT)		
HEADCHEESE (Oscar Mayer)	1-oz. serving	338
HERRING:		
Raw (USDA) Pacific, meat only	4 oz.	84
Smoked (USDA) Hard	4-oz. serving	7066
HO-HOS (Hostess)	1-oz. cake	85
HOMINY, canned (Allen's)		
solids & liq.		
Golden:		
Regular	½ cup	370
Mexican style	½ cup	430
White	½ cup	430
HOMINY GRITS:		
Dry:		
(USDA):		
Degermed	1 oz.	Tr.
Degermed	½ cup (2.8 oz.)	<1
(Albers)	¼ cup (1½ oz.)	<1
(Aunt Jemima)	3 T. (1 oz.)	<1
(Quaker):		
Regular	1 T. (.33 oz.)	Tr.
Instant:		
Regular	.8-oz. packet	385
With imitation bacon bits	1-oz. packet	544
With artificial cheese flavor	1-oz. packet	497
With imitation ham bits	1-oz. packet	544
(3-Minute Brand) quick, enriched	⅙ cup (1 oz.)	<1
Cooked (USDA) degermed	⅔ cup (5.6 oz.)	336
HONEY, strained:		
(USDA)	½ cup (5.7 oz.)	8
(USDA)	1 T. (.7 oz.)	1
HONEYCOMB, cereal (Post):		
Regular	1⅓ cups	214
Strawberry	1⅓ cups	160
HONEYDEW, fresh (USDA):		
Whole	1 lb. (weighed whole)	34

Food and Description	Measure or Quantity	Sodium (milligrams)
Wedge	2" × 7" wedge (5.3 oz.)	11
Flesh only	4 oz.	14
Flesh only, diced	1 cup (5.9 oz.)	20
HONEY SMACKS, cereal (Kellogg's)	¾ cup	70
HOPPING JOHN, frozen (Green Giant) Southern recipe	⅓ of 10-oz. pkg.	419
HORSERADISH:		
Raw (USDA):		
Whole	1 lb. (weighed unpared)	26
Pared	1 oz.	2
Prepared (USDA)	1 oz.	27
HOSTESS O's	1 piece	428
HYACINTH BEAN (USDA)		
Young bean, raw:		
Whole	1 lb. (weighed untrimmed)	8
Trimmed	4 oz.	2

I

ICE CREAM and FROZEN CUSTARD:		
(USDA):		
10% fat	1 cup (4.7 oz.)	84
12% fat	1 cup (5 oz.)	57
12% fat, brick-type	2½-oz. slice	28
12% fat	small container (3½ fl. oz)	25
16% fat	1 cup (5.2 oz.)	49
Almond Amaretto (Baskin-Robbins)	4 fl. oz.	30

Food and Description	Measure or Quantity	Sodium (milligrams)
Bon-Bon (Carnation):		
Chocolate	1 piece	11
Vanilla	1 piece	8
Brandied black cherry		
(Häagen-Dazs)	4 fl. oz.	55
Butter almond (Breyer's)	½ cup	125
Butter pecan:		
(Breyer's)	½ cup	125
(Häagen-Dazs)	4 fl. oz.	100
(Lady Borden)	½ cup	65
Cappuccino:		
(Baskin-Robbins) chip	4 fl. oz.	40
(Häagen-Dazs)	4 fl. oz.	65
Cherry vanilla (Häagen-Dazs)	4 fl. oz.	68
Chip crunch bar (Good Humor)	3-fl.-oz. bar	35
Chocolate:		
(Baskin-Robbins):		
Plain	1 scoop (4 fl.oz.)	128
Mousse Royale	1 scoop (4 fl. oz.)	150
(Borden) old fashioned or		
swirl	½ cup	65
(Breyer's)	½ cup	35
(Häagen-Dazs):		
Regular:		
Plain	4 fl. oz.	50
Chip	4 fl. oz.	55
Mint	4 fl. oz.	60
Bar, dark chocolate coating	1 bar	50
Chocolate Eclair Bar (Good Humor)	3-fl.-oz. bar	70
Chocolate fudge cake (Good Humor)	3-fl.-oz. piece	95
Chocolate malt bar (Good Humor)	3-fl.-oz. bar	50
Chocolate raspberry truffle (Baskin-Robbins)	4 fl. oz.	40
Coffee:		
(Breyer's)	½ cup	50
(Häagen-Dazs):		
Plain	4 fl. oz.	65

Food and Description	Measure or Quantity	Sodium (milligrams)
Chip	4 fl. oz.	68
Cookies & cream:		
(Breyer's)	½ cup	60
(Häagen-Dazs)	4 fl. oz.	90
(Sealtest)	½ cup	75
Cookie sandwich (Good Humor)	2.7-fl.-oz. piece	195
Eskimo Pie:		
Chocolate fudge bar	1¾-fl.-oz. bar	30
Chocolate fudge bar	2½-fl.-oz. bar	45
Chocolate fudge bar	3-fl.-oz. bar	50
Dietary dairy bar, chocolate covered	2½-fl.-oz. bar	40
Old fashioned:		
Crispy	1 bar	70
Double chocolate	1 bar	150
Vanilla	1 bar	70
Pie:		
Regular:		
Chocolate	3-fl.-oz. bar	100
Crunch	3-fl.-oz. bar	55
Vanilla	3-fl.-oz. bar	45
Jr:		
Chocolate	1¾-fl.-oz. bar	60
Crunch	1¾-fl.-oz. bar	30
Vanilla	1¾-fl.-oz. bar	25
Original:		
Double chocolate	bar	75
Vanilla	1 bar	35
Thin mints	2-fl.-oz. bar	30
Twin pop	1 bar	0
Fat Frog (Good Humor)	3-fl.-oz. pop	45
Fudge royal (Sealtest)	½ cup	55
Grand Marnier (Baskin-Robbins)	4 fl. oz.	50
Heart (Good Humor)	4-fl.-oz. pop	45
Jamocha (Baskin-Robbins)	2½-fl.-oz. scoop	64
Keylime & cream (Häagen-Dazs)	4 fl. oz.	30
Macadamia brittle (Häagen-Dazs)	4 fl. oz.	60
Macadamia nut (Häagen-Dazs)	4 fl. oz.	114
Maple walnut (Häagen-Dazs)	4 fl. oz.	55

Food and Description	Measure or Quantity	Sodium (milligrams)
Mocha double nut (Häagen-Dazs)	4 fl. oz.	85
Orange & vanilla (Häagen-Dazs)	4 fl. oz.	35
Oreo, cookie & cream:		
Regular, any flavor	3 fl. oz.	100
Sandwich	1 sandwich	300
Stick	1 bar	100
Peach:		
(Breyer's)	½ cup	35
(Häagen-Dazs) elberta	4 fl. oz.	50
Peanut butter vanilla (Häagen-Dazs)	4 fl. oz.	12
Pralines'n Cream (Baskins-Robbins)	2½-fl.-oz. scoop	166
Raspberry & vanilla (Häagen-Dazs)	4 fl.oz.	35
Rocky road (Baskin-Robbins)	4-fl.-oz.	123
Rum raisin (Häagen-Dazs)	4 fl. oz.	495
Shark Bar (Good Humor)	3-fl.-oz. pop	0
Slice (Good Humor) vanilla, regular or Cal-control	3.2-fl.-oz. slice	45
Strawberry:		
(Baskin-Robbins):		
Plain	4 fl. oz.	109
Wild, light	4 fl. oz.	70
(Borden)	½ cup	55
(Breyer's) natural	½ cup	40
(Häagen-Dazs)	4 fl. oz.	55
Strawberry & cream (Borden)	½ cup	55
Swiss almond chocolate (Häagen-Dazs)	4 fl. oz.	64
Toasted almond bar (Good Humor)	3-fl.-oz. bar	30
Toasted caramel bar (Good Humor)	3-fl.-oz. bar	55
Vanilla:		
(Baskin-Robbins):		
Regular	4 fl. oz.	91
French	4 fl. oz.	95
(Borden)	½ cup	55

Food and Description	Measure or Quantity	Sodium (milligrams)
(Eagle Brand)	½ cup	55
(Good Humor):		
Bar, chocolate-coated	3-fl.-oz. piece	40
Sandwich	2½-fl.-oz. piece	120
Slice, regular or *Cal-control*	1 piece	45
(Häagen-Dazs):		
Regular:		
Plain	4 fl. oz.	65
Chip	4 fl. oz.	51
Bar, milk chocolate coating	3.55-fl.-oz. bar	60
(Sealtest)	½ cup	50
Vanilla swiss almond		
(Häagen-Dazs)	4 fl. oz.	60
Whammy (Good Humor)	1.6-oz. piece	25
ICE CREAM CONE (Baskin-Robbins):		
Cake	1 cone	26
Sugar	1 cone	45
***ICE CREAM MIX** (Salada):		
Dutch chocolate	1 cup	75
Wild strawberry	1 cup	60
ICE MILK:		
(USDA):		
Hardened	1 cup (4.6 oz.)	89
Soft serve	1 cup (6.3 oz.)	119
(Borden):		
Chocolate	½ cup	80
Strawberry or vanilla	½ cup	65
Light N' Lively, coffee	½ cup	55
ICING (See **CAKE ICING**)		
INSTANT BREAKFAST (See individual brand name or company listings)		
IRISH WHISKEY (See **DISTILLED LIQUORS**)		
ITALIAN DINNER, frozen		
(Banquet)	12-oz. dinner	1783

Food and Description	Measure or Quantity	Sodium (milligrams)

J

JACKFRUIT, fresh (USDA):

Food and Description	Measure or Quantity	Sodium (milligrams)
Whole	1 lb. (weighed with seeds & skin)	3
Flesh only	4 oz.	2
JACK IN THE BOX:		
Beef fajita pita sandwich	6.2-oz. serving	635
Breakfast Jack	4.4-oz. serving	871
Burger:		
Plain	3.6-oz. burger	556
Cheese:		
Regular	4-oz. burger	746
Bacon	8.1-oz. burger	1127
Ultimate	9.9-oz. burger	1176
Ham & swiss	9.1-oz. burger	1217
Jumbo Jack:		
Regular	7.8-oz. burger	733
Cheese	8½-oz. burger	1090
Monterey	9.9-oz. burger	1124
Mushroom	6.4-oz. burger	910
Canadian crescent	4.7-oz. serving	851
Cheesecake	3½-oz. piece	208
Chicken fajita pita sandwich	6.7-oz. sandwich	703
Chicken strips	1 piece	177
Chicken supreme sandwich	8.1-oz. sandwich	1535
Club pita sandwich, excluding sauce	6.3-oz. sandwich	931
Egg, scrambled, platter	8.8-oz. serving	1188
Egg roll	1 piece	301
Fish supreme sandwich	8-oz. sandwich	1047
French fries	2.4-oz. regular order	164
Hot club supreme sandwich	7½-oz. sandwich	1467
Jelly, grape	1 T. (.5 oz.)	3

Food and Description	Measure or Quantity	Sodium (milligrams)
Ketchup	1 serving	99
Milk shake:		
Chocolate	10-oz. serving	270
Strawberry	10-oz. serving	240
Vanilla	10-oz. serving	230
Nachos:		
Cheese	6-oz. serving	1154
Supreme	11.9-oz. serving	2914
Onion rings	3.8-oz. serving	407
Pancake platter	8.1-oz. serving	888
Salad:		
Chef	11.7-oz. salad	900
Mexican chicken	15.2-oz. salad	1530
Side	3.9-oz. salad	84
Taco	14.8-oz. salad	1670
Salad dressing:		
Regular:		
Bleu cheese	1.2-oz. serving	459
Buttermilk	1.2-oz. serving	347
Thousand Island	1.2-oz. serving	350
Dietetic, french	1.2-oz. serving	300
Sauce:		
A-1	1.8-oz. serving	809
BBQ	.9-oz. serving	300
Guacamole	.9-oz. serving	130
Mayo-mustard	.8-oz. serving	247
Mayo-onion	.8-oz. serving	140
Salsa	.9-oz. serving	129
Seafood cocktail	1-oz. serving	206
Sweet & sour	1-oz. serving	160
Sausage crescent	5½-oz. serving	1012
Shrimp	.3-oz. piece	67
Soft drink:		
Sweetened:		
Coca-Cola Classic	12 fl. oz.	14
Dr Pepper	12 fl. oz.	18
Sprite	12 fl. oz.	46
Dietetic, Coke	12 fl. oz.	26
Supreme crescent	5.1-oz. crescent	1053
Syrup, pancake	1½-oz. serving	6

Food and Description	Measure or Quantity	Sodium (milligrams)
Taco:		
Regular	2.9-oz. serving	406
Super	4.8-oz. serving	765
Turnover, hot apple	4.2-oz. piece	350
JAM, sweetened (See also individual listings by flavor):		
(USDA)	1 oz.	3
(USDA)	1 tsp.	2
JELL-O FRUIT & CREAM BAR:		
Blueberry, raspberry or strawberry	1.7-fl.-oz. bar	98
Peach	1.7-fl.-oz. bar	109
JELL-O GELATIN POPS	1.7-fl.-oz. pop	7
JELL-O PUDDING POP:		
Banana butterscotch or vanilla	2-fl.-oz. pop	63
Chocolate or chocolate fudge	2-fl.-oz. pop	99
Chocolate & caramel swirl	2-fl.-oz. pop	83
Chocolate & vanilla swirl	2-fl.-oz. pop	81
JELLY, sweetened (See also individual listings by flavor)		
(USDA)	1 T. (.6 oz.)	3
JORDAN ALMOND (See CANDY)		
JUICE (See individual flavors)		
JUJUBE or CHINESE DATE (USDA):		
Fresh, whole	1 lb. (weighed with seeds)	13
Fresh, flesh only	4 oz.	3
JUNIOR FOOD (See BABY FOOD)		

Food and Description	Measure or Quantity	Sodium (milligrams)

K

Food and Description	Measure or Quantity	Sodium (milligrams)
KABOOM, cereal (General Mills)	1 cup (1 oz.)	370
KALE:		
Raw (USDA) leaves only	1 lb. (weighed untrimmed)	218
Boiled (USDA) leaves, including stems	½ cup (1.9 oz.)	24
Canned (Sunshine) chopped, solids & liq.	½ cup (4.1 oz.)	251
Frozen:		
(Birds Eye) chopped	⅓ of pkg.	14
(McKenzie) chopped	3.3 oz.	28
(Southland) chopped	⅕ of 16-oz. pkg.	15
KETCHUP (See CATSUP)		
KIDNEY (USDA):		
Beef:		
Raw	4 oz.	200
Braised	4 oz.	287
Hog, raw	4 oz.	130
Lamb, raw	4 oz.	257
KINGFISH, raw (USDA):		
Whole	1 lb. (weighed whole)	166
Meat only	4 oz.	94
KING VITAMAN, cereal (Quaker)	1¼ cups (1 oz.)	251
KIPPERS (See HERRING)		
KIX, cereal (General Mills)	1½ cups (1 oz.)	315
KOHLRABI (USDA):		
Raw:		
Whole	1 lb. (weighed with skin, without leaves)	26
Diced	1 cup (4.8 oz.)	11

Food and Description	Measure or Quantity	Sodium (milligrams)
Boiled, without salt:		
Drained	4 oz.	7
Drained	1 cup (5.5 oz.)	9
*KOOL-AID (General Foods):		
Unsweetened (sugar to be added):		
Apple, cherry, grape, lemon-lime, orange or raspberry	8 fl. oz.	<1
Strawberry	8 fl. oz.	33
Sunshine punch	8 fl. oz.	2
Tropical punch	8 fl. oz.	5
Pre-sweetened:		
Regular, with sugar:		
Apple, grape, orange, raspberry or strawberry	8 fl. oz.	<1
Cherry	8 fl. oz.	7
Sunshine punch	8 fl. oz.	3
Tropical punch	8 fl. oz.	10
Dietetic, Sugar free:		
Cherry	8 fl. oz.	7
Grape or tropical punch	8 fl. oz.	<1
Sunshine punch	8 fl. oz.	4
KUMQUAT, fresh (USDA):		
Whole	1 lb. (weighed with seeds)	30
Flesh & skin	4 oz.	8

L

LAKE HERRING, raw (USDA):		
Whole	1 lb.	111
Meat only	4 oz.	53

Food and Description	Measure or Quantity	Sodium (milligrams)
LAMB, choice grade (USDA):		
Chop, broiled:		
Loin. One 5-oz. chop (weighed before cooking with bone) will give you:		
Lean & fat	2.8 oz.	55
Lean only	2.3 oz.	46
Rib. One 5-oz. chop (weighed before cooking with bone) will give you:		
Lean & fat	2.9 oz.	57
Lean only	2 oz.	39
Leg:		
Raw, lean & fat	1 lb. (weighed with bone)	280
Roasted, lean & fat	4 oz.	79
Roasted, lean only	4 oz.	79
Shoulder:		
Raw, lean & fat	1 lb. (weighed with bone)	270
Roasted, lean & fat	4 oz.	79
Roasted, lean only	4 oz.	79
LARD	Any quantity	0
LASAGNA:		
Canned (Hormel) *Short Order*	7½-oz. can	1083
Frozen:		
(Armour) *Dinner Classics*	10-oz. meal	1120
(Banquet) Family Entree, with meat sauce	2-lb. pkg.	6000
(Blue Star) *Dining Lite*:		
Vegetable	11-oz. meal	720
Zucchini	11-oz. meal	780
(Buitoni):		
Regular	9-oz. serving	929
Al forno	8-oz. serving	1107
Meat sauce	5-oz. serving	499
Sorrentina, cheese	8-oz. serving	728
(Celentano):		
Regular	½ of 16-oz. pkg.	410
Regular	¼ of 25-oz. pkg.	325

Food and Description	Measure or Quantity	Sodium (milligrams)
Primavera	11-oz. pkg.	500
(Conagra) *Light & Elegant*,		
florentine	11¼-oz. entree	980
(Green Giant):		
Baked:		
With meat sauce	12-oz. entree	1660
With meat sauce	21-oz. entree	3030
Chicken	12-oz. entree	1215
Spinach	12-oz. entree	1455
Boil 'n Bag	9½-oz. pkg.	1145
(Stouffer's):		
Regular	10½-oz. pkg.	1200
Lean Cuisine	11-oz. pkg.	1000
(Swanson):		
Regular, 4-compartment		
dinner	13-oz. meal	800
Hungry Man, with		
meat	18¾-oz. dinner	1510
Main Course	13¼-oz. entree	1120
(Van de Kamp's):		
Beef & mushroom	11-oz. meal	970
Creamy spinach	11-oz. meal	840
Italian sausage	11-oz. meal	1190
(Weight Watchers) 1-compartment meal:		
Regular	12-oz. meal	1097
Italian cheese	12-oz. meal	1420
LATKES, frozen (Empire Kosher):		
Mini	3-oz. serving	400
Rounds	2½-oz. serving	305
Triangles	3-oz. serving	335
LEEKS, raw (USDA):		
Whole	1 lb. (weighed untrimmed)	12
Trimmed	4 oz.	6
LEMON, fresh (USDA) peeled	1 med. (2⅛″ dia.)	1
LEMONADE:		
Canned:		
Capri Sun, natural	6¾ fl. oz.	2

Food and Description	Measure or Quantity	Sodium (milligrams)
Country Time	12-fl.-oz. can	61
(Hi-C)	6 fl. oz.	6
Ssips (Johanna Farms)	8.45-fl.-oz. container	25
Chilled (Minute Maid):		
Regular	6 fl. oz.	<1
Pink	6 fl. oz.	<1
*Frozen:		
(USDA)	½ cup (4.4 oz.)	Tr.
Country Time, regular or pink	8 fl. oz.	21
(Minute Maid)	6 fl. oz.	<1
(Sunkist)	6 fl. oz.	Tr.
*Mix, regular:		
Country Time, regular or pink	8 fl. oz.	29
(Hi-C)	6 fl. oz.	6
(Kool-Aid) unsweetened package, regular or pink	8 fl. oz.	<1
(Kool-Aid) pre-sweetened package, regular or pink	8 fl. oz.	Tr.
(Minute Maid) regular or pink	6 fl. oz.	6
*Mix, dietetic:		
Crystal Light	8 fl. oz.	<1
(Kool Aid)	8 fl. oz.	<1
(Sunkist)	8 fl. oz.	35
LEMONADE BAR (Sunkist)	3-fl.-oz. bar	5
LEMON JUICE:		
Fresh:		
(USDA)	1 cup (8.6 oz.)	2
(USDA)	1 T. (.5 oz.)	<1
Canned, unsweetened:		
(USDA)	1 cup (8.6 oz.)	2
(USDA)	1 T. (.5 oz.)	<1
Plastic container:		
(USDA)	¼ cup (2 oz.)	<1
ReaLemon	1 fl. oz.	10
Frozen, unsweetened:		
(USDA):		
Concentrate	½ cup (5.1 oz.)	7

Food and Description	Measure or Quantity	Sodium (milligrams)
Single strength (Minute Maid) full strength, already constituted	½ cup (4.3 oz.)	1
	1 fl. oz.	<1
*LEMON-LIMEADE, mix:		
Regular (Country Time)	8 fl. oz.	28
Dietetic, *Crystal Light*	8 fl. oz.	<1
LEMON LIME DRINK,		
canned, *Ssips* (Johanna Farms)	8.45-fl.-oz. container	15
LEMON & PEPPER SEASONING (French's)	1 tsp. (3.6 grams)	800
LENTIL, whole, dry:		
(USDA)	½ lb.	68
(USDA)	1 cup (6.7 oz.)	57
LETTUCE (USDA):		
Bibb, untrimmed	1 lb. (weighed untrimmed)	30
Bibb, untrimmed	7.8-oz. head (4″ dia.)	15
Boston, untrimmed	1 lb. (weighed untrimmed)	30
Boston, untrimmed	7.8-oz. head (4″ dia.)	15
Butterhead varieties (See Bibb & Boston)		
Cos (See Romaine)		
Dark green (See Romaine)		
Grand Rapids	1 lb. (weighed untrimmed)	26
Grand Rapids	2 large leaves (1.8 oz.)	4
Great Lakes	1 lb. (weighed untrimmed)	39
Great Lakes, trimmed	1-lb. head (4¾″ dia.)	41
Iceberg:		
Untrimmed	1 lb. (weighed untrimmed)	39
Trimmed	1-lb. head (4¾″ dia.)	41

Food and Description	Measure or Quantity	Sodium (milligrams)
Leaves	1 cup (2.3 oz.)	6
Chopped	1 cup (2 oz.)	5
Chunks	1 cup (2.6 oz.)	7
Looseleaf varieties (See Salad Bowl)		
New York	1 lb. (weighed untrimmed)	39
New York	1-lb. head (4¾" dia.)	41
Romaine:		
Untrimmed	1 lb. (weighed untrimmed)	26
Trimmed, shredded & broken into pieces	½ cup (.8 oz.)	2
Salad Bowl	1 lb. (weighed untrimmed)	26
Salad Bowl	2 large leaves (1.8 oz.)	4
Simpson	1 lb. (weighed untrimmed)	26
Simpson	2 large leaves (1.8 oz.)	4
White Paris (see Romaine)		
LIFE, cereal (Quaker):		
Regular	⅔ cup (1 oz.)	163
Cinnamon	⅔ cup (1 oz.)	149
LIL' ANGELS (Hostess)	1 piece	92
LIMA BEAN (See BEAN, LIMA)		
LIME, fresh (USDA):		
Whole	1 lb. (weighed with skin & seeds)	8
Whole	1 med (2" dia., 2.4 oz.)	1
*LIMEADE, frozen, sweetened: (USDA) diluted with 4⅓ parts water	½ cup (4.4 oz.)	Tr.
(Minute Maid)	6 fl. oz.	<1
LIME JUICE:		
Fresh (USDA)	1 cup (8.7 oz.)	2

Food and Description	Measure or Quantity	Sodium (milligrams)
Canned or bottled, unsweetened:		
(USDA)	1 cup (8.7 oz.)	2
(USDA)	1 fl. oz. (1.1 oz.)	<1
Plastic container, *ReaLime*	1 T. (.5 oz.)	5
LINGCOD, raw (USDA):		
Whole	1 lb. (weighed whole)	91
Meat only	4 oz.	67
LINGUINI WITH CLAM SAUCE, frozen (Stouffer's)	10½-oz. meal	1010
LITCHI NUT (USDA):		
Fresh:		
Whole	4 oz. (weighed in shell with seeds)	2
Flesh only	4 oz.	3
Dried:		
Whole	4 oz. (weighed in shell with seeds)	2
Flesh only	2 oz.	2
LIVER:		
Beef:		
(USDA):		
Raw	1 lb.	617
Fried	4 oz.	209
(Swift) packaged, *True-Tender*, sliced, cooked	⅕ of 1-lb. pkg.	70
Calf (USDA):		
Raw	1 lb.	331
Fried	4 oz.	134
Chicken (USDA):		
Raw	1 lb.	318
Simmered	4 oz.	69
Goose, raw (USDA)	1 lb.	635
Hog (USDA):		
Raw	1 lb.	331
Fried	4 oz.	126
Lamb (USDA):		
Raw	1 lb.	236
Broiled	4 oz.	96
Turkey, raw (USDA)	1 lb.	286

Food and Description	Measure or Quantity	Sodium (milligrams)
LIVER PÂTÉ (See **PÂTÉ**)		
LIVER SAUSAGE or LIVERWURST, spread (Underwood)	1 oz.	237
LOBSTER:		
Cooked, meat only (USDA)	4 oz.	238
Canned (USDA) meat only	4 oz.	238
LOBSTER NEWBURG, home recipe (USDA)	4 oz.	572
LOBSTER SALAD, home recipe (USDA)	4 oz.	141
LOGANBERRY (USDA):		
Fresh:		
Untrimmed	1 lb. (weighed with caps)	4
Trimmed	1 cup (5.1 oz.)	1
Canned, solids & liq.:		
Extra heavy syrup	4 oz.	1
Heavy syrup	4 oz.	1
Juice pack	4 oz.	1
Light syrup	4 oz.	1
LONG JOHN SILVER'S:		
Catfish fillet	2.7-oz. piece	469
Catsup	.4-oz. serving	136
Chicken Plank	1.4-oz. serving	295
Chicken sandwich	6.1-oz. serving	1159
Chowder, clam	6 fl. oz.	611
Clams, breaded	4.7-oz. order	1170
Cole slaw, drained on fork	3.5 oz.	367
Fish fillet:		
Baked, with sauce	5.5-oz. serving	361
Batter fried	3-oz. piece	673
Kitchen breaded	2-oz. piece	374
Fish sandwich	6.4-oz. sandwich	1243
French fries	3-oz. serving	6
Hush puppy	.85-oz. piece	202
Milk	8 fl. oz.	119
Oyster, breaded	.7-oz. piece	65
Peg Leg, battered	1-oz. serving	225

Food and Description	Measure or Quantity	Sodium (milligrams)
Pie:		
Apple	4-oz. piece	247
Cherry	4-oz. piece	251
Lemon meringue	3½-oz. piece	254
Pecan	4-oz. piece	435
Pumpkin	4-oz. piece	242
Scallop, battered	.7-oz. piece	201
Seafood salad	5.8-oz. serving	833
Seafood sauce	1.2-oz. serving	358
Shrimp:		
Battered	.6-oz. piece	154
Breaded	4.7-oz. serving	1229
Chilled	.2-oz. piece	19
Vegetables, mixed	4 oz.	570
LUCKY CHARMS, cereal (General Mills)	1 cup (1 oz.)	185
LUNCHEON MEAT (See also individual listings e.g., **BOLOGNA,** etc.):		
All meat (Oscar Mayer)	1-oz. slice	346
Banquet loaf (Eckrich)	¾-oz. slice	250
Bar B-Q-Loaf:		
(Eckrich)	1-oz. slice	370
(Oscar Mayer)	1-oz. slice	346
Beef, jellied loaf (Hormel)	1 slice	450
Gourmet loaf (Eckrich):		
Regular	1-oz. slice	390
Smorgas Pac	¾-oz. slice	300
Ham & cheese (See **HAM & CHEESE**)		
Ham roll sausage (Oscar Mayer)	.5-oz.slice	329
Ham roll sausage (Oscar Mayer)	1-oz. slice	329
Honey loaf:		
(Hormel)	1 slice	292
(Oscar Mayer)	1-oz. slice	366
Liver loaf (Hormel)	1 slice	352
Liver cheese (Oscar Mayer)	1.3-oz. slice	433

Food and Description	Measure or Quantity	Sodium (milligrams)
Luncheon roll sausage (Oscar Mayer)	.8-oz. slice	222
Luxury loaf:		
(Ohse)	1 oz.	320
(Oscar Mayer)	1-oz. slice	300
Macaroni-cheese loaf (Eckrich)	1-oz. slice	370
New England brand sausage (Oscar Mayer) 92% fat free	.8-oz. slice	292
Old fashioned loaf:		
(Eckrich):		
Regular	1-oz. slice	330
Smorgas Pac	¾-oz. slice	250
(Oscar Mayer)	1-oz. slice	321
Olive loaf:		
(Eckrich)	1-oz. slice	370
(Hormel)	1 slice	405
(Oscar Mayer)	1-oz. slice	395
Peppered loaf (Oscar Mayer) 93% fat free	1-oz. slice	361
Pickle loaf:		
(Eckrich):		
Regular or *Smorgas Pac*	1-oz. slice	320
Beef, *Smorgas Pac*	¾-oz. slice	260
(Hormel) regular	1 slice	376
(Ohse)	1 oz.	330
Pickle & pimiento loaf (Oscar Mayer)	1-oz. slice	394
Picnic loaf (Oscar Mayer)	1-oz. slice	330
Spiced (Hormel) regular	1 slice	351

Food and Description	Measure or Quantity	Sodium (milligrams)

M

MACARONI, Plain macaroni products are essentially the same in caloric value and carbohydrate content on the same weight basis. The longer they are cooked, the more water is absorbed and this affects the nutritive values.

Food and Description	Measure or Quantity	Sodium (milligrams)
Dry:		
(USDA):		
Elbow-type	1 cup (4.8 oz.)	3
1-inch pieces	1 cup (3.8 oz.)	2
2-inch pieces	1 cup (3 oz.)	2
(Creamette) spinach, ribbons	2 oz.	70
(Pritikin) whole wheat	2 oz.	40
Cooked (USDA):		
8–10 minutes, firm	1 cup (4.6 oz.)	1
8–10 minutes, firm	4 oz.	1
14–20 minutes, tender	1 cup (4.9 oz.)	1
14–20 minutes, tender	4 oz.	1
Canned (Franco-American) *PizzO*s, in pizza sauce	7½-oz. can	980
MACARONI & BEEF:		
Canned:		
(Bounty) *Chili Mac,* in tomato sauce	7¾-oz. can	1209
(Franco-American) *BeefyO*s, in tomato sauce	7½-oz. can	1250
Frozen:		
(Morton)	10-oz. dinner	800
(Stouffer's) with tomatoes	5¾-oz. serving	810
(Swanson)	12-oz. dinner	850

Food and Description	Measure or Quantity	Sodium (milligrams)
MACARONI & CHEESE:		
Home recipe (USDA) baked	1 cup (7.1 oz.)	1086
Canned:		
(USDA)	1 cup	730
(Franco-American):		
Regular	7⅜-oz. can	960
Elbow	7⅜-oz. can	910
(Hormel) *Short Orders*	7½-oz. can	917
Frozen:		
(Banquet):		
Casserole	8-oz. pkg.	930
Dinner	9-oz. pkg.	940
(Celentano) baked	½ of 12-oz. pkg.	425
(Conagra) *Light & Elegant*	9 oz. entree	1010
(Green Giant) *Boil 'N Bag*	9-oz. entree	1115
(Morton):		
Casserole	20-oz. casserole	2600
Dinner	11-oz. dinner	1000
(Stouffer's)	6-oz. serving	780
(Swanson) 3-compartment:		
Dinner	12¼-oz. dinner	970
Entree	12-oz. entree	824
(Swanson):		
Entree	12-oz. entree	1850
Dinner	12¼-oz. dinner	980
Mix:		
(Golden Gram)	¼ of pkg.	430
*(Kraft):		
Regular:		
Plain	¼ of pkg.	420
Spiral	⅓ of pkg.	400
Velveeta, shells	¼ of pkg.	720
*(Prince)	¾ cup	574
Packaged (Ohse)	1 oz.	310
MACARONI & CHEESE PIE, frozen (Swanson)	7-oz. pie	880
***MACARONI, SHELLS, AND SAUCE,** mix (Lipton):		
Creamy garlic	½ cup	535
Herb tomato	½ cup	435

Food and Description	Measure or Quantity	Sodium (milligrams)
MACE (French's)	1 tsp. (1.8 grams)	1
MAGIC SHELL (Smucker's)	1 T.	12–25
MAI TAI COCKTAIL MIX (Holland House):		
Instant	.56-oz. packet	4
Liquid	1 oz.	60
MALTED MILK MIX:		
(USDA) dry powder	1 oz.	125
(Carnation):		
Chocolate	3 heaping tsps. (.7 oz.)	47
Natural	3 heapings tsps. (.7 oz.)	98
MALT EXTRACT, dried (USDA)	1 oz.	23
MALT LIQUOR, *Champale,* 6¼% alcohol	12 fl. oz.	64
MALT-O-MEAL, cereal:		
Regular	1 T. (.3 oz.)	<1
Chocolate flavored	1 T. (.3 oz.)	<1
MAMEY or MAMMEE APPLE, fresh (USDA)	1 lb. (weighed with skin & seeds)	42
MANDARIN ORANGE (See **TANGERINE**)		
MANGO, fresh (USDA):		
Whole	1 lb. (weighed with seeds & skin)	21
Whole	1 med. (7 oz.)	9
Flesh only, diced or sliced	½ cup (2.9 oz.)	6
MANGO NECTAR, canned (Libby's)	6 fl. oz.	5
MANHATTAN COCKTAIL:		
Canned (Mr. Boston)	3 fl. oz.	4
Mix (Holland House) liquid	1 oz.	5
MANICOTTI frozen:		
(Buitoni):		
Cheese	5½-oz. serving	432

Food and Description	Measure or Quantity	Sodium (milligrams)
Florentine (Celentano):	2 pieces (5½ oz.)	396
Without sauce	2 pieces (7 oz.)	420
With sauce	2 pieces (8 oz.)	435
*MANWICH (Hunt's):		
Original	5.8 oz.	630
Mexican	5.8 oz.	690
MAPLE SYRUP (See SYRUP)		
MARGARINE:		
Salted:		
Regular:		
(USDA)	1 lb.	4477
(USDA)	1 cup (8 oz.)	2239
(USDA)	1 T. (.5 oz.)	138
Autumn, soft or stick	1 T.	109
(Blue Bonnet) soft or stick	1 T. (.5 oz.)	95
(Fleischmann's) soft or stick	1 T. (.5 oz.)	95
Holiday	1 T. (.5 oz.)	165
(Imperial) soft	1 T. (.5 oz.)	96
(Mazola) regular	1 T. (.5 oz.)	116
(Nucoa):		
Regular	1 T. (.5 oz.)	165
Soft	1 T. (.4 oz.)	130
(Promise) soft or stick	1 T. (.5 oz.)	96
Unsalted, regular:		
(USDA)	1 T.	1
Mazola	1 T.	<1
Imitation or dietetic:		
(Blue Bonnet)	1 T.	99
(Imperial) diet	1 T. (.5 oz.)	136
(Mazola)	1 T.	130
(Mazola)	½ cup	1066
Whipped:		
(USDA) salted	½ cup	750
(USDA) unsalted	½ cup	<8
(Blue Bonnet)	1 T. (9 g.)	99
Fleischmann's, soft, unsalted	1 T.	7
Imperial, spread	1 T. (9 g.)	70

Food and Description	Measure or Quantity	Sodium (milligrams)
(Parkay) cup	1 T.	74
MARGARITA COCKTAIL		
MIX (Holland House):		
Instant:		
Regular	.5-oz. packet	4
Strawberry	.56-oz. packet	<1
Liquid:		
Regular	1 oz.	92
Strawberry	1 oz.	3
MARINADE MIX:		
(Adolph's):		
Chicken	1-oz. pkg.	4105
Meat	.8-oz. pkg.	4636
(Durkee) meat	1-oz. pkg.	4104
(French's) meat	1-oz. pkg.	4320
(Kikkomon) meat	1-oz. pkg.	4000
MARJORAM (French's)	1 tsp. (1.2 g.)	1
MARMALADE:		
Sweetened:		
(USDA)	1 T. (.7 oz.)	3
(Home Brands)	1 T.	7
(Smucker's)	1 T. (.7 oz.)	Tr.
Dietetic:		
(Estee)	1 T.	<3
(Featherweight)	1 T.	40–50
(Louis Sherry)	1 T.	<3
MARSHMALLOW FLUFF	1 heaping tsp. (.6 oz.)	5
MARSHMALLOW KRISPIES,		
cereal (Kellogg's)	1¼ cups	285
MASA HARINA (Quaker)	⅓ cup (1.3 oz.)	2
MASA TRIGO (Quaker)	⅓ cup (1.3 oz.)	294
MATZO:		
(Goodman's) *Diet-10*'s	1 sq.	<1
(Horowitz-Margareten) unsalted	1 matzo (1.2 oz.)	<1
(Manischewitz):		
Regular	1 piece (1 oz.)	<5
American	1 piece	175
Dietetic:		
Tam Tams, unsalted	1 piece	Tr.

Food and Description	Measure or Quantity	Sodium (milligrams)
Thins	1 piece (.8 oz.)	<5
Egg	1 piece	<10
Egg & onion	1 piece	180
Miniatures	1 piece	Tr.
Tea, thin	1 piece	Tr.
Tam Tams:		
Regular	1 piece	17
Garlic or onion	1 piece	16
Wheat	1 piece	18
MATZO MEAL (Manischewitz)	1 cup (4.1 oz.)	2
MAYONNAISE:		
Real:		
(Bama)	1 T.	65
(Bennett's)	1 T.	65
(Hellmann's)	1 T. (.5 oz.)	80
(Hellmann's)	½ cup (3.9 oz.)	624
(Kraft)	1 T.	65
Dietetic or imitation:		
(Diet Delight) *Mayo-Lite*	1 T.	75
(Featherweight) *Soyamaise*	1 T.	3
(Kraft) light	1 T.	90
McDONALD'S:		
Big Mac	1 hamburger	979
Biscuit:		
Plain	3-oz. biscuit	786
With bacon, egg & cheese	5.1-oz. sandwich	1269
With sausage	4.3-oz. sandwich	1147
With sausage & egg	6.2-oz. sandwich	1301
Cheeseburger	1 cheeseburger	743
Chicken McNuggets	1 serving (4.3 oz.)	623
Chicken McNugget Sauce:		
Barbecue	1.1-oz. serving	309
Honey	.5-oz. serving	2
Hot mustard	1.1-oz. serving	259
Sweet & sour	1.1-oz. serving	186
Cookie:		
Chocolate chip	2.4-oz. pkg.	313

Food and Description	Measure or Quantity	Sodium (milligrams)
McDonaldland	2.4-oz. pkg.	358
Egg McMuffin	1 serving	885
Egg, scrambled	1 serving	205
English muffin, buttered	2.2-oz. muffin	310
Filet-o-Fish sandwich	1 sandwich	799
Grapefruit juice	6 fl. oz.	2
Hamburger	1 hamburger	506
Hot cakes, with butter & syrup	1 serving	1070
Orange juice	6 fl. oz.	2
Pie:		
Apple	3-oz. pie	398
Cherry	3.1-oz. pie	427
Potato:		
French fries	1 regular order	109
Hash browns	1 regular order	325
Quarter Pounder:		
Regular	1 burger	718
With cheese	1 burger with cheese	1220
Sausage, pork	1.9-oz. serving	423
Sausage McMuffin:		
Plain	4.1-oz. sandwich	942
With egg	5.8-oz. sandwich	1044
Shake:		
Chocolate	10.3-oz. serving	300
Strawberry	10.2-oz. serving	207
Vanilla	10.3-oz. serving	201
Sundae:		
Caramel	5.8-oz. serving	145
Hot fudge	5.8-oz. serving	170
Strawberry	5.8-oz. serving	90
MEATBALL DINNER or ENTREE, frozen (Swanson) with brown gravy	8½-oz. meal	900
MEATBALL SEASONING MIX:		
*(Durkee) Italian	½ cup	503
(French's)	1½-oz. pkg.	3300

Food and Description	Measure or Quantity	Sodium (milligrams)
MEATBALL STEW:		
Canned:		
(Libby's)	⅓ of 24-oz. can	1083
(Morton House)	⅓ of 24-oz. can	1100
Frozen (Stouffer's) *Lean Cuisine*	10-oz. meal	1260
MEATBALL, SWEDISH, frozen		
(Armour) *Dinner Classics*	11½-oz. meal	1560
MEAT LOAF DINNER or ENTREE, frozen:		
(Banquet):		
Dinner	11-oz. dinner	1333
Entree for One	5-oz. entree	827
(Morton) dinner:	11-oz. dinner	1300
(Swanson):		
Dinner	11-oz. dinner	970
Entree, with tomato sauce	9-oz. entree	950
MEAT LOAF SEASONING MIX:		
(Contadina)	3¾-oz. pkg.	4301
(French's)	1½-oz. pkg.	4920
MEAT, POTTED:		
(Hormel)	1 T.	145
(Libby's)	⅓ of 5-oz. can	297
MEAT TENDERIZER		
(French's) unseasoned or seasoned	1 tsp. (5 g.)	1760
MELBA TOAST (Old London):		
Garlic rounds	1 piece (2 g.)	22
Pumpernickel	1 piece (5 g.)	39
Rye:		
Regular	1 piece (5 g.)	39
Unsalted	1 piece (5 g.)	<1
Sesame rounds	1 piece (2 g.)	28
Wheat:		
Regular	1 piece (5 g.)	39
Unsalted	1 piece (5 g.)	<1
White:		
Regular	1 piece (5 g.)	39
Rounds	1 piece (2 g.)	22

Food and Description	Measure or Quantity	Sodium (milligrams)
Unsalted	1 piece (5 g.)	<1
MELON (See individual listings such as **CANTALOUPE, WATERMELON**, etc.)		
MELON BALLS (cantaloupe & honeydew) in syrup, frozen (USDA)	½ cup (4.1 oz.)	10
MENUDO, canned (Hormel)		
Casa Grande	7½-oz. can	1097
MEXICALI DOGS, frozen (Hormel)	5 oz.	952
MEXICAN DINNER, frozen:		
(Banquet) dinner:		
Regular	12-oz. dinner	1995
Combination	12-oz. dinner	1978
Extra Helping	21¼-oz. dinner	4778
(Morton)	11-oz. dinner	1242
(Swanson):		
Regular	16-oz. dinner	1780
Hungry Man	22-oz. dinner	2430
(Van de Kamp's)	11½-oz. dinner	1040
MILK BREAK BARS (Pillsbury):		
Chocolate or natural	1 bar	75
Chocolate mint	1 bar	80
Peanut butter	1 bar	115
MILK, CONDENSED (Carnation) sweetened, canned	1 cup (10.8 oz.)	392
MILK, DRY:		
Whole (USDA) packed cup	1 cup (5.1 oz.)	587
*Nonfat, instant:		
(Alba):		
Regular	8 fl. oz.	120
Chocolate flavor	8 fl. oz.	114
(Carnation)	8 fl. oz.	125
Sanalac (Sanna)	1 cup	<1
MILK, EVAPORATED, canned:		
Regular:		
(USDA) unsweetened	1 cup (8.9 oz.)	297
(Carnation)	1 fl. oz.	33
(Pet)	1 fl. oz.	35

Food and Description	Measure or Quantity	Sodium (milligrams)
Buttermilk (Borden) *Golden Churn Brand*	1 fl. oz.	31
Low fat (Carnation)	1 fl. oz.	34
Skimmed (Carnation)	1 fl. oz.	35
MILK, FRESH:		
Buttermilk, cultured, fresh (Friendship) no salt added	8 fl. oz.	125
Chocolate milk drink, fresh:		
(USDA)	1 cup (8.8 fl. oz.)	118
(Borden) *Dutch Brand*	8 fl. oz.	180
(Hershey's)	1 cup	130
(Johanna):		
Regular	1 cup	200
Low fat	1 cup	210
Lowfat:		
(Borden):		
1% milkfat	8 fl. oz.	130
2% milkfat, *Hi-Protein Brand*	8 fl. oz.	150
(Johanna):		
Regular:		
1% milkfat	1 cup	125
2% milkfat:		
Regular	1 cup	125
Mighty Milk	1 cup	150
Buttermilk	1 cup	250
Skim:		
(USDA)	1 cup (8.6 oz.)	127
(Borden):		
Regular	8 fl. oz.	130
Skim-Line	8 fl. oz.	150
(Dean)	1 cup (8.2 oz.)	130
Whole:		
(USDA)	1 cup (8.6 oz.)	122
(Borden) regular or hi-calcium	8 fl. oz.	130
(Dean)	1 cup (8.6 oz.)	112
MILK, GOAT (USDA)	1 cup (8.6 oz.)	83
MILK, HUMAN (USDA)	1 oz. (by wt.)	5
***MILK MAKERS** (Swiss Miss):		
Chocolate	8 fl. oz.	230
Malted	8 fl. oz.	220

Food and Description	Measure or Quantity	Sodium (milligrams)
Strawberry	8 fl. oz.	170
MILNOT, dairy vegetable blend	1 fl. oz.	35
MINCEMEAT (See PIE FILLING)		
MINERAL WATER (Schweppes)	6 fl. oz.	3
MINESTRONE SOUP (See SOUP, Minestrone)		
MINI-WHEATS, cereal (Kellogg's) brown-sugar cinnamon or sugar frosted	1 biscuit (.25 oz.)	<10
MINT LEAVES (HEW/FAO):		
Raw, untrimmed	1 lb. (weighed with tough stems & branches)	1
Raw, trimmed	½ oz.	Tr.
MOLASSES:		
(USDA):		
Blackstrap	1 T. (.7 oz.)	18
Light	1 T. (.7 oz.)	3
Dark	1 T. (.7 oz.)	7
Medium	1 T. (.7 oz.)	8
(Grandma's) unsulphured	1 T.	8
MOST, cereal (Kellogg's)	½ cup (1 oz.)	30
MOSTACCIOLI, frozen (Banquet) *Buffet Supper*, & sauce	2-lb. pkg.	5681
MUFFIN (See also MUFFIN MIX):		
Blueberry:		
Home recipe (USDA)	3″ muffin (1.4 oz.)	253
(Hostess)	1¾-oz. muffin	149
(Pepperidge Farm)	1.9-oz. muffin	250
Frozen (Morton):		
Regular	1.6-oz. muffin	130
Rounds	1.6-oz. muffin	180
Bran:		
(USDA) home recipe	3″ muffin (1.4 oz.)	179
(Arnold) *Bran'nola*	2.3-oz. muffin	260
(Pepperidge Farm) with raisins	2.1-oz. muffin	295

Food and Description	Measure or Quantity	Sodium (milligrams)
Corn:		
Home recipe (USDA) prepared with whole-ground cornmeal	1.4-oz. muffin	198
(Pepperidge Farm)	1.9-oz. muffin	260
Frozen (Morton)	1.7-oz. muffin	280
English:		
(Pepperidge Farm):		
Regular	1 muffin	180
Cinnamon raisin	1 muffin	180
(Thomas') regular	2-oz. muffin	207
(Wonder)	2-oz. muffin	284
Plain, home recipe (USDA)	1.4-oz. muffin (3″ dia.)	176
Raisin:		
(Arnold)	2½-oz. muffin	350
(Wonder)	2-oz. muffin	227
Sourdough (Wonder)	2-oz. muffin	128
MUFFIN MIX:		
*Apple (Betty Crocker) spiced	¹⁄₁₂ pkg.	135
*Blueberry (Betty Crocker) wild	1 muffin	150
Bran (Duncan Hines)	¹⁄₁₂ pkg.	161
Corn:		
*Home recipe (USDA) prepared with egg & milk	1.4-oz. muffin	136
*Home recipe (USDA) prepared with egg and water	1.4-oz. muffin	138
*(Betty Crocker)	1 muffin	315
*(Flako)	1 muffin	370
MULLET, raw (USDA):		
Whole	1 lb. (weighed whole)	195
Meat only	4 oz.	92
MUNG BEAN SPROUT (See **BEAN SPROUT**)		
MUSCATEL WINE (Gold Seal)		
19% alcohol	3 fl. oz.	3

Food and Description	Measure or Quantity	Sodium (milligrams)
MUSHROOM:		
Raw (USDA):		
Whole	½ lb. (weighed untrimmed)	33
Trimmed, slices	½ cup (1.2 oz.)	5
Canned, solids & liq.:		
(USDA)	½ cup (4.3 oz.)	488
(Green Giant)	2-oz. serving	260
(Shady Oak)	4-oz. can	452
Frozen:		
(Green Giant) in butter sauce	½ cup	240
(Larsen)	3.5 oz.	15
MUSHROOM, CHINESE		
(HEW/FAO):		
Dried	1 oz.	11
Dried, soaked, drained	1 oz.	Tr.
MUSKMELON (See CANTA-LOUPE, CASABA or HONEYDEW)		
MUSSEL (USDA) Atlantic & Pacific, raw, Meat only	4 oz.	328
MUSTARD POWDER		
(French's)	1 tsp.	Tr.
MUSTARD, PREPARED:		
Brown:		
(USDA)	1 tsp.	118
(French's) *'N Spicy*	1 tsp.	50
Chinese (La Choy) hot	1 tsp. (2. oz.)	130
Grey Poupon	1 tsp.	149
Horseradish (French's)	1 tsp.	93
Hot, *Mr. Mustard*	1 tsp.	90
Medford (French's)	1 tsp.	83
Onion (French's)	1 tsp.	67
Unsalted (Featherweight)	1 tsp.	1
Yellow (French's)	1 tsp.	60
MUSTARD GREENS:		
Raw (USDA) whole	1 lb. (weighed untrimmed)	102
Boiled (USDA) drained	1 cup (7.8 oz.)	40

Food and Description	Measure or Quantity	Sodium (milligrams)
Canned (Sunshine) chopped, solids & liq.	½ cup (4.1 oz.)	371
Frozen:		
(USDA) boiled, drained	½ cup (3.8 oz.)	11
(Birds Eye) chopped	⅓ of 10-oz. pkg.	27
(McKenzie) chopped	3.3 oz.	37
(Southland) chopped	⅕ of 16-oz. pkg.	20

N

NATHAN'S:

French fries	1 regular order	151
Hamburger	4½-oz. sandwich	203
Hot dog	1 order	675

NATURAL CEREAL:

Familia:

Regular	½ cup	8
Bran	½ cup	90
Granola	½ cup	67
No added sugar	½ cup	2
Heartland (Pet)	¼ cup	80

(Quaker):

100% natural:

Regular	¼ cup (1-oz.)	11
With apples & cinnamon	¼ cup (1 oz.)	15
With raisins & dates	¼ cup (1 oz.)	11
Whole wheat, hot	⅓ cup (1 oz.)	1

NATURE SNACKS (Sun-Maid):

Carob crunch	1-oz. serving	13
Carob peanut	1¼-oz. serving	16
Carob raisin	1¼-oz. serving	21
Raisin crunch	1-oz. serving	41
Rocky road	1-oz. serving	4

Food and Description	Measure or Quantity	Sodium (milligrams)
Sesame nut crunch	1-oz. serving	159
Tahitian treat	1-oz. serving	7
Yogurt crunch	1-oz. serving	28
Yogurt peanut	1¼-oz. serving	25
Yogurt raisin	1¼-oz. serving	20
NECTARINE, fresh (USDA):		
Whole	1 lb. (weighed with pits)	25
Flesh only	4 oz.	7
NEW ZEALAND SPINACH (USDA):		
Raw	1 lb.	721
Boiled, drained	4 oz.	104
NOODLE. Plain noodle products are essentially the same in caloric value and carbohydrate content on the same weight basis. The longer they are cooked, the more water is absorbed and this affects the nutritive values (USDA):		
Dry	1 oz.	1
Dry, 1½" strips	1 cup (2.6 oz.)	4
Cooked	1 oz.	<1
NOODLE & BEEF:		
Canned (Hormel) *Short Orders*	7½-oz. can	974
Frozen (Banquet) *Buffet Supper*	2-lb. pkg.	5581
NOODLE & CHICKEN:		
Canned (Hormel) *Dinty Moore, Short Orders*	7½-oz. can	1144
Frozen (Swanson) 3-compartment	10½-oz. dinner	820
NOODLE, CHOW MEIN, canned (La Choy)	½ cup (1. oz.)	230
NOODLE MIX:		
*(Betty Crocker):		
Fettucini Alfredo	¼ pkg.	490
Parisienne	¼ pkg.	540
Romanoff	¼ pkg.	705
Stroganoff	¼ pkg.	605

Food and Description	Measure or Quantity	Sodium (milligrams)
*(Lipton) & sauce:		
Regular:		
Beef	½ cup	595
Butter	½ cup	565
Butter & herb	½ cup	525
Cheese	½ cup	540
Chicken	½ cup	465
Sour cream & chive	½ cup	455
Deluxe:		
Alfredo	½ cup	560
Chicken Bombay	½ cup	515
Parmesano	½ cup	445
Stroganoff	½ cup	510
(Noodle Roni) parmesano	⅕ pkg.	270
*NOODLE, RAMEN, canned		
(La Choy):		
Beef	½ of 3-oz. pkg.	1040
Chicken	½ of 3-oz. pkg.	1159
Oriental	½ of 3-oz. pkg.	742
NOODLE, RICE, canned (La Choy)	⅓ of 3-oz. can	420
NOODLE ROMANOFF, frozen (Stouffer's)	4 oz.	675
NUT, MIXED (See also individual kinds):		
(Adams) *All America Nut*	1 oz.	85
(Fisher):		
Dry, salted	1 oz.	110
Honey roasted & cashews	1 oz.	90
Oil:		
Salted:		
Regular	1 oz.	85
Cashews & peanuts	1 oz.	80
No peanuts	1 oz.	70
Lightly salted	1 oz.	45
(Guy's) with peanuts	1 oz.	140
(Planters):		
Dry:		
Salted	1 oz.	270
Unsalted	1 oz.	0

Food and Description	Measure or Quantity	Sodium (milligrams)
Oil:		
Regular	1 oz.	130
Deluxe	1 oz.	135
Unsalted	1 oz.	0
NUTMEG (French's)	1 tsp.	Tr.
NUT*Os (General Mills)	1 T.	55
NUTRI-GRAIN, cereal (Kellogg's):		
Barley	⅔ cup (1 oz.)	190
Corn	½ cup (1 oz.)	185
Rye or wheat	⅔ cup (1 oz.)	195

O

OAT FLAKES, cereal (Post)	⅔ cup (1 oz.)	254
OATMEAL:		
Regular, dry:		
(USDA)	1 T.	<1
(Elam's) Scotch style	1 oz.	3
(H-O):		
Old fashioned	1 T. (5 g.)	<1
Old fashioned	1 cup (2.6 oz.)	<1
(Quaker)	⅓ cup (1 oz.)	1
(Ralston Purina)	⅓ cup (1 oz.)	1
*Regular, cooked (USDA)	1 cup (8.5 oz.)	523
Instant, dry:		
(Harvest Brand):		
Regular	1 oz.	230
Apple & cinnamon	1¼ oz.	242
Cinnamon & spice	1⅝ oz.	307
Maple & brown sugar	1½ oz.	295
Peaches & cream	⅓ cup (1¼ oz.)	199
(H-O):		
Regular, box	1 T. (4 g.)	Tr.
Regular	1-oz. packet	230

Food and Description	Measure or Quantity	Sodium (milligrams)
With bean & spice	1½-oz. packet	297
With cinnamon & spice	1.6-oz. packet	306
With country apple & brown sugar	1.1-oz. packet	222
With maple & brown sugar flavor	1½-oz. packet	286
Sweet & mellow	1.4-oz. packet	270
(Quaker):		
Regular	1-oz. packet	281
Apple & cinnamon	1¼-oz. packet	181
Bran & raisins	1½-oz. packet	240
Cinnamon & spice	1⅝-oz. packet	258
Honey & graham	1¼-oz. packet	224
Maple & brown sugar	1½-oz. packet	228
Raisins & spice	1½-oz. packet	217
Quick, dry:		
(Harvest Brand)	⅓ cup (1 oz.)	<5
(H-O)	1 cup (2.5 oz.)	2
(Quaker)	⅓ cup	1
(Ralston Purina)	⅓ cup (1 oz.)	3
(3-Minute Brand)	⅓ cup (1 oz.)	3
OCEAN PERCH, fresh (USDA):		
Atlantic:		
Raw, whole	1 lb. (weighed whole)	111
Fried	4 oz.	174
Pacific:		
Raw, whole	1 lb. (weighed whole)	77
Raw, meat only	4 oz.	71
OIL, SALAD or COOKING	Any quantity	0
OKRA:		
Raw (USDA) whole	1 lb. (weighed untrimmed)	12
Boiled (USDA) drained:		
Whole	½ cup (3.1 oz.)	2
Pods	8 pods, 3″ × ⅝″ (3 oz.)	2
Slices	½ cup (2.8 oz.)	2

Food and Description	Measure or Quantity	Sodium (milligrams)
Frozen:		
(USDA) boiled, drained:		
Cut	½ cup (3.2 oz.)	2
Whole	½ cup (2.4 oz.)	1
(Birds Eye):		
Cut	⅓ of 10-oz. pkg.	3
Whole	⅓ of 10-oz. pkg.	3
(Frosty Acres)	3.3 oz.	0
(Larsen) cut or whole	3.3 oz.	5
(McKenzie)	3.3 oz.	19
(Southland):		
Cut	⅕ of 16-oz. pkg.	0
Whole	⅕ of 16-oz. pkg.	0
OLD FASHIONED COCKTAIL MIX (Holland House) liquid	1 oz.	6
OLEOMARGARINE (See MARGARINE)		
OLIVE:		
Green style (USDA):		
With pits, drained	1 oz.	748
Pitted, drained	1 oz.	932
Green (USDA)	1 oz.	680
Ripe, by variety:		
(USDA):		
Ascalano, any size, pitted & drained	1 oz.	230
Manzanilla, any size	1 oz.	230
Mission, any size	1 oz.	213
Mission	3 small or 2 large	75
Mission, slices	½ cup (2.2 oz.)	465
Sevillano, any size	1 oz.	235
ONION (See also ONION, GREEN and ONION, WELCH):		
Raw (USDA):		
Whole	1 lb. (weighed untrimmed)	41
Whole	3.9-oz. onion (2½" dia.)	10
Chopped	½ cup (3 oz.)	9

Food and Description	Measure or Quantity	Sodium (milligrams)
Chopped	1 T. (.4 oz.)	1
Grated	1 T. (.5 oz.)	1
Slices	½ cup (2 oz.)	6
Boiled, drained (USDA):		
Whole	½ cup (3.7 oz.)	7
Whole, pearl onions	½ cup (3.7 oz.)	6
Halves or pieces	½ cup (3.2 oz.)	6
Canned, *O & C* (Durkee):		
Boiled	1-oz. serving	2
In cream sauce	1-oz. serving	2854
Dehydrated:		
Flakes:		
(USDA)	1 tsp. (1.3 g.)	1
(Gilroy)	1 tsp.	<1
Powder (Gilroy)	1 tsp.	1
Frozen:		
(Birds Eye):		
Chopped	1 oz.	2
Small, whole	⅓ of 12-oz. pkg.	9
Small, with cream sauce	⅓ of 9-oz. pkg.	333
(Frosty Acres) chopped	1 oz.	5
(Green Giant) cheese sauce	½ cup	400
(Larsen):		
Diced	1 oz.	Tr.
Whole	3.3 oz.	10
(McKenzie) chopped	1 oz.	2
(Mrs. Paul's) rings, breaded & fried	½ of 5-oz. pkg.	305
(Southland) chopped	⅕ of 10-oz. pkg.	0
ONION BOUILLON:		
(Herb-Ox):		
Regular	1 cube	560
Instant	1 packet	800
MBT	1 packet	795
(Wyler's) instant	1 tsp.	670
ONION, COCKTAIL (Vlasic) lightly spiced	1 oz.	371
ONION, GREEN, raw (USDA):		
Whole	1 lb. (weighed untrimmed)	22

Food and Description	Measure or Quantity	Sodium (milligrams)
Bulb & entire top	1 oz.	1
Bulb without green top	3 small onions (.9 oz.)	1
Slices, bulb & white portion of top	½ cup (1.8 oz.)	2
Tops only	1 oz.	1
ONION SALAD SEASONING		
(French's) instant	1 T.	2
ONION SOUP (See SOUP, Onion)		
*ON*YOS* (General Mills)	1 T.	45
ORANGE, fresh (USDA):		
California Navel:		
Whole	1 lb. (weighed with rind & seeds)	3
Whole	6.3-oz orange (2⅘″ dia.)	1
Sections	1 cup (8.5 oz.)	2
California Valencia:		
Whole	1 lb. (weighed with rind & seeds)	3
Fruit including peel	6.3-oz. orange (2⅝″ dia.)	4
Sections	1 cup (8.5 oz.)	2
Florida, all varieties:		
Whole	1 lb. (weighed with rind & seeds)	3
Whole	7.4-oz. orange (3″ dia.)	2
Sections	1 cup (8.5 oz.)	2
ORANGE-APRICOT JUICE DRINK, canned (USDA)		
40% fruit juices	1 cup (8.8 oz.)	Tr.
ORANGE DRINK:		
Canned:		
Bama (Borden)	8.45-fl.-oz. container	60
Capri Sun, natural	6¾ fl. oz.	2

Food and Description	Measure or Quantity	Sodium (milligrams)
(Hi-C)	6 fl. oz.	43
Ssips (Johanna Farms)	8.45-fl.-oz. container	<10
Chilled (Sealtest)	6 fl. oz.	Tr.
*Mix:		
Regular (Hi-C)	6 fl. oz.	<1
Dietetic:		
Crystal Light	6 fl. oz.	<1
(Sunkist)	6 fl. oz.	52
ORANGE EXTRACT (Virginia Dare) 79% alcohol	1 tsp.	0
ORANGE-GRAPEFRUIT JUICE:		
Canned, unsweetened:		
(USDA)	1 cup (8.7 oz.)	2
(Borden) *Sippin' Pak*	8.45-fl.-oz. container	25
(Del Monte)	6 fl. oz.	2
(Libby's)	6 fl. oz.	5
Canned, sweetened:		
(USDA)	1 cup (8.9 oz.)	3
(Del Monte)	6 fl. oz. (6.5 oz.)	2
*Frozen:		
(USDA) unsweetened	½ cup (4.4 oz.)	Tr.
(Minute Maid) unsweetened	6 fl. oz.	<1
ORANGE JUICE:		
Fresh (USDA):		
California Navel	½ cup (4.4 oz.)	1
California Valencia	½ cup (4.4 oz.)	1
Florida, early or midseason	½ cup (4.4 oz.)	1
Florida Temple	½ cup (4.4 oz.)	1
Florida Valencia	½ cup (4.4 oz.)	1
Canned, unsweetened:		
(USDA)	½ cup (4.4 oz.)	1
(Del Monte)	6 fl. oz. (6.5 oz.)	<10
(Libby's)	6 fl. oz.	5
(Texsun)	6 fl. oz.	2
Canned, sweetened:		
(USDA)	½ cup (4.4 oz.)	1

Food and Description	Measure or Quantity	Sodium (milligrams)
(Borden) *Sippin' Pak*	8.45-fl.-oz. container	25
(Del Monte)	6 fl. oz.	2
(Libby's)	6 fl. oz.	5
Chilled (Citrus Hill)	6 fl. oz.	10
*Dehydrated crystals (USDA)	½ cup (4.4 oz.)	1
*Frozen:		
(USDA)	½ cup (4.4 oz.)	1
(Citrus Hill)	6 fl. oz.	10
(Minute Maid)	6 fl. oz.	1
(Snow Crop)	6 fl. oz.	1
(Sunkist)	6 fl. oz.	Tr.
ORANGE JUICE BAR, frozen (Sunkist)	3-fl.-oz. bar	5
ORANGE JUICE DRINK, canned (Sunkist)	8.45 fl. oz.	0
ORANGE, MANDARIN (See **TANGERINE**)		
ORANGE-PINEAPPLE JUICE, canned (Texsun) unsweetened	6 fl. oz.	2
ORANGE SPREAD, dietetic (Estee)	1 tsp. (5.7 grams)	<1
OREGANO, dried (French's)	1 tsp.	Tr.
OVALTINE, dry:		
Chocolate flavor	4 heaping tsps. (¾ oz.)	146
Malt flavor	4 heaping tsps. (¾ oz.)	92
OVEN FRY (General Foods):		
Crispy crumb for chicken	4.2-oz. envelope	3308
Crispy crumb for pork	4.2-oz. envelope	2780
Home style flour recipe	3.2-oz. envelope	3955
OYSTER:		
Raw (USDA) meat only:		
Eastern	13–19 med. oysters (1 cup, 8.5 oz.)	175
Eastern	4 oz.	83
Fried (USDA) dipped in egg, milk & breadcrumbs	4 oz.	234
OYSTER CRACKER (See **CRACKER**)		

Food and Description	Measure or Quantity	Sodium (milligrams)
OYSTER STEW (USDA):		
Home recipe:		
1 part oysters to 2 parts milk by volume	1 cup (8.5 oz.)	814
1 part oysters to 3 parts milk by volume	1 cup (8.5 oz.)	487
*Frozen:		
Prepared with equal volume milk	1 cup (8.5 oz.)	878
Prepared with equal volume water	1 cup (8.5 oz.)	816

P

PAC-MAN cereal (General Mills)	1 cup (1 oz.)	195
PANCAKE, home recipe (USDA)	4″ pancake (1 oz.)	115
PANCAKE & WAFFLE		
BATTER, frozen (Aunt Jemima):		
Plain	4″ pancake	286
Blueberry	4″ pancake	233
Buttermilk	4″ pancake	244
PANCAKE DINNER OR		
ENTREE, frozen (Swanson):		
& blueberry sauce	7-oz. meal	800
& sausage	6-oz. meal	940
PANCAKE & WAFFLE MIX:		
Plain:		
(USDA)	1 oz.	406
(USDA)	1 cup (4.8 oz.)	1935
*(USDA) prepared with milk	4″ pancake (1 oz.)	122
*(USDA) prepared with egg & milk	4″ pancake	152
*(Aunt Jemima):		
Complete	4″ pancake	290

Food and Description	Measure or Quantity	Sodium (milligrams)
Original	4″ pancake	183
*(Log Cabin) complete	4″ pancake	203
*(Pillsbury) *Hungry Jack:*		
Complete:		
Bulk	4″ pancake	243
Packets	4″ pancake	225
Extra Lights	4″ pancake	163
Golden Blend:		
Regular	4″ pancake	167
Complete	4″ pancake	305
Panshakes	4″ pancake	293
*Blueberry (Pillsbury) *Hungry Jack*	4″ pancake	273
Buckwheat:		
(USDA)	1 cup (4.8 oz.)	1801
*(USDA) prepared with egg & milk	4″ pancake	125
Buttermilk:		
(USDA)	1 cup (4.8 oz.)	1935
*(USDA) prepared with egg & milk	4″ pancake	152
*(Aunt Jemima):		
Regular	4″ pancake	330
Complete	4″ pancake	290
*(Betty Crocker):		
Regular	4″ pancake	270
Complete	4″ pancake	193
*(Log Cabin)	4″ pancake	242
*(Pillsbury) *Hungry Jack,* regular	4″ pancake	190
*Whole wheat (Aunt Jemima)	4″ pancake	242
*Dietetic:		
(Dia-Mel)	3″ pancake	58
(Featherweight)	4″ pancake	23
PANCAKE & WAFFLE SYRUP (See **SYRUP**)		
PANCREAS, raw (USDA):		
Beef, lean only	4 oz.	76
Hog or hog sweetbread	4 oz.	50

Food and Description	Measure or Quantity	Sodium (milligrams)
PAPAYA, fresh (USDA):		
Whole	1 lb. (weighed with skin & seeds)	9
Cubed	1 cup (6.4 oz.)	5
PAPAYA JUICE, canned (HEW/FAO)	4 oz.	12
PAPRIKA, domestic (French's)	1 tsp.	Tr.
PARSLEY, fresh (USDA):		
Whole	½ lb.	102
Chopped	1 T. (4 g.)	2
PARSLEY FLAKES, dehydrated (French's)	1 tsp. (1.1 g.)	6
PARSNIP (USDA):		
Raw, whole	1 lb. (weighed unprepared)	46
Boiled, drained, cut in pieces	½ cup (3.7 oz.)	8
PASTINA, DRY (USDA) egg	1 oz.	1
PASTRAMI, packaged:		
(Carl Buddig)	1 oz.	320
(Eckrich)	1 oz.	360
PASTRY POCKETS (Pillsbury)	1 piece	550
PASTRY SHEET, PUFF, frozen (Pepperidge Farm)	1 sheet	1160
PASTRY SHELL (See also **PIE CRUST**):		
Home recipe (USDA) baked	1 shell (1.5 oz.)	260
Frozen (Pepperidge Farm)	1 shell	180
PÂTÉ, liver (Sell's)	4.8-oz. can	1142
PEA, green:		
Raw (USDA):		
In pod	1 lb. (weighed in pod)	3
Shelled	1 lb.	9
Shelled	½ cup (2.4 oz.)	1
Boiled (USDA) drained	½ cup (2.9 oz.)	<1
Canned, regular pack:		
(USDA):		
Alaska, early or June:		
Solids & liq.	½ cup (4.4 oz.)	293

Food and Description	Measure or Quantity	Sodium (milligrams)
Solids only	½ cup (3 oz.)	203
Sweet:		
Solids & liq.	½ cup (4.4 oz.)	293
Solids only	½ cup (3 oz.)	203
Drained liquid	4 oz.	268
(Comstock) solids & liq.	½ cup	400
(Del Monte) solids & liq:		
Seasoned	½ cup	355
Sweet	½ cup	355
(Festal):		
Early garden, solids & liq.	½ cup	333
Seasoned, solids only	½ cup	226
Sweet, tiny size, solids only	½ cup	313
(Green Giant) solids & liq.:		
Early, with onion	¼ of 17-oz. can	535
Sweet:		
Regular	½ of 8½-oz. can	375
Small,	¼ of 17-oz. can	349
With onion	¼ of 17-oz. can	665
(Kounty Kist): solids & liq.:		
Early	½ of 8½-oz. can	453
Sweet	½ of 8½-oz. can	333
(Larsen) *Freshlike*	½ cup	370
(Le Sueur) sweet, mini, solids & liq.	¼ of 17-oz. can	425
(Libby's) sweet, solids & liq.	½ cup (4.2 oz.)	337
(Stokely-Van Camp) solids & liq.:		
Early	½ cup (4.4 oz.)	375
Sweet	½ cup (4.4 oz.)	375
Canned, dietetic or low calorie:		
(USDA):		
Alaska, early or June:		
Solids & liq.	4 oz.	3
Solids only	4 oz.	3

Food and Description	Measure or Quantity	Sodium (milligrams)
Sweet:		
Solids & liq.	4 oz.	3
Solids only	4 oz.	3
(Blue Boy) sweet, solids & liq.	½ cup	8
(Del Monte) no salt added, solids & liq.	½ cup	<10
(Diet Delight) solids & liq.	½ cup (4.3 oz.)	5
(Featherweight) sweet, solids & liq.	½ cup	<10
(Larsen) *Fresh-Lite*, sweet, solids & liq.	½ cup	10
(S&W) *Nutradiet*, sweet, solids & liq.	½ cup	<10
Frozen:		
(USDA) boiled, drained	½ cup (3 oz.)	97
(Birds Eye):		
With butter sauce	⅓ of 10-oz. pkg.	641
With cream sauce	⅓ of 8-oz. pkg.	446
Sweet, 5-minute style	⅓ of 10-oz. pkg.	131
Tender tiny, deluxe	⅓ of 10-oz. pkg.	121
(Frosty Acres):		
Regular	3.3 oz.	90
Tiny	3.3 oz.	130
(Green Giant):		
In cream sauce	½ cup	320
Early June or sweet, polybag	½ cup	25
Early & sweet in butter sauce	½ cup	490
Sweet, *Harvest Fresh*	½ cup	280
(Larsen)	3.3 oz.	75
(Le Sueur) early, in butter sauce	⅓ of 10-oz. pkg.	411
(McKenzie):		
Regular	3.3 oz.	122
Tiny	3.3 oz.	47
PEA & CARROT:		
Canned, regular pack, solids & liq.:		
(Comstock)	½ cup	430

Food and Description	Measure or Quantity	Sodium (milligrams)
(Del Monte)	½ cup (4 oz.)	355
(Larsen) *Freshlike*	½ cup	340
(Libby's) solids & liq.	½ cup (4.2 oz.)	315
(Veg-All)	½ cup	340
Canned, dietetic or low calorie, solids & liq.:		
(Blue Boy)	½ cup	4
(Diet Delight)	½ cup (4.3 oz.)	5
(Larsen) *Fresh-Lite*	½ cup	30
(S&W) *Nutradiet*	½ cup	<10
Frozen:		
(USDA) boiled, without salt, drained	½ cup (3.1 oz.)	73
(Birds Eye)	⅓ pkg.	92
(Frosty Acres)	3.3 oz.	75
(McKenzie)	3.3 oz.	75
PEA, CROWDER, frozen (Birds Eye)	⅕ of 16-oz. pkg.	6
PEA, MATURE SEED, dry (USDA):		
Whole	1 lb.	159
Whole	1 cup	70
Split	1 lb.	181
Split	1 cup (7.2 oz.)	81
Cooked, split, drained solids	½ cup (3.4 oz.)	13
PEA & ONION:		
Canned (Larsen) *Freshlike*	½ cup	440
Frozen:		
(Frosty Acres)	3.3 oz.	80
(Larsen)	3.3 oz.	100
PEA POD, frozen (La Choy)	6 oz.	<20
PEA PUREE, canned (Larsen) low sodium	½ cup	7
PEACH:		
Fresh (USDA):		
Whole, without skin	1 lb. (weighed unpeeled)	4
Whole	4-oz. peach (2″ dia.)	1
Diced	½ cup (4.7 oz.)	1

Food and Description	Measure or Quantity	Sodium (milligrams)
Sliced	½ cup (3 oz.)	1
Canned, regular pack, solids & liq.:		
(USDA):		
Extra heavy syrup	4 oz.	2
Heavy syrup	2 med. halves & 2 T. syrup (4.1 oz.)	2
Juice pack	4 oz.	2
Light syrup	4 oz.	2
(Del Monte):		
Cling halves or slices	½ cup	<10
Freestone, halves or slices	½ cup	<10
Spiced	½ of 7¼-oz. can	<10
(Hunt's) *Snack Pack*	5-oz. container	5
(Libby's) heavy syrup:		
Halves	½ cup (4.5 oz.)	9
Slices	½ cup (4.5 oz.)	10
(Stokely-Van Camp):		
Halves	½ cup (4.4 oz.)	23
Slices	½ cup (4.5 oz.)	23
Canned, dietetic or low calorie, solids & liq.:		
(USDA) water pack	½ cup (4.3 oz.)	2
(Del Monte) *Lite*	½ cup	<10
(Diet Delight) Cling or Freestone, juice pack	½ cup (4.4 oz.)	7
(Featherweight):		
Cling or Freestone, halves or slices, juice pack	½ cup	<10
Cling, halves or slices, water pack	½ cup	<10
(Libby's water pack, sliced	½ cup (4.3 oz.)	3
Dehydrated (USDA):		
Uncooked	1 oz.	6
Cooked, with added sugar, solids & liq.	½ cup (5.4 oz.)	8
Dried (USDA):		
Uncooked	½ cup	14

Food and Description	Measure or Quantity	Sodium (milligrams)
Cooked:		
Unsweetened	½ cup	7
Sweetened	½ cup (5.4 oz.)	6
Frozen:		
(USDA) unthawed, slices, sweetened	½ cup	2
(Birds Eye) quick thaw	½ of 10-oz. pkg.	9
Canned	6 fl. oz.	<1
*Mix	6 fl. oz.	17
PEACH NECTAR, canned		
(Libby's)	6 fl. oz.	5
PEACH PRESERVE or JAM:		
Sweetened (Smucker's)	1 T. (.7 oz.)	4
Dietetic, (Tillie Lewis) *Tasti Diet*	1 T.	<1
PEACH, STRAINED, canned		
(Larsen) low sodium	½ cup	6
PEANUT:		
Raw (USDA):		
In shell	1 lb. (weighed in shell)	17
With skins	1 oz.	1
Without skins	1 oz.	1
Roasted:		
(USDA):		
Whole	1 lb. (weighed in shell)	25
Chopped	½ cup	288
Halves	½ cup	301
(Adams) *All American Nut*	1 oz.	85
(Eagle) *Honey Roast*	1 oz.	170
(Fisher):		
Dry:		
Lightly salted	1 oz.	85
Salted	1 oz.	220
Unsalted	1 oz.	0
Honey roasted:		
Regular	1 oz.	100
Dry	1 oz.	90

Food and Description	Measure or Quantity	Sodium (milligrams)
Oil:		
Salted:		
Blanched	1 oz.	125
Party	1 oz.	140
Lightly salted, blanched	1 oz.	35
(Frito-Lay's):		
In shell, salted	1 oz. shelled	267
Shelled	1 oz.	169
(Guy's) dry roasted	1 oz.	310
(Planter's):		
In shell, roasted:		
Salted	1 oz.	160
Unsalted	1 oz.	0
Shelled:		
Dry:		
Salted	1 oz.	250
Unsalted	1 oz.	0
Lite	1 oz.	180
Honey	1 oz.	180
Oil:		
Regular or cocktail:		
Salted	1 oz.	160
Unsalted	1 oz.	0
Sweet 'N Crunchy	1 oz.	20
Tavern nuts	1 oz.	65
(Tom's):		
In shell	1 oz.	3
Shelled:		
Dry roasted	1 oz.	170
Hot flavored	1 oz.	230
Redskin	1 oz.	130
Toasted	1 oz.	110
Spanish, roasted:		
(Adams) *All American Nut*	1 oz.	85
(Fisher):		
Raw	1 oz.	0
Oil roasted:		
Salted	1 oz.	115
Lightly salted	1 oz.	50

Food and Description	Measure or Quantity	Sodium (milligrams)
(Frito-Lay's)	1 oz.	161
(Planter's):		
Raw, unsalted	1 oz.	0
Roasted:		
Dry	1 oz.	200
Oil	1 oz.	150
PEANUT BUTTER:		
(Adams)	1 T.	65
(Bama):		
Creamy	1 T.	70
Crunchy	1 T.	57
(Elam's) natural, with defatted wheat germ	1 T. (.6 oz.)	4
(Holsum)	1 T. (.6 oz.)	82
(Home Brands) real	1 T.	56
(Jif) creamy	1 T.	89
(Laura Scudder's)	1 T.	62
(Peter Pan):		
Crunchy	1 T.	60
Smooth	1 T. (.6 oz.)	75
(Planter's) creamy or crunchy	1 T. (.6 oz.)	94
(Skippy):		
Creamy	1 T. (.6 oz.)	80
Old fashioned, creamy or super chunk	1 T.	75
Low sodium:		
(Adams)	1 T.	<3
(Featherweight)	1 T.	<5
(Home Brands):		
Lightly salted or no added sugar	1 T.	62
Unsalted	1 T.	<4
(Peter Pan)	1 T.	0
(Smucker's)	1 T.	0
(S&W) *Nutradiet*	1 T.	<10
PEANUT BUTTER BAKING CHIPS (Nestlé)	3 T. (1 oz.)	60
PEANUT BUTTER AND JELLY (Bama)	1 T.	37

Food and Description	Measure or Quantity	Sodium (milligrams)
PEAR:		
Fresh (USDA):		
Whole	1 lb. (weighed with stems & core)	8
Whole	6.4-oz. pear (3″ × 2½″ × 2½″dia.)	3
Quartered	1 cup (6.8 oz.)	4
Slices	½ cup (6.8 oz.)	2
Canned, regular pack, solids & liq.:		
(USDA):		
Extra heavy syrup	4 oz.	1
Heavy syrup	½ cup	1
Juice pack	4 oz.	1
Light syrup	4 oz.	<1
(Del Monte) Bartlett halves or slices, regular or chunky	½ cup (4 oz.)	<10
(Libby's) halves, heavy syrup	½ cup (4.5 oz.)	6
(Stokely-Van Camp):		
Halves	½ cup (4.5 oz.)	15
Slices	½ cup (4.5 oz.)	10
Canned, unsweetened or dietetic, solids & liq.:		
(USDA) water pack	½ cup (4.3 oz.)	1
(Del Monte) *Lite*, Bartlett halves	½ cup	<10
(Diet Delight)	½ cup (4.4 oz.)	5
(Featherweight) Bartlett halves:		
Juice pack	½ cup	<10
Water pack	½ cup	<10
(Libby's)	½ cup (4.3 oz.)	10
Dried (USDA):		
Uncooked	1 lb.	32
Cooked:		
Without added sugar	4 oz.	3
With added sugar, solids & liq.	4 oz.	3

Food and Description	Measure or Quantity	Sodium (milligrams)
PEAR NECTAR, canned:		
(Del Monte)	6 fl. oz.	6
(Libby's)	6 fl. oz.	5
PEBBLES, cereal (POST):		
Cocoa	⅞ cup (1 oz.)	136
Fruity	⅞ cup (1 oz.)	158
PECAN:		
In shell (USDA)	1 lb. (weighed in shell)	Tr.
Shelled (USDA):		
Whole	1 lb.	Tr.
Chopped	½ cup (1.8 oz.)	Tr.
Chopped	1 T. (7 g.)	Tr.
Halves	12–14 halves (.5 oz.)	Tr.
Halves	½ cup (1.9 oz.)	Tr.
Oil dipped (Fisher) salted	¼ cup	126
Roasted, dry:		
(Fisher) salted	¼ cup (1.1 oz.)	110
(Flavor House)	1 oz.	32
(Planters) salted	1 oz.	222
PECTIN, FRUIT:		
Certo	1 T.	<1
Certo	6-oz. pkg.	5
Sure-Jell:		
Regular	1¾-oz. pkg.	12
Light	1¾-oz. pkg.	5
PEP, cereal (Kellogg's)	¾ cup (1 oz.)	200
PEPPER, BLACK (French's):		
Regular	1 tsp. (2.3 g.)	Tr.
Seasoned	1 tsp. (2.9 g.)	5
PEPPER, BANANA (Vlasic)	1 oz.	465
PEPPER, CHERRY (Vlasic)	1 oz.	410
PEPPER, HOT CHILI:		
Green:		
Canned:		
(Del Monte) whole or diced	1 oz.	172
(Old El Paso):		
Chopped	1 T.	35

Food and Description	Measure or Quantity	Sodium (milligrams)
Whole	1 pepper	105
(Ortega) diced, strips or whole	1 oz.	22
Jalapeno, canned:		
(Del Monte) whole or sliced	1 oz.	422
(Old El Paso)	1 pepper	239
(Ortega) diced or whole	1 oz.	6
(Vlasic)	1 oz.	380
PEPPERONCINI (Vlasic)		
Greek, mild	1 oz.	450
PEPPERONI (Hormel):		
Regular	1 oz.	462
Chub, Chunk	1 oz.	423
Leoni Brand	1 oz.	508
Packaged, sliced	1 slice	140
Rosa	1 oz.	626
Rosa Grande	1 oz.	512
PEPPER STEAK DINNER:		
*Canned:		
(Chun King)	6 oz.	1003
(La Choy)	¾ cup	960
Frozen:		
(Armour) *Classic Lites* beef	10-oz. meal	1020
(Blue Star) *Dining Lite*, with rice	9¼-oz. meal	1400
(Le Menu)	11½-oz. meal	1110
(Stouffer's) with rice	10½-oz. meal	1500
PEPPER, STUFFED:		
Home recipe (USDA) with beef & crumbs	2¾″ × 2½″ pepper with 1⅛ cups stuffing (6.5 oz.)	581
Frozen:		
(Armour) *Dinner Classics*	12-oz. meal	1750
(Celentano) red, with beef, in sauce	12½-oz. pkg.	530
(Green Giant) with beef, in creole sauce, green	½ of pkg.	785

Food and Description	Measure or Quantity	Sodium (milligrams)
(Stouffer's)	7¾ oz.)	960
(Weight Watchers) with veal stuffing	11¾-oz. meal	1180
PEPPER, SWEET:		
Green:		
Raw (USDA):		
Whole	1 lb. (weighed untrimmed)	48
Without stems & seeds	1 med. pepper (2.6 oz.)	8
Chopped	½ cup (2.6 oz.)	10
Slices	½ cup (1.4 oz.)	5
Strips	½ cup (1.7 oz.)	6
Boiled (USDA) strips, drained	½ cup (2.4 oz.)	6
Boiled (USDA) whole, drained	1 med. pepper (2.6 oz.)	8
Frozen:		
(Frosty Acres) diced:		
Green	1 oz.	1
Red & green	1 oz.	22
(Larsen) green or red	1 oz.	0
(Southland) dried	2 oz.	0
PERCH, raw (USDA):		
Yellow, whole	1 lb. (weighed whole)	120
Yellow, meat only	4 oz.	77
PERCH DINNER or ENTREE,		
frozen:		
(Banquet) ocean	8¾-oz. dinner	1416
(Mrs. Paul's) fillets, breaded & fried, crispy, crunchy	2-oz. fillet	240
(Van de Kamp's) *Today's Catch*	4 oz.	180
PERSIMMON (USDA):		
Japanese or Kaki, fresh:		
With seeds	1 lb. (weighed with skin, calyx & seeds)	22

Food and Description	Measure or Quantity	Sodium (milligrams)
With seeds	4.4-oz. persimmon	6
Seedless	1 lb. (weighed with skin & calyx)	23
Seedless	4.4-oz. persimmon (2½" dia.)	6
Native, fresh:		
Whole	1 lb. (weighed with seeds & calyx)	4
Flesh only	4 oz.	1
PICKLE:		
Chowchow (See **CHOWCHOW**)		
Cucumber, fresh or bread & butter:		
(USDA)	3 slices (¼" × 1½")	141
(Fanning's)	1 fl. oz.	189
(Featherweight) dietetic, slices	1 oz.	3
(Vlasic):		
Chips, sweet butter	1 oz.	160
Chunks, deli or old fashioned	1 oz.	120
Stix, sweet butter	1 oz.	110
Dill:		
(USDA)	4.8-oz. pickle	1928
(Featherweight) low sodium	1 oz.	<5
(Smucker's):		
Candied stick	4" pickle (.8 oz.)	182
Hamburger	1 slice (.13 oz.)	<141
(Vlasic):		
Original	1 oz.	375
No garlic	1 oz.	210
Hamburger (Vlasic) chips, dill	1 oz.	175
Hot & Spicy (Vlasic) garden mix	1 oz.	380

Food and Description	Measure or Quantity	Sodium (milligrams)
Kosher dill:		
(Claussen):		
Halves	2 oz.	599
Whole	2 oz.	581
(Featherweight) low sodium	1 oz.	<5
(Smucker's) whole	2½"-long pickle	642
(Vlasic):		
Baby, crunchy or gherkins	1 oz.	210
Crunchy, half-the-salt	1 oz.	125
Deli	1 oz.	290
Spear:		
Regular	1 oz.	175
Half-the-Salt	1 oz.	120
Sour:		
(USDA) cucumber	1¾" × 4" (4.8 oz.)	384
(Aunt Jane's)	2-oz. pickle	769
Sweet:		
(Aunt Jane's)	1.5-oz. pickle	420
(Smucker's) whole	2½"-long pickle (.4 oz.)	119
(Vlasic) butter chips, half-the-salt	1 oz.	80
Sweet & Sour (Claussen) slices	1 slice	25
PIE:		
Commercial type, non-frozen:		
Apple:		
Home recipe (USDA) 2-crust	⅙ of 9" pie (5.6 oz.)	476
(Hostess)	4½-oz. pie	563
Banana, home recipe		
(USDA) cream or custard, unenriched or enriched	⅙ of 9" pie (5.4 oz.)	295
Berry (Hostess)	4½-oz. pie	415
Blackberry, home recipe		
(USDA) 2-crust, made with vegetable shortening	⅙ of 9" pie (5.6 oz.)	423
Blueberry:		
Home recipe (USDA) 2-crust, made with lard	⅙ of 9" pie (5.6 oz.)	423

Food and Description	Measure or Quantity	Sodium (milligrams)
(Hostess)	4½-oz. pie	415
Boston cream, home recipe (USDA)	1/12 of 8″ pie (2.4 oz.)	128
Butterscotch, home recipe (USDA)	⅙ of 9″ pie (5.4 oz.)	325
Cherry:		
Home recipe (USDA) 2-crust	⅙ of 9″ pie (5.6 oz.)	480
(Hostess)	4½-oz. pie	537
Chocolate chiffon, home recipe (USDA) made with lard	⅙ of 9″ pie (3.8 oz.)	353
Chocolate meringue, home recipe (USDA) made with vegetable shortening	⅙ of 9″ pie (4.9 oz.)	358
Coconut custard, home recipe (USDA)	⅙ of 9″ pie (5.4 oz.)	375
Custard, home recipe (USDA) enriched or unenriched	⅙ of 9″ pie (5.4 oz.)	436
Lemon:		
Chiffon, home recipe (USDA) made with lard or vegetable shortening	⅙ of 9″ pie	282
Meringue, home recipe, (USDA) 1-crust	⅙ of 9″ pie (4.9 oz.)	395
(Hostess)	4½-oz. pie	422
Mince, home recipe (USDA) 2-crust, enriched or unenriched	⅙ of 9″ pie (5.6 oz.)	708

Food and Description	Measure or Quantity	Sodium (milligrams)
Peach:		
Home recipe (USDA)		
2-crust	⅙ of 9″ pie	
	(5.6 oz.)	423
(Hostess)	4½-oz. pie	447
Pecan:		
Home recipe (USDA)		
1-crust, made with lard		
or vegetable shortening	⅙ of 9″ pie	305
(Frito-Lay's)	3-oz. serving	453
Pineapple, home recipe		
(USDA) 2-crust, made with		
lard or vegetable shortening	⅙ of 9″ pie	
	(5.6 oz.)	428
Pineapple custard, home		
recipe (USDA) made with		
lard or vegetable shortening	⅙ of 9″ pie	
	(5.4 oz.)	283
Pumpkin, home recipe		
(USDA) 1 crust, made with		
lard or vegetable shortening	⅙ of 9″ pie	
	(5.4 oz.)	325
Raisin, home recipe (USDA)		
2-crust, made with lard or		
vegetable shortening	⅙ of 9″ pie	
	(5.6 oz.)	450
Rhubarb, home recipe		
(USDA) 2-crust, made with		
lard or vegetable shortening	⅙ of 9″ pie	
	(5.6 oz.)	427
Strawberry, home recipe		
(USDA) made with lard or		
vegetable shortening	⅙ of 9″ pie	
	(5.6 oz.)	307
Frozen:		
Apple:		
(USDA) baked	5-oz. serving	302
(Banquet):		
Regular	8-oz. pie	598
Family Size	⅙ of 20-oz. pie	282

Food and Description	Measure or Quantity	Sodium (milligrams)
(Morton):		
Regular	⅙ of 24-oz. pie	240
Great Little desserts:		
Plain	8-oz. pie	510
Dutch	7¾-oz. pie	470
(Sara Lee):		
Regular	⅙ of 31-oz. pie	280
Dutch apple	⅙ of 31-oz. pie	282
(Weight Watchers)	3 oz.	290
Banana:		
(Banquet) cream	⅙ of 14-oz. pie	146
(Morton):		
Regular	⅙ of 14-oz. pie	130
Great Little Desserts,		
cream	3½-oz. pie	200
Blackberry (Banquet)	⅙ of 20-oz. pie	342
Blueberry:		
(Banquet)	⅙ of 20-oz. pie	342
(Morton):		
Regular	⅙ of 24-oz. pie	250
Great Little Desserts	8-oz. pie	525
(Sara Lee)	⅙ of 31-oz. pie	220
Cherry:		
(Banquet) Family Size	⅙ of 20-oz. pie	258
(Morton);		
Regular	⅙ of 24-oz. pie	240
Great Little Desserts	8-oz. pie	520
(Sara Lee)	⅙ of 31-oz. pie	233
(Weight Watchers)	3 oz.	190
Chocolate (Morton)	⅙ of 14-oz. pie	140
Chocolate cream:		
(Banquet)	⅙ of 14-oz. pie	106
(Morton) *Great Little*		
Desserts	3½-oz. pie	200
Coconut:		
Plain (Morton)	⅙ of 14-oz. pie	130
Cream:		
(Banquet)	⅙ of 14-oz. pie	113
(Morton) *Great Little*		
Desserts	3½ oz. pie	190

Food and Description	Measure or Quantity	Sodium (milligrams)
Custard (Morton) *Great Little Desserts*)	6½-oz. pie	495
Lemon (Morton)	⅙ of 14-oz. pie	130
Lemon, cream:		
(Banquet)	⅙ of 14-oz. pie	111
(Morton) *Great Little Desserts*	3½-oz. pie	200
Mince:		
(Banquet)	⅙ of 20-oz. pie	364
(Morton)	⅙ of 24-oz. pie	355
Peach:		
(Banquet) Family Size	⅙ of 20-oz. pie	275
(Morton):		
Regular	⅙ of 24-oz. pie	260
Great Little Desserts	8-oz. pie	520
(Sara Lee)	⅙ of 31-oz. pie	253
Pumpkin:		
(Banquet)	⅙ of 20-oz. pie	341
(Morton)	⅙ of 24-oz. pie	310
(Sara Lee)	⅛ of 45-oz. pie	403
Strawberry cream, (Banquet)	⅙ of 14-oz. pie	112
PIE CRUST (See also **PASTRY SHELL**):		
Home recipe (USDA) baked	9″ pie crust (6.3 oz.)	1100
Mix:		
(USDA) dry	10-oz. pkg.	1968
(USDA) prepared with water, baked	4 oz.	922
(Betty Crocker):		
Regular	⅟₁₆ of pkg.	140
Stick	⅛ of stick	140
*(Flako)	⅙ of 9″ pie shell	314
*(Pillsbury) mix or stick	⅙ of 2-crust pie	420
Refrigerated (Pillsbury) 2-crust shell	2 shells	2220
PIE FILLING (See also **PUDDING or PIE FILLING**)		
Apple:		
(Comstock)	21-oz. can	900

Food and Description	Measure or Quantity	Sodium (milligrams)
(Thank You Brand)	3½-oz.	94
Apricot (Comstock)	21-oz. can	1500
Banana cream (Comstock)	21-oz. can	3600
Blueberry (Comstock)	21-oz. can	2100
Cherry:		
(Comstock)	21-oz. can	2400
(Thank You Brand):		
Regular	3½ oz.	15
Sweet	3½ oz.	20
Chocolate cream (Comstock)	21-oz. can	3600
Coconut cream (Comstock)	21-oz. can	3900
Lemon (Comstock)	21-oz. can	1800
Peach (Comstock)	21-oz. can	1500
Pineapple (Comstock)	21-oz. can	900
Pumpkin (See also **PUMPKIN**, canned) (Comstock)	4½-oz. serving	3600
Raisin (Comstock)	21-oz. can	1200
Strawberry (Comstock)	21-oz. can	1200
Dietetic (Thank You Brand):		
Apple	3½ oz.	42
Cherry	3⅓ oz.	9
*PIE MIX:		
(Betty Crocker) Boston cream	⅛ of pie	405
(Royal) *No Bake*, chocolate mint	⅛ of pie	280
PIEROGIES, frozen:		
(Empire Kosher):		
Cheese	1½ oz.	120
Onion	1½ oz.	158
(Mrs. Paul's) potato & cheese	1.7-oz. piece	260
PIGEONPEA (USDA):		
Raw, immature seeds in pods	1 lb.	9
Dry seeds	1 lb.	118
PIGNOLIA (See **PINE NUT**)		
PIKE, raw (USDA) Walleye:		
Whole	1 lb. (weighed whole)	132
Meat only	4 oz.	58
PILI NUT (USDA):		
In shell	1 lb. (weighed in shell)	2

Food and Description	Measure or Quantity	Sodium (milligrams)
Shelled	4 oz.	3
PIMIENTO, canned (Sunshine) diced or sliced, drained	1 T. (.6 oz.)	3
PINA COLADA COCKTAIL		
Canned (Mr. Boston)	3 fl. oz.	29
Mix:		
*(Bar-Tender's)	5 fl. oz.	45
(Holland House):		
Instant	.56-oz. packet	<1
Liquid	1 oz.	4
PINEAPPLE:		
Fresh (USDA):		
Whole	1 lb. (weighed untrimmed)	2
Diced	½ cup (2.8 oz.)	<1
Sliced	¾" × 3½" slice (3 oz.)	<1
Canned, regular pack, solids & liq.:		
(USDA):		
Heavy syrup:		
Crushed	½ cup (5.6 oz.)	1
Slices	1 large slice & 2 T. syrup (4.3 oz.)	1
Tidbits	½ cup (4.6 oz.)	1
Juice pack	4 oz.	1
Light syrup	5 oz.	1
(Del Monte):		
Chunks	½ cup	<10
Crushed	½ cup (4 oz.)	<10
Slices:		
Medium	½ cup	2
Large	½ cup	3
Tidbits	½ cup	2
(Dole) heavy syrup, chunks, crushed, slices or tidbits	½ cup	1
Canned, dietetic or low calorie, solids & liq.:		
(USDA)	4 oz.	1

Food and Description	Measure or Quantity	Sodium (milligrams)
(Diet Delight) juice pack	½ cup (4.4 oz.)	5
(Featherweight) chunks or slices:		
Juice pack	½ cup	<10
Water pack	½ cup	<10
(Libby's) *Lite*	½ cup	10
PINEAPPLE-GRAPEFRUIT JUICE, canned (Texsun)	6 fl. oz.	2
PINEAPPLE & GRAPEFRUIT JUICE DRINK, canned:		
(USDA) 40% fruit juices	½ cup (4.4 oz.)	Tr.
(Del Monte):		
Regular	6 fl. oz.	50
Pink	6 fl. oz.	50
(Dole) pink	6 fl. oz.	Tr.
PINEAPPLE JUICE:		
Canned, unsweetened:		
(Del Monte)	6 fl. oz.	<10
(Dole)	6 fl. oz.	2
(Texsun)	6 fl. oz.	2
*Frozen, unsweetened:		
(USDA)	½ cup (4.4 oz.)	1
(Minute Maid)	6 fl. oz.	2
PINEAPPLE & ORANGE JUICE DRINK:		
Canned:		
(USDA) 40% fruit juices	½ cup (4.4 oz.)	Tr.
(Del Monte)	6 fl. oz.	6
(Hi-C)	6 fl. oz.	<1
Tree Ripe (Johanna Farms)	8.45-fl.-oz. container	3
*Frozen (Minute Maid)	6 fl. oz.	2
PINEAPPLE PRESERVE, unsweetened (Smucker's)	1 T.	2
PISTACHIO NUT, roasted:		
(Fisher) salted:		
In shell	1 oz.	50
Shelled	1 oz.	100
(Flavor House) dry roasted	1 oz.	32
(Frito-Lay's)	1 oz.	213

Food and Description	Measure or Quantity	Sodium (milligrams)
(Planters)	1 oz.	250
PIZZA PIE (See also **PIZZA PIE MIX** and *SHAKEY'S*):		
Regular:		
Domino's:		
Beef, ground:		
Plain:		
Small	⅛ of 12″ pizza	390
Large	1/12 of 16″ pizza	399
Pepperoni:		
Small	⅛ of 12″ pizza	410
Large	1/12 of 16″ pizza	979
Cheese:		
Plain:		
Small	⅛ of 12″ pizza	255
Large	1/12 of 16″ pizza	335
Double:		
Small	⅛ of 12″ pizza	318
Large	1/12 of 16″ pizza	421
Double with pepperoni:		
Small	⅛ of 12″ pizza	429
Large	1/12 of 16″ pizza	561
Mushroom & sausage:		
Small	⅛ of 12″ pizza	301
Large	1/12 of 16″ pizza	396
Pepperoni:		
Plain:		
Small	⅛ of 12″ pizza	365
Large	1/12 of 16″ pizza	474
With mushroom:		
Small	⅛ of 12″ pizza	366
Large	1/12 of 16″ pizza	475
With sausage:		
Small	⅛ of 12″ pizza	411
Large	1/12 of 16″ pizza	534
Sausage:		
Small	⅛ of 12″ pizza	300
Large	1/12 of 16″ pizza	395

Food and Description	Measure or Quantity	Sodium (milligrams)
Godfather's:		
Cheese:		
Original:		
Mini	¼ of pizza	260
Small	⅙ of pizza	400
Medium		
Stuffed:		
Small	⅙ of pizza	560
Medium	⅛ of pizza	610
Large	⅒ of pizza	677
Thin crust:		
Small	⅙ of pizza	370
Medium	⅛ of pizza	410
Large	⅒ of pizza	464
Combo:		
Original:		
Mini	¼ of pizza	450
Small	⅙ of pizza	830
Medium	⅛ of pizza	930
Large:		
Regular	⅒ of pizza	1019
Hot Slice	⅛ of pizza	1270
Stuffed:		
Small	⅙ of pizza	1000
Medium	⅛ of pizza	1105
Large	⅒ of pizza	1205
Thin crust:		
Small	⅙ of pizza	710
Medium	⅛ of pizza	790
Large	⅒ of pizza	870
Frozen:		
Cheese:		
(Celentano):		
Mini slice	2.7-oz. slice	166
Thick crust	⅓ of 13-oz. pizza	252
(Celeste):		
Small	7-oz. pie	1310
Large	¼ of 19-oz. pie	803
(Stouffer's) French Bread Pizza	½ of 10⅜-oz. pkg.	850

Food and Description	Measure or Quantity	Sodium (milligrams)
(Weight Watchers)	6-oz. pie	670
Combination:		
(Celeste) Chicago style	¼ of 24-oz. pie	1156
(Weight Watchers) deluxe	7¼-oz. pie	944
Deluxe:		
(Celeste):		
Small	9-oz. pie	1588
Large	¼ of 23½-oz. pie	1049
(Stouffer's) French Bread		
Pizza	½ of 12⅜-oz. pie	1150
Hamburger (Stouffer's)		
French Bread Pizza	½ of 12¼-oz. pie	1100
Mushroom (Stouffer's)		
French Bread Pizza	½ of 12-oz. pkg.	1755
Pepperoni:		
(Celeste):		
Regular:		
Small	7¼-oz. pie	1776
Large	¼ of 20-oz. pie	1082
Chicago, style, deluxe	¼ of 24-oz. pie	1389
(Stouffer's) French Bread		
Pizza	½ of 11¼-oz. pkg.	1190
(Weight Watchers)	6½-oz. pie	802
Sausage:		
(Celeste):		
Regular:		
Small	8-oz. pie	1528
Large	¼ of 22-oz. pie	1227
Chicago style-deluxe	¼ of 24-oz. pie	1153
(Stouffer's) French Bread		
Pizza	½ of 12-oz. pkg.	1320
Sausage, veal (Weight		
Watchers)	6¾-oz. pie	936
Sausage & mushroom		
(Celeste):		
Small	9-oz. pie	1576
Large	¼ of 24-oz. pie	1195
Sicilian style (Celeste)		
deluxe	¼ of 26-oz. pie	1190
PIZZA PIE CRUST, refrigerated		
(Pillsbury)	⅛ of crust	170

Food and Description	Measure or Quantity	Sodium (milligrams)
PIZZA PIE MIX (Ragú)		
Pizza Quick:		
Crust only	1/12 of pkg.	360
*Pizza, cheese	1/4 of pie	810
PIZZA SAUCE, canned:		
(Contadina):		
Regular	1/2 cup	790
With cheese	1/2 cup	760
With pepperoni	1/2 cup	72(
With tomato chunks	1/2 cup	600
(Ragú)		
Regular, with extra tomatoes	1/4 of 15½-oz. jar	475
Pizza Quick:		
Chunky	1/3 of 14-oz. jar	786
Mushroom, sausage or traditional	1/3 of 14-oz. jar	824
Pepperoni	1/3 of 14-oz. jar	906
PIZZA SEASONING SPICE		
(French's)	1 tsp. (.1 oz.)	390
PLANTAIN, raw (USDA):		
Whole	1 lb. (weighed with skin)	16
Flesh only	4 oz.	6
PLUM:		
Fresh (USDA):		
Damson:		
Whole	1 lb. (weighed with pits)	8
Flesh only	4 oz.	2
Japanese & hybrid:		
Whole	1 lb. (weighed with pits)	4
Whole	2.1-oz. plum (2″ dia.)	<1
Diced	1/2 cup (2.9 oz.)	<1
Halves	1/2 cup (3.1 oz.)	<1
Slices	1/2 cup (3 oz.)	<1
Prune type:		
Whole	1 lb. (weighed with pits)	4

Food and Description	Measure or Quantity	Sodium (milligrams)
Halves	½ cup (2.8 oz.)	<1
Canned, purple, regular pack, solids & liq.:		
(USDA):		
Extra heavy syrup	4 oz.	1
Light syrup	4 oz.	1
(Stokely-Van Camp)	½ cup	28
(Thank You Brand):		
Heavy syrup	½ cup (4.8 oz.)	14
Light syrup	½ cup (4.7 oz.)	13
Canned, unsweetened or low calorie, solids & liq.:		
(Diet Delight) purple, juice pack	½ cup (4.4 oz.)	5
(Featherweight) purple:		
Juice pack	½ cup	<10
Water pack	½ cup	<10
(Thank You Brand) water pack	½ cup (4.8 oz.)	<5
PLUM JELLY, sweetened:		
(Home Brands)	1 T.	15
(Smucker's)	1 T. (.7 oz.)	7
PLUM PRESERVE or JAM, sweetened (Smucker's)	1 T. (.7 oz.)	3
PLUM PUDDING, canned (Richardson & Robbins)	2″ wedge (3.6 oz.)	150
POLISH-STYLE SAUSAGE (See **SAUSAGE**)		
POLYNESIAN STYLE DINNER, frozen (Swanson)	12-oz. dinner	1430
POMEGRANATE, raw (USDA):		
Whole	1 lb. (weighed whole)	8
Pulp only	4 oz.	3
POMPANO, raw (USDA):		
Whole	1 lb. (weighed whole)	119
Meat only	4 oz.	53
PONDEROSA RESTAURANT:		
A-1 Sauce	1 tsp.	82

Food and Description	Measure or Quantity	Sodium (milligrams)
Beef, chopped (patty only):		
Regular	3½ oz.	58
Double Deluxe	5.9 oz.	99
Junior (*Square Shooter*)	1.6 oz.	27
Steakhouse Deluxe	2.96 oz.	50
Beverages:		
Coca-Cola	8 fl. oz.	1
Coffee	6 fl. oz.	26
Dr. Pepper	8 fl. oz.	18
Milk, chocolate	8 fl. oz.	149
Orange drink	8 fl. oz.	12
Root beer	8 fl. oz.	18
Sprite,	8 fl. oz.	31
Tab	8 fl. oz.	18
Bun:		
Regular	2.4-oz. bun	334
Hot dog	1 bun	263
Junior	1.4-oz. bun	197
Steakhouse deluxe	2.4-oz bun	334
Chicken strips:		
Adult portion	2¾ oz.	420
Child	1.4 oz.	210
Cocktail sauce	1½ oz.	143
Filet Mignon	3.8 oz. (edible portion)	82
Filet of sole, fish only (See also Bun)	3-oz. piece	46
Fish, baked	4.9-oz. serving	363
Gelatin dessert	½ cup	55
Gravy, au jus	1 oz.	125
Ham & cheese:		
Bun (See Bun)		
Cheese, Swiss	2 slices (.8 oz.)	310
Ham	2½ oz.	724
Hot dog, child's, meat only (See also Bun)	1.6-oz. hot dog	542
Margarine:		
Pat	1 tsp.	49
On potato, as served	½ oz.	138

Food and Description	Measure or Quantity	Sodium (milligrams)
New York strip steak	6.1 oz. (edible portion)	79
Onion, chopped	1 T.	1
Pickle, dill	3 slices (.7 oz.)	279
Potato:		
Baked	7.2-oz. potato	6
French fries	3-oz. serving	5
Prime ribs:		
Regular	4.2 oz. (edible portion)	71
Imperial	8.4 oz. (edible portion)	141
King	6 oz. (edible portion)	101
Pudding, chocolate	4½ oz.	177
Ribeye	3.2 oz. (edible portion)	271
Ribeye & Shrimp:		
Ribeye	3.2 oz.	271
Shrimp	2.2 oz.	114
Roll, kaiser	2.2-oz. roll	311
Salad bar:		
Beets	1 oz.	56
Broccoli	1 oz.	4
Cabbage, red	1 oz.	7
Carrots	1 oz.	13
Cauliflower	1 oz.	4
Celery	1 oz.	36
Chickpeas (Garbanzos)	1 oz.	7
Cucumber	1 oz.	2
Mushrooms	1 oz.	4
Onion, white	1 oz.	3
Pepper, green	1 oz.	4
Radish	1 oz.	5
Tomato	1 oz.	Tr.
Salad dressing:		
Blue cheese	1 oz.	265
Italian, creamy	1 oz.	419
Low calorie	1 oz.	220
Oil & vinegar	1 oz.	Tr.

Food and Description	Measure or Quantity	Sodium (milligrams)
Thousand Island	1 oz.	170
Shrimp dinner	7 pieces (3½ oz.)	182
Sirloin:		
Regular	3.3 oz. (edible portion)	372
Super	6½ oz. (edible portion)	695
Tips	4 oz. (edible portion)	375
Steak sauce	1 oz.	329
Tartar sauce	1.5 oz.	300
T-Bone	4.3 oz. (edible portion)	545
Tomato (See also Salad Bar):		
Slices	2 slices (.9 oz.)	7
Whole, small	3.5 oz.	3
Topping, whipped	¼ oz.	4
POPCORN:		
Unpopped, (USDA)	1 oz.	<1
Popped, fresh:		
(USDA):		
Plain	1 oz.	<1
Plain, large kernel	1 cup (6 g.)	<1
Butter or oil & salt added	1 oz.	550
Butter or oil & salt added	1 cup (9 g.)	175
Sugar coated	1 cup (1.2 oz.)	<1
(Jiffy Pop):		
Plain	½ pkg. (2½ oz.)	936
Buttered	½ pkg. (2½ oz.)	936
(Jolly Time):		
Regular	1 cup	Tr.
Microwave:		
Natural	1 cup	60
With real butter	1 cup	68
(Orville Reddenbacher's)		
Gourmet:		
Original, plain	1 cup	0
Caramel crunch	1 oz.	100
Hot air corn	1 cup	0

Food and Description	Measure or Quantity	Sodium (milligrams)
Microwave:		
Regular:		
Butter flavored:		
Salted	1 cup	50
Without salt	1 cup	0
Natural:		
Salted	1 cup	65
Without salt	1 cup	0
Flavored:		
Caramel	1 cup	36
Cheese:		
Cheddar	1 cup	93
Nacho	1 cup	133
Sour cream & onion	1 cup	87
(Pillsbury) Microwave Popcorn:		
Regular	1 cup	129
Butter flavor	1 cup	176
Packaged:		
Cracker Jack (Borden)	1 oz.	85
(Tom's):		
Regular	1 oz.	300
Cheese flavored	1 oz.	460
(Snyder's) cheese flavored	1 oz.	250
(Wise) butter flavored	1 oz.	440
POPCORN POPPING OIL		
(Orville Reddenbacher's)		
Gourmet, buttery flavor	1 T. (.5 oz.)	0
POPOVER:		
Home recipe (USDA)	1 average popover (2 oz.)	125
*Mix (Flako)	1 popover	355
POPPY SEED (French's)	1 tsp.	Tr.
PORGY, raw (USDA):		
Whole	1 lb. (weighed whole)	117
Meat only	4 oz.	71
PORK, medium-fat:		
Fresh (USDA):		
Boston butt:		
Raw	1 lb. (weighed with bone & skin)	260

Food and Description	Measure or Quantity	Sodium (milligrams)
Roasted, lean & fat	4 oz.	74
Roasted, lean only	4 oz.	74
Chop:		
Broiled, lean & fat	1 chop (4 oz., weighed with bone)	49
Broiled, lean & fat	1 chop (3 oz., weighed with bone)	55
Broiled, lean only	1 chop (3 oz. weighed without bone)	55
Ham (See also **HAM**):		
Raw	1 lb. (weighed with bone & skin)	320
Roasted, lean & fat	4 oz.	74
Roasted, lean only	4 oz.	74
Loin:		
Raw	1 lb. (weighed with bone)	260
Roasted, lean only	4 oz.	74
Picnic:		
Raw	1 lb. (weighed with bone & skin)	260
Simmered, lean & fat	4 oz.	74
Simmered, lean only	4 oz.	74
Spareribs:		
Raw, with bone	1 lb. (weighed with bone)	775
Braised, lean & fat	4 oz.	74
Cured, light commercial cure:		
Bacon (See **BACON**)		
Bacon butt (USDA), roasted, lean only	4 oz.	1055
Ham (See also **HAM**) roasted, lean only (USDA)	4 oz.	1055
Picnic:		
Raw (Wilson) smoked	4 oz.	1247

Food and Description	Measure or Quantity	Sodium (milligrams)
Roasted, lean only (USDA)	4 oz.	1055
PORK & BEANS (See **BEAN, BAKED**)		
PORK, CANNED, chopped luncheon meat (USDA):		
Regular	1 oz.	350
Chopped	1 cup (4.8 oz.)	1678
Diced	1 cup	1740
PORK DINNER:		
*Canned (Hunt's) *Minute Gourmet Microwave Entree Maker,* Cajun	6.6 oz.	1270
Frozen (Swanson) loin of	11¼-oz. dinner	710
PORK, PACKAGED (Eckrich) slender sliced	1 oz.	350
PORK RINDS, fried (Tom's):		
Regular	.6 oz.	220
BBQ	.6 oz.	260
PORK SAUSAGE (See **SAUSAGE**)		
PORK, SWEET & SOUR, frozen (La Choy)	½ of 15-oz. entree	1586
PORT WINE:		
(Gold Seal)	3 fl. oz.	3
(Great Western) Solera, Tawny,	3 fl. oz.	34
POSTUM, cereal beverage (General Foods)	6 fl. oz.	3
POTATO (See also **POTATO CHIP, POTATO MIX, POTATO SALAD, POTATO STICK,** etc.):		
Raw (USDA):		
Whole	1 lb. (weighed unpared)	11
Pared, chopped	1 cup (5.2 oz.)	4
Pared, diced	1 cup (5.5 oz.)	5
Pared, sliced	1 cup (5.2 oz.)	4

Food and Description	Measure or Quantity	Sodium (milligrams)
Cooked (USDA):		
Au gratin or scalloped, with cheese	½ cup (4.3 oz.)	433
Au gratin or scalloped, without cheese	½ cup (4.3 oz.)	545
Baked, peeled after baking	2½"-dia. potato (3 raw to 1 lb.)	4
Boiled, peeled after boiling	1 med. (3 raw to 1 lb.)	2
Boiled, peeled before boiling:		
Whole	1 med (3 raw to 1 lb.)	2
Diced	½ cup (2.8 oz.)	2
Mashed	½ cup (3.7 oz.)	2
Riced	½ cup (4 oz.)	2
Sliced	½ cup (2.8 oz.)	2
French fried in deep fat	10 pieces (2" × ½" × ½", 2 oz.)	3
Hash browned, after holding overnight	½ cup (3.4 oz.)	281
Mashed, milk added	½ cup (3.5 oz.)	295
Mashed, milk & butter added	½ cup (3.4 oz.)	324
Pan fried from raw	½ cup (3 oz.)	190
Scalloped (See Au Gratin)		
Canned, solids & liq.:		
(USDA) solids & liq.	1 cup (8.8 oz.)	2
(Allen's) *Butterfield*	½ cup (4 oz.)	360
(Del Monte) white, sliced or whole	½ cup	355
(Larsen) *Freshlike*	½ cup (4½ oz.)	260
(Stokely-Van Camp) whole	½ cup (4.4 oz.)	335
(Sunshine) whole	½ cup	377
Dehydrated, mashed (see also **POTATO MIX**) (USDA):		
Flakes, dry, without milk	½ cup (.8 oz.)	20
*Flakes, prepared with water, milk & fat	½ cup (3.8 oz.)	247
Granules, dry, without milk	½ cup	84
*Granules, prepared with water, milk & butter	½ cup (3.7 oz.)	256

Food and Description	Measure or Quantity	Sodium (milligrams)
Frozen (See also **POTATO, STUFFED**):		
(USDA):		
French-fried, heated	10 pieces (2″ × ½″, 2 oz.)	2
Mashed, heated	4 oz.	407
(Birds Eye):		
Cottage fries	⅕ of 14-oz. pkg.	14
Crinkle cuts:		
Regular	⅓ of 9-oz. pkg.	36
Deep Gold	¼ of 12-oz. pkg.	12
Farm style wedge	⅛ of 24-oz. pkg.	25
French fries:		
Regular	3-oz. serving	23
Deep Gold	3-oz. serving	280
Hash browns:		
Regular	4-oz. serving	54
Shredded	3-oz. serving	21
Shoestring	3-oz. serving	45
Steak fries	3-oz. serving	25
Tasti Fries	2½-oz. serving	268
Tasti Puffs	2½-oz. serving	401
Tiny Taters	3.2-oz. serving	282
Triangles	1½-oz. piece	167
Whole, peeled	⅒ of 32-oz. pkg.	5
(Empire Kosher) french fries	3 oz.	35
(Green Giant):		
& sweet peas in bacon cream sauce	½ cup	400
Slices in butter sauce	½ cup	470
(Larsen) diced	4 oz.	40
(McKenzie) whole, white, boiled	3.5-oz. serving	20
(Stouffer's) au gratin	⅓ of 11½-oz. pkg.	480
POTATO & BACON, canned		
(Hormel) *Short Orders*	7½-oz. can	942
POTATO CHIP:		
(USDA)	1 oz.	284
(Cottage Fries) no salt added	1 oz.	5
Delta Gold:		
Regular or dip style	1 oz.	160

Food and Description	Measure or Quantity	Sodium (milligrams)
Mesquite flavored Bar-B-Q	1 oz.	240
(Featherweight) unsalted	1 oz.	6
(Frito-Lay's) natural style	1 oz.	262
(Laura Scudder's):		
Barbecue	1 oz.	200
Sour cream & onion	1 oz.	170
Lay's:		
Regular	1 oz.	200
Bar-B-Q	1 oz.	310
Italian cheese	1 oz.	210
Jalapeño & cheddar	1 oz.	290
Salt & vinegar	1 oz.	460
Sour cream & onion	1 oz.	250
Unsalted	1 oz.	10
(New York Deli)	1 oz.	120
O'Grady's:		
Regular	1 oz.	210
Au gratin cheese	1 oz.	330
Pringle's:		
Regular	1 oz.	216
Cheez-Ums	1 oz.	240
Light	1 oz.	152
Rippled	1 oz.	250
Ruffles:		
Regular, bacon & sour cream or light	1 oz.	190
Bar-B-Q	1 oz.	320
Cajun Spice or sour cream & onion	1 oz.	240
Cheddar & sour cream	1 oz.	260
Cottage Fries:		
Regular	1 oz.	240
Unsalted	1 oz.	10
Ridgies:		
Natural flavor	1 oz.	150
Sour cream & onion	1 oz.	240
(Toms):		
Regular	1 oz.	200
BBQ, sour cream & onion or vinegar & salt	1 oz.	280

Food and Description	Measure or Quantity	Sodium (milligrams)
Hot	1 oz.	310
(Wise):		
Barbecue	1 oz.	240
Garlic & onion	1 oz.	250
Lightly salted	1 oz.	100
Natural	1 oz.	150
Salt & vinegar	1 oz.	350
POTATO & HAM canned		
(Hormel) *Short Orders*	7½-oz. can	1189
POTATO MIX:		
*Au Gratin:		
(Betty Crocker)	½ cup (⅙ of pkg.)	605
(French's) tangy	½ cup	460
*Creamed (Betty Crocker)	½ cup (⅙ of pkg.)	385
*Hash brown, (Betty Crocker)		
with onion	½ cup (⅙ of pkg.)	460
*Julienne (Betty Crocker)	½ cup (⅙ of pkg.)	570
*Mashed:		
(Betty Crocker) *Buds*	½ cup	355
(French's):		
Regular	½ cup	320
Spuds	½ cup	380
(Pillsbury) *Hungry Jack,*		
flakes	½ cup	380
*Scalloped:		
(Betty Crocker)	½ cup	570
(French's):		
Cheese	½ cup	540
Crispy top	½ cup	520
*Sour cream & chive (Betty		
Crocker)	½ cup (⅙ of pkg.)	495
*POTATO PANCAKE MIX		
(French's)	3″ pancake	130
POTATO SALAD, home recipe		
(USDA):		
With cooked salad dressing &		
seasonings	4 oz.	599
With mayonnaise & French		
dressing, hard-cooked eggs,		
seasonings	4 oz.	544

Food and Description	Measure or Quantity	Sodium (milligrams)
POTATO STICK, *O&C* (Durkee)	1½-oz. can	383
POTATO, STUFFED, BAKED,		
frozen (Green Giant):		
With cheese flavored topping	½ of 10-oz. pkg.	520
With sour cream & chives	½ of 10-oz. pkg.	580
PRETZEL:		
(Eagle)	1 oz.	570
(Estee) unsalted	1 piece	<1
(Featherweight) unsalted	1 piece	1
(Nabisco) *Mister Salty:*		
Regular:		
Dutch	1 piece	220
Logs	1 piece	57
Mini	1 piece	28
Nuggets	1 piece	26
Rings, regular	1 piece	23
Rods	1 piece (.5 oz.)	250
Sticks, regular	1 piece	7
Twists	1 piece	118
Juniors	1 piece	18
(Pepperidge Farm):		
Nuggets	1½ oz.	497
Sticks, thin	1¼ oz.	492
Twist, tiny	1 oz.	366
(Planters)	1 oz.	700
Rold Gold:		
Rods	1 oz.	550
Sticks	1 oz.	760
Tiny Tim	1 oz.	610
Twists	1 oz.	470
(Seyfert's) rods, butter	1 oz.	530
(Snyder's) hard:		
Hard	1 oz.	548
Stix	1 oz.	386
Thins	1 oz.	655
(Tom's) twists	1 oz.	430
(Wise) nugget	1 oz.	600
PRICKLY PEAR, fresh (USDA):		
Whole	1 lb. (weighed with rind & seeds)	4

Food and Description	Measure or Quantity	Sodium (milligrams)
Flesh only	4 oz.	2
PRODUCT 19, cereal (Kellogg's)	1 cup (1 oz.)	290
PROSCIUTTO (Hormel) boneless	1 oz.	502
PRUNE:		
Canned, regular pack (Sunsweet) stewed	½ cup	2
Canned, dietetic (Featherweight) stewed, water pack, solids & liq.	½ cup	<10
Dried:		
(USDA) dried, cooked, with sugar	1 cup (16–18 prunes & ⅔ cup liq.)	9
(Del Monte)	2 oz.	<10
(Sunsweet):		
With pits	2 oz.	5
Pitted	2 oz.	3
PRUNE JUICE, canned:		
(USDA)	½ cup (4.5 oz.)	2
(Del Monte)	6 fl. oz.	<10
(Sunsweet):		
Regular	6 fl. oz.	4
Home style, with pulp	6 fl. oz.	12
PRUNE WHIP, home recipe (USDA)	1 cup (4.8 oz.)	221
PUDDING or PIE FILLING:		
Home recipe (USDA):		
Rice, made with raisins	½ cup (4.7 oz.)	94
Tapioca:		
Apple	½ cup (4.4 oz.)	64
Cream	½ cup (2.9 oz.)	128
Vanilla, with starch base	½ cup (4.5 oz.)	83
Canned, regular pack:		
Banana:		
(Del Monte) *Pudding Cup*	5-oz. container	277
(Hunt's) *Snack Pack*	4¼-oz. container	180
(Thank You Brand)	½ cup (4.6 oz.)	182
Butterscotch:		
(Del Monte) *Pudding Cup*	5-oz. container	277

Food and Description	Measure or Quantity	Sodium (milligrams)
(Hunt's) *Snack Pack*	4¼-oz. container	200
(Swiss Miss)	4-oz. container	210
(Thank You Brand)	½ cup (4.6 oz.)	221
Chocolate:		
(Betty Crocker)	½ cup (5 oz.)	260
(Del Monte) *Pudding Cup:*		
Regular	5-oz. container	327
Fudge	5-oz. container	297
(Hunt's) *Snack Pack:*		
Regular, German or marshmallow	4¼-oz. container	135
Fudge	4¼-oz. container	140
(Swiss Miss):		
Regular:		
Plain	4-oz. container	200
Fudge	4-oz. container	190
Fruit on bottom:		
Black cherry	4-oz. container	150
Strawberry	4-oz. container	160
(Thank You Brand):		
Regular	½ cup (4.6 oz.)	117
Fudge	½ cup (4.6 oz.)	130
Lemon:		
(Hunt's) *Snack Pack*	4¼-oz. container	70
(Thank You Brand)	½ cup (4.6 oz.)	195
Rice:		
(Betty Crocker)	½ cup (4¼ oz.)	150
(Comstock)	½ of 7½-oz. can	450
(Hunt's) *Snack Pack*	4¼-oz. container	200
(Menner's)	½ of 7½-oz. can	450
Tapioca:		
(Betty Crocker)	½ cup (4¼ oz.)	170
(Del Monte) *Pudding Cup*	5-oz. container	253
(Hunt's) *Snack Pack*	4¼-oz. container	140
(Swiss Miss)	4-oz. container	190
(Thank You Brand)	½ cup (4.6 oz.)	169
Vanilla:		
(Del Monte) *Pudding Cup*	5-oz. container	320
(Hunt's) *Snack Pack*	4¼-oz. container	160
(Swiss Miss)	4-oz. container	200

Food and Description	Measure or Quantity	Sodium (milligrams)
(Thank You Brand)	½ cup (4.6 oz.)	182
Canned, dietetic (Estee):		
Butterscotch	½ cup	80
Chocolate or vanilla	½ cup	75
Chilled, *Swiss Miss:*		
Butterscotch	4-oz. container	175
Chocolate:		
Regular	4-oz. container	176
Malt	4-oz. container	175
Sundae	4-oz. container	166
Double rich	4-oz. container	173
Rice	4-oz. container	296
Tapioca	4-oz. container	170
Vanilla:		
Regular	4-oz. container	175
Sundae	4-oz. container	166
Frozen (Rich's):		
Banana	3-oz. container	118
Butterscotch	4½-oz. container	192
Chocolate	4½-oz. container	205
Vanilla	4½-oz. container	243
*Mix, regular pack:		
Banana:		
(Jell-O) cream:		
Regular	½ cup	257
Instant	½ cup	445
(Royal) cream:		
Regular	½ cup	210
Instant	½ cup	390
Butter pecan (Jell-O) instant	½ cup	442
Butterscotch:		
(Jell-O):		
Regular	½ cup	247
Instant	½ cup	483
(Royal):		
Regular	½ cup	210
Instant	½ cup	390
Chocolate:		
(Jell-O):		
Regular:		
Plain	½ cup	170

Food and Description	Measure or Quantity	Sodium (milligrams)
Fudge	½ cup	171
Milk	½ cup	173
Instant:		
Plain or milk	½ cup	507
Fudge	½ cup	482
(Royal):		
Regular, plain or *Dark N' Sweet*	½ cup	150
Instant, plain, chocolate chip mint or *Dark N' Sweet*	½ cup	390
Coconut:		
(Jell-O) cream:		
Regular	⅙ of 8″ pie (excluding crust)	140
Regular	½ cup	216
Instant	½ cup	358
(Royal) instant	½ cup	350
Custard:		
Jell-O Americana, golden egg	½ cup	222
(Royal) regular	½ cup	115
Flan (Royal) regular	½ cup	115
Lemon:		
(Jell-O):		
Regular	⅙ of 9″ pie (excluding crust)	91
Regular	½ cup	94
Instant	½ cup	397
(Royal):		
Regular	½ cup	120
Instant	½ cup	350
Lime (Royal) regular, Key Lime	½ cup	120
Pineapple (Jell-O) cream, instant	½ cup	400
Pistachio:		
(Jell-O) instant	½ cup	445
(Royal) instant	½ cup	350

Food and Description	Measure or Quantity	Sodium (milligrams)
Raspberry (Salada) *Danish Dessert*	½ cup	5
Rice, *Jell-O Americana*	½ cup	158
Strawberry (Salada) *Danish Dessert*	½ cup	5
Tapioca:		
Jell-O Americana chocolate or vanilla	½ cup	170
(Royal) Vanilla	½ cup	150
Vanilla:		
(Jell-O):		
Regular:		
Plain	½ cup	198
French	½ cup	201
Instant, French	½ cup	442
(Royal):		
Regular	½ cup	210
Instant	½ cup	390
*Mix, dietetic pack:		
Butterscotch:		
(Dia-Mel)	½ cup	80
(D-Zerta)	½ cup	115
(Estee)	½ cup	80
(Featherweight), artificially sweetened	4-oz. serving	70
(Royal) instant	½ cup	470
Chocolate:		
(Dia-Mel)	½ cup	80
(D-Zerta)	4-oz. serving	116
(Estee) instant	½ cup	75
(Featherweight) artificially sweetened	½ cup	78
(Louis Sherry)	½ cup	80
(Royal) instant	½ cup	470
Lemon (Estee) instant	½ cup	75
Vanilla:		
(Dia-Mel)	½ cup	80
(D-Zerta)	½ cup	105
(Estee) instant	½ cup	75
(Featherweight) artificially sweetened	½ cup	70

Food and Description	Measure or Quantity	Sodium (milligrams)
(Royal) instant	½ cup	470
PUDDING STIX (Good Humor)	1¾-fl.-oz. pop	65
PUDDING SUNDAE (Swiss Miss):		
Caramel, mint or peanut butter	4-oz. container	180
Chocolate or vanilla	4-oz. container	200
PUFFED CORN, cereal (USDA) with added nutrients	1 oz.	301
PUFFED OAT, cereal (USDA):		
Plain, added nutrients	1 oz.	359
Sugar coated, added nutrients	1 oz.	167
PUFFED RICE, cereal:		
(Malt-O-Meal)	1 cup (½ oz.)	1
(Quaker)	1 cup (½ oz.)	1
PUFFED WHEAT, cereal:		
(Malt-O-Meal)	1 cup (½ oz.)	1
(Quaker)	1 cup (½ oz.)	1
PUFFS, frozen (Rich's) vanilla	1.8-oz. puff	117
PUMPKIN:		
Fresh (USDA):		
Whole	1 lb. (weighed with rind & seeds)	3
Flesh only	4 oz.	1
Canned:		
(USDA) salted	½ cup (4.3 oz.)	288
(Del Monte)	½ cup (4.3 oz.)	<10
(Festal)	½ cup	6
(Libby's) solid pack	½ cup	5

Food and Description	Measure or Quantity	Sodium (milligrams)

Q

QUAIL, raw (USDA) meat & skin only	4 oz.	45
QUIK (Nestlé):		
Chocolate flavor	1 T. (.4 oz.)	18
Strawberry flavor	1 T. (.4 oz.)	0
QUINCE, fresh (USDA):		
Untrimmed	1 lb. (weighed with skin & seeds)	11
Flesh only	4 oz.	5
QUISP, cereal (Quaker)	1⅙ cups (1 oz.)	189

R

RABBIT (USDA) domesticated:		
Raw, ready-to-cook	1 lb. (weighed with bones)	154
Stewed, flesh only	4 oz.	46
RADISH (USDA) common, raw:		
Without tops	½ lb. (weighed untrimmed)	36
Trimmed, whole	4 small radishes (1.4 oz.)	7
Trimmed, sliced	½ cup (2 oz.)	10
RAISIN:		
Dried:		
(USDA):		
Whole, pressed down	½ cup (2.9 oz.)	22

Food and Description	Measure or Quantity	Sodium (milligrams)
Chopped	½ cup (2.9 oz.)	22
Ground	½ cup (4.7 oz.)	36
(Del Monte):		
Golden	3 oz.	<10
(Sun-Maid) seedless, natural,	3 oz.	15
Thompson	½ cup (3 oz.)	12
Cooked (USDA) added sugar, solids & liq.	½ cup (4.3 oz.)	16
RAISINS, RICE & RYE, cereal (Kellogg's)	¾ cup (1 oz.)	235
RALSTON cereal, instant and regular	¼ cup (1 oz.)	3
RASPBERRY:		
Black (USDA):		
Fresh:		
Whole	1 lb. (weighed with caps & stems)	2
Without caps & stems	½ cup (2.4 oz.)	<1
Canned, water pack, unsweetened, solids & liq.	4 oz.	1
Red:		
Fresh (USDA):		
Whole	1 lb. (weighed with caps & stems)	2
Without caps & stems	½ cup (2.5 oz.)	<1
Canned, water pack, unsweetened or low calorie, solids & liq. (USDA)	4 oz.	1
Frozen (Birds Eye) quick thaw	½ of 10-oz. pkg.	1
RASPBERRY JELLY, sweetened:		
(Home Brands)	1 T.	15
(Smucker's) black or red	1 T.	2
RASPBERRY PRESERVE or JAM sweetened (Smucker's) black or red	1 T.	2
RATATOUILLE, frozen (Stouffer's)	5 oz.	1320

Food and Description	Measure or Quantity	Sodium (milligrams)
RAVIOLI:		
Canned, regular pack (Franco-American) beef:		
In meat sauce	7½-oz. serving	1090
In meat sauce, *RavioliOs*	7½-oz. serving	890
Canned, dietetic or low calorie:		
(Dia-Mel) beef, in sauce	8-oz. can	75
(Estee)	7½-oz. can	110
(Featherweight)	8-oz. can	68
Frozen:		
(Buitoni):		
Cheese:		
Ravioletti	2.6 oz.	217
Square	4.8 oz.	237
Meat:		
Ravioletti	2.6 oz.	244
Square	4.8 oz.	371
(Celentano) cheese:		
Regular	½ of 13-oz. pkg.	360
Mini	½ of 8-oz. box	180
(Weight Watchers) cheese, baked	8¹⁄₁₆-oz. serving	685
RED & GRAY SNAPPER, raw (USDA):		
Whole	1 lb. (weighed whole)	158
Meat only	4 oz.	76
RED LOBSTER RESTAURANT		
(lunch portion refers to cooked 5-oz. portion, weighed raw, before cooking unless otherwise noted):		
Calamari, breaded & fried	lunch portion	1150
Catfish	lunch portion	50
Chicken breast	4-oz. serving	60
Crab legs:		
King	16-oz. serving	900
Snow	16-oz. serving	1630
Flounder	lunch portion	95
Grouper	lunch portion	70

Food and Description	Measure or Quantity	Sodium (milligrams)
Hamburger, without bun	5.3-oz. burger	70
Lobster, tail	1 tail	1090
Monkfish	lunch portion	95
Munch	3-oz.	150
Oyster	6 raw oysters	90
Salmon	lunch portion	60
Shrimp	8–12 pieces	110
Steak:		
Porterhouse	18-oz. serving	150
Sirloin	7-oz. serving	85
Strip	7-oz. serving	70
RELISH:		
Dill (Vlasic)	1 oz.	415
Hamburger (Vlasic)	1 oz.	255
Hot dog (Vlasic)	1 oz.	255
Sweet:		
(USDA) finely chopped	1 T. (.5 oz.)	107
(Aunt Jane's)	1 rounded tsp. (.4 oz.)	71
(Smucker's)	1 T. (.6 oz.)	158
(Vlasic)	1 oz.	220
RENNET MIX (Junket):		
*Powder:		
Chocolate:		
Made with skim milk	½ cup	70
Made with whole milk	½ cup	65
Raspberry or strawberry:		
Made with skim milk	½ cup	65
Made with whole milk	½ cup	60
Vanilla:		
Made with skim milk	½ cup	70
Made with whole milk	½ cup	65
Tablet	1 tablet	165
RHINE WINE:		
(Gold Seal) 12% alcohol	3 fl. oz.	3
(Great Western):		
Regular, 12% alcohol	3 fl. oz.	25
Dutchess, 12% alcohol	3 fl. oz.	27

Food and Description	Measure or Quantity	Sodium (milligrams)
RHUBARB (USDA):		
Fresh:		
Partly trimmed	1 lb. (weighed with part leaves, ends & trimmings)	7
Trimmed	4 oz.	2
Diced	½ cup (2.2 oz.)	1
Cooked, sweetened, solids & liq.	½ cup (4.2 oz.)	2
Frozen, sweetened, cooked, added sugar	½ cup (4.4 oz.)	4
RICE:		
Brown:		
Raw (USDA)	½ cup (3.7 oz.)	9
Dry, parboiled (Uncle Ben's) long-grain	1 oz.	4
*(Uncle Ben's) parboiled:		
No added butter or salt	⅔ cup	5
Added butter & salt	⅔ cup (4.2 oz.)	458
White:		
Dry:		
(USDA) long grain, instant or precooked	1 oz.	<1
(USDA) regular	½ cup (3.3 oz.)	5
*Cooked:		
(USDA) long grain	⅔ (3.3 oz.)	254
(Minute Rice) no butter:		
With salt	⅔ cup	268
Without salt	⅔ cup	2
(Uncle Ben's):		
Long grain, no added butter or salt	⅔ cup (4.2 oz.)	13
Long grain, with butter or salt couverted, no butter or salt	⅔ cup (4.3 oz.)	233
Converted, no butter or salt	⅔ cup (4.6 oz.)	2
RICE BRAN (USDA)	1 oz.	Tr.
RICE CAKE, dietetic (Pritikin):		
Plain:		
Low sodium	1 cake	30

Food and Description	Measure or Quantity	Sodium (milligrams)
Sodium free	1 cake	0
Sesame or 7-Grain:		
Low sodium	1 cake	35
Sodium free	1 cake	0
RICE, FRIED:		
*Canned, (La Choy)	⅓ of 11-oz. can	965
Frozen:		
(Birds Eye)	⅓ of 11-oz. pkg.	432
(Green Giant) *Boil 'N Bag*	10-oz. entree	1130
(La Choy) meat	8-oz. entree	1770
*Seasoning mix (Durkee)	1 cup	1597
RICE, FRIED, & PORK ENTREE, frozen (La Choy)	½ of 12-oz. entree	1716
RICE KRINKLES, cereal (Post)	⅞ cup (1 oz.)	179
RICE KRISPIES, cereal (Kellogg's):		
Regular	1 cup (1 oz.)	285
Cocoa	¾ cup (1 oz.)	195
Frosted	¾ cup (1 oz.)	200
Marshmallow	1¼ cups	285
Strawberry	¾ cup (1 oz.)	200
RICE MIX:		
Beef:		
*(Lipton) & sauce	½ cup	665
*(Minute Rice) rib roast	½ cup	720
(Rice-A-Roni)	⅙ of pkg.	780
*(Uncle Ben's):		
With butter	½ cup	506
Without butter	½ cup	474
Chicken:		
*(Lipton) & sauce	½ cup	525
*(Minute Rice) drumstick	½ cup	694
(Rice-A-Roni)	⅙ of pkg.	800
*Fried (Minute Rice)	½ cup	549
*Herb & butter (Lipton) & sauce	½ cup	500
*Long grain & wild:		
(Minute Rice)	½ cup	578

Food and Description	Measure or Quantity	Sodium (milligrams)
(Uncle Ben's):		
Regular:		
With butter	½ cup	442
Without butter	½ cup	420
Fast cooking:		
With butter	½ cup	430
Without butter	½ cup	387
*Medley (Lipton) & sauce	½ cup	400
*Mushroom (Lipton) & sauce	½ cup	560
Spanish:		
*(Minute Rice)	½ cup	839
(Rice-A-Roni)	⅐ of pkg.	720
RICE PUDDING (See **PUDDING or PIE FILLING**)		
***RICE SEASONING** (French's)		
Spice Your Rice:		
Beef flavor & onion	½ cup	560
Buttery herb	½ cup	430
Cheese & chives	½ cup	400
Chicken flavor & herb or parmesan	½ cup	440
RICE, SPANISH:		
Home recipe (USDA)	4 oz.	358
Canned, regular pack:		
(Comstock)	½ of 7½-oz. can	850
(Libby's)	½ of 15-oz. can	1108
(Menner's)	½ of 7½-oz. can	850
Canned, dietetic (Featherweight)	7½-oz. can	32
Frozen (Birds Eye)	⅓ of 11-oz. pkg.	495
*Mix (Lipton) & sauce	½ cup	520
RICE & VEGETABLES,		
frozen:		
(Birds Eye) rice, peas & mushrooms	⅓ of 7-oz. pkg.	322
(Green Giant) *Rice Originals:*		
& broccoli in flavored cheese sauce	½ cup	405
With herb butter sauce	½ cup	420
Italian blend & spinach in cheese sauce	½ cup	460
Long grain & white	½ cup	565

Food and Description	Measure or Quantity	Sodium (milligrams)
Medley	½ cup	280
Pilaf	½ cup	520
ROCKFISH (USDA):		
Raw, meat only	1 lb.	272
Oven steamed, with onion	4 oz.	77
ROE (USDA) baked or broiled, cod & shad, prepared with butter or margarine & lemon juice or vinegar	4 oz.	83
ROLL or BUN (See also **ROLL DOUGH** and **ROLL MIX**):		
Commercial type:		
Biscuit (Wonder)	1¼-oz. roll	188
Brown & serve:		
(USDA) browned	1-oz. roll	159
(Pepperidge Farm) club	1.3-oz. roll	220
(Wonder):		
Buttermilk	1-oz. roll	142
French	1-oz. roll	151
Gem Style	1-oz. roll	156
Half & half	1-oz. roll	72
Home bake	1-oz. roll	114
Cloverleaf (USDA) home recipe	1 cloverleaf (1.2 oz.)	98
Crescent, butter (Pepperidge Farm)	1 roll	160
Croissant (Pepperidge Farm):		
Almond	2-oz. roll	260
Butter	2-oz. roll	310
Chocolate	2.4-oz. roll	325
Cinnamon	2-oz. roll	280
Honey sesame	2-oz. roll	270
Raisin	2-oz. roll	265
Walnut	2-oz. roll	275
Dinner:		
Home Pride	1-oz. roll	170
(Wonder)	1¼-oz. roll	188
Dinner Party Rounds (Arnold)	.7-oz. roll	140

Food and Description	Measure or Quantity	Sodium (milligrams)
Frankfurter:		
(USDA)	1.4-oz. roll	202
(Arnold)	1.3-oz. roll	290
(Pepperidge Farm)	1¾-oz. roll	240
(Wonder)	2-oz. roll	153
French:		
(Arnold) Francisco, sour-		
dough	1.1-oz. roll	160
(Pepperidge Farm):		
Regular	1.3-oz. roll	250
Sourdough	1 roll	240
Golden twist (Pepperidge		
Farm)	1 roll	160
Hamburger:		
(USDA)	1.4-oz. roll	202
(Arnold)	1.4-oz. roll	285
(Pepperidge Farm)	1½-oz. roll	260
(Wonder)	2-oz. roll	153
Hard (USDA) round or		
rectangular	1.8-oz. roll	312
Hoggie (Wonder)	6-oz. roll	869
Honey (Hostess)	3¾ oz. roll	522
Kaiser (Wonder)	6-oz. roll	869
Old fashioned (Pepperidge		
Farm)	.6-oz. roll	95
Pan (Wonder)	1¼-oz. roll	188
Parkerhouse:		
(Arnold) *Dinner Party*	.7-oz. roll	63
(Pepperidge Farm)	1 roll	90
Party pan (Pepperidge Farm)	1 roll	50
Plain (USDA)	1-oz. roll	143
Raisin (USDA)	1-oz. roll	109
Sandwich:		
(Arnold):		
Francisco	2-oz. roll	325
Soft, plain	1.3-oz. roll	260
Soft, sesame seeds	1.3-oz. roll	260
(Pepperidge Farm):		
Regular with poppy or		
sesame seeds	1.6-oz. roll	210

Food and Description	Measure or Quantity	Sodium (milligrams)
Onion, with poppy seeds	1.9-oz. roll	240
Sourdough French (Pepperidge Farm)	1.3-oz. roll	255
Sweet (USDA)	1.5-oz. bun	167
Whole wheat (USDA)	1⅓-oz. roll	214
Frozen:		
Apple crunch (Sara Lee)	1-oz. roll	105
Caramel pecan (Sara Lee)	1.3-oz. roll	148
Caramel sticky (Sara Lee)	1-oz. bun	110
Cinnamon (Sara Lee)	.9-oz. roll	96
Croissant (Sara Lee)	.9-oz. roll	140
Crumb (Sara Lee):		
Blueberry	1¾-oz. bun	191
French	1.7-oz. bun	170
Danish (Sara Lee)		
Apple	1⅓-oz. roll	110
Apple country	1.8-oz. roll	214
Cheese	1⅓-oz. roll	124
Cheese country	1½-oz. roll	166
Cherry	1⅓-oz. roll	103
Cherry country	1.6-oz. roll	127
Cinnamon raisin	1⅓-oz. roll	132
Pecan	1⅓-oz. roll	119
Honey:		
(Morton):		
Regular	2.3-oz. roll	150
Mini	1.3-oz. roll	90
(Sara Lee)	1-oz. roll	119
ROLL DOUGH:		
*Frozen (Rich's):		
Cinnamon	1 roll	226
Danish, round	1 roll	417
Frankfurter	1 roll	238
Hamburger:		
Regular	1 roll	227
Deluxe	1 roll	256
Onion:		
Regular	1 roll	215
Deluxe	1 roll	294
Parkerhouse	1 roll	133

Food and Description	Measure or Quantity	Sodium (milligrams)
Refrigerated (Pillsbury):		
Apple danish	1 roll	260
Butterflake	1 roll	520
Caramel danish with nuts	1 roll	245
Cinnamon:		
Regular	1 roll	260
With icing:		
Regular	1 roll	260
Hungry Jack, Butter Tastin'	1 roll	285
& raisin danish	1 roll	225
Crescent	1 roll	230
Orange danish with icing	1 roll	245
*ROLL MIX (Pillsbury) hot roll	1 roll	215
ROMAN MEAL CEREAL:		
Regular, 2- or 5-minute	⅓ cup (1 oz.)	2
With oats, 5-minute	⅓ cup (1 oz.)	6
ROSEMARY LEAVES		
(French's)	1 tsp.	<1
ROSÉ WINE (Great Western) 12% alcohol:		
Regular	3 fl. oz.	38
Isabella	3 fl. oz.	<1
ROTINI, canned (Franco-American):		
In tomato sauce	½ of 15-oz. can	625
& meatballs in tomato sauce	½ of 14¾-oz. can	1170
ROY ROGERS:		
Bar Burger, R.R.	1 burger	1826
Biscuit	1 biscuit	575
Breakfast crescent sandwich:		
Regular	4.5-oz. sandwich	867
With bacon	4.7-oz. sandwich	1035
With ham	5.8-oz. sandwich	1192
With sausage	5.7-oz. sandwich	1289
Brownie	1 piece	150
Cheeseburger:		
Regular	1 burger	1404
With bacon	1 burger	1535
Chicken:		
Breast	1 piece	609

Food and Description	Measure or Quantity	Sodium (milligrams)
Leg	1 piece	190
Thigh	1 piece	406
Wing	1 piece	285
Coleslaw	3⅝-oz. serving	261
Danish:		
Apple	1 piece	255
Cheese	1 piece	260
Cherry	1 piece	242
Drinks:		
Coffee, black	6 fl. oz.	2
Coke:		
Regular	12 fl. oz.	22
Diet	12 fl. oz.	52
Hot chocolate	6 fl. oz.	124
Milk	8 fl. oz.	120
Orange juice:		
Regular	7 fl. oz.	2
Large	10 fl. oz.	3
Shake:		
Chocolate	1 shake	290
Vanilla	1 shake	261
Strawberry	1 shake	282
Tea, iced, plain	8 fl. oz.	Tr.
Egg & biscuit platter:		
Regular	1 meal	734
With bacon	1 meal	957
With ham	1 meal	1156
With sausage	1 meal	1059
Hamburger	1 burger	495
Pancake platter, with syrup & butter:		
Plain	1 order	842
With bacon	1 order	1065
With ham	1 order	1264
With sausage	1 order	1167
Potato:		
Baked, *Hot Topped:*		
Plain	1 potato	10
With bacon & cheese	1 potato	778
With broccoli & cheese	1 potato	523

Food and Description	Measure or Quantity	Sodium (milligrams)
With margarine	1 potato	106
With sour cream & chives	1 potato	138
With taco beef & cheese	1 potato	726
French fries:		
Regular	3 oz.	165
Large	4 oz.	220
Potato salad	3½-oz. order	696
Roast beef sandwich:		
Plain:		
Regular	1 sandwich	785
Large	1 sandwich	1044
With cheese:		
Regular	1 sandwich	1694
Large	1 sandwich	1953
Salad bar:		
Bacon bits	1 T.	210
Beets, sliced	¼ cup	100
Broccoli	½ cup	7
Carrot, shredded	¼ cup	7
Cheese, cheddar	¼ cup	195
Croutons	1 T.	130
Cucumber	1 slice	Tr.
Egg, chopped	1 T.	21
Lettuce	1 cup	7
Macaroni salad	1 T.	155
Mushrooms	¼ cup	3
Noodle, Chinese	¼ cup	100
Pea, green	¼ cup	66
Pepper, green	1 T.	1
Potato salad	1 T.	175
Sunflower seeds	1 T.	4
Tomato	1 slice	1
Salad dressing:		
Regular:		
Bacon & tomato	1 T.	75
Bleu cheese	1 T.	76
Ranch	1 T.	50
1,000 Island	1 T.	75
Low calorie, Italian	1 T.	50
Strawberry shortcake	7.2-oz. serving	674

Food and Description	Measure or Quantity	Sodium (milligrams)
Sundae:		
Caramel	1 sundae	193
Hot fudge	1 sundae	230
Strawberry	1 sundae	99
RUM (See **DISTILLED LIQUOR**)		
RUTABAGA:		
Raw (USDA):		
Without tops	1 lb. (weighed with skin)	19
Diced	½ cup (2.5 oz.)	4
Boiled (USDA) drained, diced	½ cup (3 oz.)	3
Canned (Sunshine) solids & liq.	½ cup (4.2 oz.)	393
Frozen (Southland)	4 oz.	20
RYE, whole grain (USDA)	1 oz.	<1
RYE FLOUR (See flour)		
RYE WHISKEY (See **DISTILLED LIQUOR**)		

S

Food and Description	Measure or Quantity	Sodium (milligrams)
SABLEFISH, raw (USDA):		
Whole	1 lb. (weighed whole)	107
Meat only	4 oz.	64
SAGE (French's)	1 tsp. (.9 grams)	<1
SALAD DRESSING (See also **SALAD DRESSING MIX**):		
Regular:		
Bacon & tomato (Henri's)	1 T.	150
Blue or bleu cheese:		
(USDA)	1 T. (.5 oz.)	164
(Henri's)	1 T.	220
(Wish-Bone) chunky	1 T. (.5 oz.)	150
Boiled, home recipe (USDA)	1 T. (.6 oz.)	116
Caesar (Wish-Bone)	1 T.	250

Food and Description	Measure or Quantity	Sodium (milligrams)
Cheddar & Bacon (Wish-Bone)	1 T.	110
Cucumber (Wish-Bone)	1 T.	125
French:		
Home recipe (USDA) made with corn or cottonseed oil	1 T. (.6 oz.)	105
(USDA) commercial type	1 T. (.6 oz.)	219
(Bernstein's):		
Creamy	1 T. (.5 oz.)	224
Chutney	1 T. (.5 oz.)	292
(Henri's):		
Hearty	1 T.	95
Original	1 T.	110
Sweet & Saucy Frontier	1 T.	100
(Wish-Bone):		
Deluxe	1 T.	80
Garlic or Sweet & Spicy	1 T.	150
Herbal	1 T.	130
Garlic (Wish-Bone)	1 T.	170
Italian:		
(USDA)	1 T. (.5 oz.)	314
(Bernstein's) regular	1 T. (.5 oz.)	184
(Henri's):		
Authentic	1 T.	260
Creamy garlic	1 T.	140
(Wish-Bone):		
Regular or herbal	1 T. (.5 oz.)	240
Creamy	1 T. (.5 oz.)	145
Robusto	1 T. (.5 oz.)	285
Mayonnaise-type (USDA)	1 T. (.5 oz.)	88
Ranchouse (Henri's) *Chef's Recipe*	1 T.	135
Roquefort (Bernstein's)	1 T. (.5 oz.)	142
Russian:		
(USDA)	1 T. (.5 oz.)	130
(Henri's)	1 T.	90
(Wish-Bone)	1 T.	140
Sour cream & bacon (Wish-Bone)	1 T.	95

Food and Description	Measure or Quantity	Sodium (milligrams)
Spin Blend (Hellman's)	1 T. (.6 oz.)	112
Sweet'n Sour (Dutch Pantry):		
Regular	1 T.	63
Creamy	1 T.	62
Tas-Tee (Henri's)	1 T.	95
Thousand Island:		
(USDA)	1 T. (.6 oz.)	112
(Bernstein's)	1 T. (.5 oz.)	127
(Henri's)	1 T.	130
(Wish-Bone):		
Regular	1 T.	130
Southern recipe:		
Plain	1 T.	90
With bacon	1 T.	95
Vinaigrette (Bernstein's) French	1 T. (.5 oz.)	180
Dietetic or low calorie:		
Bacon & tomato (Dia-Mel)	1 T.	0
Bleu or blue cheese:		
(USDA)	1 T. (.6 oz.)	177
(Dia-Mel)	1 T. (.5 oz.)	20
(Henri's)	1 T.	200
(Walden Farms) chunky	1 T.	270
(Wish-Bone) chunky	1 T. (.5 oz.)	190
Buttermilk (Wish-Bone)	1 T.	150
Caesar (Estee) garlic	1 T. (.5 oz.)	150
Catalina (Kraft)	1 T.	125
Chef's Recipe Ranchouse (Henri's)	1 T.	115
Cucumber, creamy:		
(Dia-Mel)	1 T.	30
(Featherweight)	1 T.	12
(Wish-Bone)	1 T. (.5 oz.)	165
Cucumber & onion (Featherweight)	1 T.	128
French:		
(USDA)	1 T. (.6 oz.)	126
(Dia-Mel)	1 T.	10

Food and Description	Measure or Quantity	Sodium (milligrams)
(Featherweight) imitation:		
Low calorie	1 T.	163
Low sodium	1 T.	4
(Henri's):		
Original	1 T.	130
Hearty	1 T.	95
(Pritikin)	1 T.	0
(Walden Farms) creamy	1 T.	132
(Wish-Bone):		
Regular	1 T.	70
Sweet & spicy	1 T.	150
Garlic (Dia-Mel) creamy	1 T.	10
Herb Garden (Estee)	1 T.	150
Herb & spice (Featherweight)	1 T.	5
Italian:		
(USDA)	1 T.	118
(Estee) spicy	1 T. (.5 oz.)	150
(Henri's) authentic	1 T.	260
(Pritikin) regular or creamy	1 T.	0
Mayonnaise, imitation		
(USDA)	1 T. (.6 oz.)	19
Ranch (Pritikin)	1 T.	0
Russian (Pritikin)	1 T.	20
Tas-Tee (Henri's)	1 T.	95
Thousand Island:		
(USDA)	1 T. (.5 oz.)	105
(Henri's)	1 T.	160
(Walden Farms) tangy	1 T.	600
(Wish-Bone)	1 T.	110
Tomato (Pritikin) zesty	1 T.	0
2-calorie low sodium		
(Featherweight)	1 T.	6
Vinaigrette (Pritikin)	1 T.	0
Whipped (Dia-Mel)	1 T.	100
SALAD DRESSING MIX:		
*Regular (Good Seasons):		
Bleu or blue cheese	1 T.	216
Buttermilk, farm style	1 T.	137
Classic herb	1 T.	147

Food and Description	Measure or Quantity	Sodium (milligrams)
Farm style	1 T.	124
French, old fashioned	1 T.	185
Garlic, with cheese	1 T.	173
Garlic & herbs	1 T.	187
Italian:		
Regular	1 T.	172
Cheese	1 T.	134
Mild	1 T.	192
Zesty	1 T.	122
Tomato & herb	1 T.	87
Dietetic or low calorie:		
*Blue cheese (Weight Watchers)	1 T.	108
*French (Weight Watchers)	1 T.	164
Italian:		
*(Good Seasons):		
Regular	1 T.	161
Lite:		
Plain	1 T.	177
Cheese	1 T.	181
*(Weight Watchers):		
Regular	1 T.	175
Creamy	1 T.	224
*Russian (Weight Watchers)	1 T.	128
*Thousand Island (Weight Watchers)	1 T.	265
SALAD LIFT, spice (French's)	1 tsp. (4 grams)	640
SALAD SEASONING (Durkee):		
Regular	1 tsp.	1151
Cheese	1 tsp.	786
SALAMI:		
(Eckrich):		
For beer	1-oz. slice	350
Cooked, chub	1 oz.	360
Cotto:		
Beef	.7-oz. slice	240
Meat	1-oz. slice	340
Hard	1 oz.	600
(Hormel):		
Beef	1 slice	110

Food and Description	Measure or Quantity	Sodium (milligrams)
Cotto:		
Chub	1 oz.	385
Sliced, regular	1 slice	375
Genoa:		
Regular	1 oz.	456
Di Lusso	1 oz.	443
Gran Valore	1 oz.	453
San Remo Brand	1 oz.	544
Hard:		
Packaged, whole	1 slice	169
Whole:		
Regular	1 oz.	468
National Brand	1 oz.	463
Party, sliced	1 oz.	399
(Ohse) cooked	1 oz.	330
(Oscar Mayer):		
For beer:		
Regular	.8-oz. slice	282
Beef	.8-oz. slice	279
Cotto:		
Regular	.8-oz. slice	290
Regular	1-oz. slice	369
Beef	.5-oz. slice	179
Beef	.8-oz. slice	294
Hard, all meat	.3-oz. slice	163
(Swift):		
Genoa	1 oz.	642
Hard	1 oz.	562
SALISBURY STEAK:		
Canned (Morton House)	⅓ of 12½-oz. can	512
Frozen:		
(Armour) *Dinner Classics*	11-oz. meal	1460
(Banquet):		
Dinner:		
American Favorite	11-oz. dinner	1333
Extra Helping	19-oz. dinner	2175
Entree for One	5 oz.	766
Family Entree	2-lb. pkg.	5100
(Blue Star) *Dining Lite*, with creole sauce	9½-oz. meal	1460

Food and Description	Measure or Quantity	Sodium (milligrams)
(Green Giant):		
Baked, with gravy	½ of entree	1095
Boil'N Bag, with creole sauce	9-oz. entree	910
Twin pouch, with mashed potatoes	11-oz. entree	1515
(Stouffer's) *Lean Cuisine,* with Italian style sauce & vegetables	9½-oz. meal	820
(Swanson):		
Regular:		
Dinner	11-oz. dinner	1050
Entree	5½-oz. entree	650
Hungry Man:		
Dinner:	16½-oz. dinner	1630
Entree	11¾-oz. entree	1340
Main Course	8½-oz. entree	1400
(Weight Watchers) beef, Romana	8¾-oz.	990
SALMON:		
Chinook or King (USDA):		
Raw:		
Steak	1 lb. (weighed whole)	180
Meat only	4 oz.	51
Canned, solids & liq., including bones	4 oz.	51
Chum, canned (USDA) solids & liq., including bones	4 oz.	60
Coho, canned (USDA) solids & liq., including bones, no salt added	4 oz.	54
Keta, canned (Bumble Bee) solids & liq.	½ cup	536
Pink or Humpback (USDA):		
Raw:		
Steak	1 lb. (weighed whole)	255
Meat only	4 oz.	73

Food and Description	Measure or Quantity	Sodium (milligrams)
Canned, solids & liq.:		
(USDA) including bones, not salted	4 oz.	73
(USDA) salted	4 oz.	439
(Bumble Bee)	½ cup	542
(Del Monte)	7¾-oz. can	1220
(Featherweight) pink, low sodium	3⅞-oz. can	77
Sockeye or Red or Blueback, canned, solids & liq.:		
(USDA) not salted	4 oz.	54
(Bumble Bee) including bones	½ cup (4 oz.)	455
Del Monte) salted	7¾-oz. can	1169
Unspecified kind of salmon (USDA) baked or broiled with vegetable shortening	4.2-oz. steak (approx. 4″ × 3″ × ½″)	139
Dietetic, canned (S&W) *Nutradiet*	½ cup	45
SALT:		
Regular:		
Butter-flavored (French's) imitation	1 tsp. (3.6 g.)	1090
Hickory smoke (French's)	1 tsp. (4 g.)	1170
Seasoned (French's)	1 tsp.	1230
Table:		
(USDA)	1 tsp. (5.5 g.)	2132
(Morton) iodized	1 tsp. (6.5 g.)	2544
Lite Salt (Morton) iodized	1 tsp. (6 g.)	1188
Substitute:		
(Adolph's):		
Regular	1 tsp. (6 g.)	<1
Packet	8-g. packet	Tr.
Seasoned	1 tsp.	<1
(Dia-Mel) *Salt-It*	1 tsp.	2
(Estee)	1 tsp.	<2
(Morton):		
Regular	1 tsp. (6 g.)	<1

Food and Description	Measure or Quantity	Sodium (milligrams)
Seasoned	1 tsp. (6 g.)	<1
SALT PORK, raw (USDA):		
With skin	1 lb. (weighed with skin)	5278
Without skin	1 oz.	344
SAND DAB (USDA) raw:		
Whole	1 lb. (weighed whole)	117
Meat only	4 oz.	88
SANDWICH SPREAD:		
Regular:		
(USDA)	1 T. (.5 oz.)	94
(Best Foods/Hellmann's)	1 T. (.5 oz.)	191
(Best Foods/Hellmann's)	½ cup (4.2 oz.)	1526
(Oscar Mayer)	1-oz. serving	261
Dietetic or low calorie (USDA)	1 T. (.5 oz.)	94
SARDINE:		
Raw (HEW/FAO):		
Whole	1 lb. (weighed whole)	249
Meat only	4 oz.	113
Canned:		
Atlantic:		
(USDA) in oil:		
Solids & liq.	3¾-oz. can	541
Drained solids, with skin & bones	3¾-oz. can	757
(Del Monte) in tomato sauce, solids & liq.	7½-oz. can	827
Imported (Underwood):		
In mustard sauce	3¾-oz. can	850
In tomato sauce	3¾-oz. can	850
Norwegian:		
(Granadaisa Brand) in tomato sauce	3¾-oz. can	434
(King David Brand) in olive oil	3¾-oz. can	842
(Queen Helga Brand) in sild oil	3¾-oz. can	603
(Underwood) in oil	3¾-oz. can	800

Food and Description	Measure or Quantity	Sodium (milligrams)
Pacific (USDA) in brine or mustard, solids & liq.	4 oz.	862
SAUCE (See also **SAUCE MIX**):		
A-1	1 T. (.6 oz.)	275
Barbecue:		
(USDA)	1 T. (.6 oz.)	130
Chris & Pitt's	1 T.	141
(Estee) dietetic	1 T.	3
(French's):		
Regular or hot	1 T. (.6 oz.)	250
Smoky	1 T. (.6 oz.)	280
(Hunt's) all natural, any flavor	1 T.	190
Open Pit:		
Regular	1 T. (.6 oz.)	236
Hot & spicy	1 T.	163
Hickory smoked flavor	1 T.	232
With minced onions	1 T.	252
Burrito (Del Monte)	¼ cup	355
Cheese (Snow's) welsh rarebit	½ cup	460
Chili (See **CHILI SAUCE**)		
Cocktail (See Seafood)		
Escoffier Sauce:		
Diable	1 T. (.6 oz.)	160
Robert	1 T.	70
Famous (Durkee)	1 T.	67
Hot (Gebhardt)	1 tsp.	90
H.P. Steak Sauce (Lea & Perrins)	1 T.	280
Italian (Contadina)	4 fl. oz.	601
Mexican (Pritikin) dietetic	1 oz.	9
Newberg (Snow's)	⅓ cup	520
Salsa Mexicana (Contadina)	4 fl. oz.	570
Salsa Picante, hot table sauce (Del Monte)	¼ cup (2 oz.)	405
Salsa Roja, mild table sauce (Del Monte)	¼ cup (2 oz.)	510
Seafood (Del Monte) cocktail	1 T. (.6 oz.)	228
Soy:		
(USDA)	1 oz.	2077

Food and Description	Measure or Quantity	Sodium (milligrams)
(USDA)	1 T. (.6 oz.)	1246
(Kikkoman)	1 T.	921
(La Choy)	1 T. (.5 oz.)	974
Steak (Dawn Fresh) with mushrooms	2 oz.	300
Steak Supreme	1 T.	125
Sweet & sour:		
(Contadina)	2 fl. oz.	250
(La Choy)	1 T.	320
Tabasco	¼ tsp.	9
Taco:		
(El Molino) red, mild	1 T.	85
(Old El Paso):		
Hot	1 T.	66
Mild	1 T.	63
(Ortega) hot	1 oz.	207
Tartar:		
(USDA)	1 T. (.5 oz.)	99
Hellmann's (Best Foods)	1 T. (.5 oz.)	182
Teriyaki (Kikkoman)	1 T. (.6 oz.)	612
Tomato (See **TOMATO SAUCE**)		
White (USDA) medium	1 cup (9 oz.)	966
Worcestershire:		
(French's) regular or smoke	1 T.	200
(Lea & Perrins)	1 T. (.6 oz.)	175
SAUCE MIX:		
Regular:		
A la King (Durkee)	1.1-oz. pkg.	1384
*Cheese:		
(Durkee)	½ cup	446
(French's)	½ cup	850
Hollandaise:		
(Durkee)	1-oz. pkg.	548
*(French's)	1 T.	97
*Sour cream:		
(Durkee)	⅔ cup	727
(French's)	2½ T.	130
*Stroganoff (French's)	⅓ cup	490

Food and Description	Measure or Quantity	Sodium (milligrams)
*Sweet & sour:		
(Durkee)	½ cup	526
(French's)	½ cup	135
(Kikkoman)	1 T.	63
*Teriyaki (French's)	1 T.	590
*White (Durkee)	1 cup	696
Dietetic, lemon butter (Weight Watchers)	1 pkg.	1895
SAUERKRAUT, canned:		
(USDA) solids & liq.	1 cup (8.3 oz.)	1755
(Claussen) drained	½ cup (2.7 oz.)	491
(Comstock) solids, & liq.:		
Regular	½ cup	800
Bavarian	½ cup	600
(Del Monte) solids & liq.	1 cup (8 oz.)	1550
(Silver Floss):		
Regular:		
Can	½ cup (4 oz.)	750
Jar	½ cup	750
Polybag	½ cup (4 oz.)	750
Bavarian Kraut	½ cup	750
Krispy Kraut	½ cup (4 oz.)	750
(Vlasic) old fashioned, solids & liq.	1 oz.	284
SAUERKRAUT JUICE, canned		
(USDA)	½ cup (4.3 oz.)	952
SAUSAGE:		
Brown & serve:		
*(Hormel)	1 link	215
*(Swift):		
Bacon & sausage	.7-oz. link	173
Beef	.7-oz. link	169
Kountry Kured	.7-oz. link	171
Original flavor	.7-oz. link	169
Links (Ohse) hot	1 oz.	310
Patty (Hormel):		
Hot	1 patty	549
Mild	1 patty	541
Polish-style:		
(Eckrich) meat:		
Regular	1 oz.	260

Food and Description	Measure or Quantity	Sodium (milligrams)
Skinless	1 oz.	250
(Hormel):		
Regular	1 sausage	287
Kielbasa	½ link	826
Kolbase	3 oz.	904
(Ohse):		
Regular	1 oz.	290
Hot	1 oz.	270
Pork:		
(USDA) link or bulk:		
Uncooked	1-oz. serving	210
Cooked	1-oz. serving	272
*(Hormel) *Little Sizzlers*	1 sausage	96
(Jimmy Dean) uncooked	2-oz. serving	338
*(Oscar Mayer):		
Little Friers	1 link	206
Patties, Southern Brand:		
1-oz. patty	.7 oz. cooked	185
2-oz. patty	1.3 oz. cooked	370
Roll (Eckrich)	1 oz.	340
Smoked:		
(Eckrich):		
Beef:		
Regular	2 oz.	520
Smok-Y-Links	.8-oz. link	200
Cheese	2 oz.	500
Ham, *Smok-Y-Links*	.8 oz.	280
Maple flavor, *Smok-Y-Links*	.8 oz.	200
Meat	2 oz.	530
Meat, skinless	2 oz.	490
(Hormel) Smokies:		
Regular	1 sausage	298
Cheese	1 sausage	311
(Ohse)	1 oz.	320
(Oscar Mayer):		
Regular	1½-oz. link	432
Regular	4-oz. link	1135
Beef	1½-oz. link	425
Cheese	1½-oz. link	448
Summer (See **THURINGER**)		

Food and Description	Measure or Quantity	Sodium (milligrams)
Turkey (Ohse)	1 oz.	180
Vienna:		
(Hormel) regular	1 sausage	120
(Libby's) in beef broth:		
5-oz. can	1 link	94
9-oz. can	1 link	86
SAUTERNES:		
(B&G) 13% alcohol	3 fl. oz.	3
SAVORY (French's)	1 tsp. (1.4 grams)	Tr.
SCALLION (See **ONION, GREEN**)		
SCALLOP:		
Raw (USDA) muscle only	4 oz.	289
Steamed (USDA)	4 oz.	301
Frozen:		
(Mrs. Paul's):		
breaded & fried	½ of 7-oz. pkg.	545
Mediterrean	11-oz. entree	775
(Stouffer's) *Lean Cuisine,* oriental	11-oz. meal	1325
SCALLOP & SHRIMP		
SCOTCH (See **DISTILLED LIQUOR**)		
MARINER, frozen (Stouffer's) with rice	10¼-oz. meal	1120
SCREWDRIVER COCKTAIL (Mr. Boston)	3 fl. oz.	104
SCROD, frozen (Gorton's) *Light Recipe,* stuffed	1 pkg.	490
SEAFOOD DINNER OR ENTREE, frozen (Armour) *Classic Lites*	11½-oz. meal	1240
SEAFOOD NEWBERG, frozen:		
(Armour) *Dinner Classics*	10½-oz. meal	1780
(Mrs. Paul's)	8½-oz. entree	610
SEAFOOD PLATTER, frozen (Mrs. Paul's) combination, breaded & fried	9-oz. pkg.	1340

Food and Description	Measure or Quantity	Sodium (milligrams)
SEGO DIET FOOD, canned:		
Regular:		
Very banana, strawberry & vanilla	1 can	360
Very chocolate, chocolate malt & Dutch chocolate	1 can	445
Lite:		
Chocolate, chocolate jamocha almond, chocolate malt, double chocolate & Dutch chocolate	1 can	475
French vanilla, strawberry & vanilla	1 can	390
SESAME NUT MIX, canned (Planters) oil roasted	1 oz.	220
SESAME SEEDS, dry (USDA) whole	1 oz.	17
7-GRAIN CEREAL (Loma Linda):		
Crunchy	1 oz.	90
No sugar	1 oz.	75
SHAD (USDA):		
Raw:		
Whole	1 lb. (weighed whole)	118
Meat only	4 oz.	61
Cooked, home recipe:		
Baked with butter or margarine & bacon slices	4 oz.	90
Creole	4 oz.	83
SHAKE 'n BAKE:		
Chicken:		
Regular	2.4-oz. pkg.	2363
Barbecue style	3½ oz. pkg.	3280
Crispy country mild	2.4-oz. pkg.	2041
Fish	2-oz. pkg.	1049
Italian	2.4-oz. pkg.	2098
Pork	2.4-oz. pkg.	2541
Pork & ribs, barbecue style	2.9-oz. pkg.	2644
SHAKEY'S:		
Chicken & potatoes:		
3-piece meal	1 order	2293

Food and Description	Measure or Quantity	Sodium (milligrams)
5-piece meal	1 order	5327
Ham & cheese, hot	1 sandwich	2135
Pizza:		
Thick:		
Cheese	13″ pie	5740
Onion, green pepper, olive, mushroom	13″ pie	3950
Pepperoni	13″ pie	4940
Sausage, mushroom	13″ pie	4450
Sausage, pepperoni	13″ pie	6260
Special	13″ pie	6060
Thin:		
Cheese	13″ pie	3160
Onion, green pepper, olive, mushroom	13″ pie	3950
Pepperoni	13″ pie	4550
Sausage, mushroom	13″ pie	4160
Sausage, pepperoni	13″ pie	5870
Special	13″ pie	5670
Potatoes	15-piece order	3703
Spaghetti with meat sauce & garlic bread	1 order	1904
SHALLOT, raw (USDA):		
With skin	1 oz.	3
With skin removed	1 oz.	3
SHELLS, PASTA, STUFFED, frozen:		
(Buitoni) jumbo:		
Cheese	5½ oz.	483
Florentine	5½ oz.	323
(Celentano):		
Broccoli & cheese	11½-oz. pkg.	480
Cheese:		
Without sauce	½ of 12½-oz. box	265
With sauce	½ of 16-oz. box	425
(Stouffer):		
Beef & spinach with tomato sauce	9-oz. pkg.	1315
Cheese with meat sauce	9-oz. pkg.	1310
Chicken with cheese sauce	9-oz. pkg.	1060

Food and Description	Measure or Quantity	Sodium (milligrams)
*SHELLS & SAUCE (Lipton):		
creamy garlic	½ cup	535
Herb tomato	½ cup	435
SHERBET OR SORBET:		
Cassis (Häagen-Dazs)	4 fl. oz.	11
Daiquiri Ice (Baskin-Robbins)	4 fl. oz.	18
Lemon (Häagen-Dazs)	4 fl. oz.	22
Orange:		
(Baskin-Robbins)	4 fl. oz.	46
(Borden)	½ cup	40
(Häagen-Dazs)	4 fl. oz.	22
Raspberry:		
(Baskin-Robbins)	4 fl. oz.	42
(Häagen-Dazs)	4 fl. oz.	17
(Sealtest)	½ cup	30
SHERRY:		
Regular:		
(Gold Seal) 19% alcohol	3 fl. oz.	3
(Great Western) Solera, 18% alcohol	3 fl. oz.	31
Cocktail (Gold Seal) 19% alcohol	3 fl. oz.	3
Cream:		
(Gold Seal) 19% alcohol		
(Great Western) Solera, 18% alcohol	3 fl. oz.	32
Dry (Great Western) Solera, 18% alcohol	3 fl. oz.	34
SHREDDED WHEAT:		
(USDA):		
Plain, without salt	1 oz.	<1
With malt, salt & sugar	1 oz.	198
(Nabisco)	Any amount	0
(Quaker)	.7-oz. biscuit	<1
(Sunshine) regular or bite size	Any quantity	0
SHRIMP:		
Raw (USDA):		
Whole	1 lb. (weighed in shell)	438
Meat only	4 oz.	159

Food and Description	Measure or Quantity	Sodium (milligrams)
Cooked, french fried (USDA) dipped in egg, breadcrumbs and flour or in batter	4 oz.	211
Frozen (San-Sea) cooked	5 oz.	330
SHRIMP COCKTAIL (Sau-Sea) canned or frozen	4 oz.	1020
SHRIMP DINNER OR ENTREE, frozen:		
(Armour) *Classic Lites*, in sherried cream sauce	10½-oz. meal	1220
(Blue Star) *Dining Lite*, creole with rice	10-oz. meal	820
(Conagra) *Light & Elegant*	10-oz. meal	1050
(Gorton's) *Light Recipe*:		
Oriental	1 pkg.	740
& pasta medley	1 pkg.	550
Scampi	1 pkg.	420
Stuffed, baked	1 pkg.	950
(Mrs. Paul's):		
Oriental	11-oz. meal	940
Parmesan	11-oz. meal	1185
(Stouffer's) Newberg	6½-oz. serving	555
SLENDER (Carnation):		
Bar:		
Chocolate	1 bar	142
Chocolate chip	1 bar	157
Chocolate peanut butter	1 bar	142
Vanilla	1 bar	160
Canned:		
Banana & strawberry	1 can	430
Chocolate	1 can	515
Chocolate fudge or vanilla	1 can	550
Chocolate Malt	1 can	530
Milk chocolate	1 can	520
Mix	1 pkg.	110
SLOPPY JOE:		
Canned:		
(Libby's) beef	⅓ cup (2½ oz.)	190
(Morton House) barbecue sauce with beef	⅓ of 15-oz. can	919

Food and Description	Measure or Quantity	Sodium (milligrams)
Frozen (Banquet) *Cookin' Bag*	5-oz. pkg.	730
SLOPPY JOE SAUCE (Ragú)		
Joe Sauce	3½ oz.	645
SLOPPY JOE SEASONING MIX:		
*(Durkee):		
Regular	1¼ cup	1788
Pizza flavor	1¼ cup	1515
(French's)	1½-oz. pkg.	3040
*(Hunt's) *Manwich*	5.9-oz. serving	590
SMOKED SAUSAGE (See SAUSAGE)		
SMURF BERRY CRUNCH, cereal (Post)	1 cup (1 oz.)	65
SNACK BAR (Pepperidge Farm):		
Apple nut, apricot raspberry, blueberry or date nut	1 piece	90
Brownie nut	1 piece	100
Chocolate chip macaroon, coconut macaroon or raisin spice	1 piece	80
SNACK (See **CRACKER, POPCORN, POTATO CHIP,** etc.)		
SNO BALLS (Hostess)	1½-oz. piece	170
SOFT DRINK:		
Sweetened:		
Aspen	6 fl. oz.	5
Birch beer (Canada Dry)	6 fl. oz.	14
Bitter lemon:		
(Canada Dry)	6 fl. oz.	13
(Schweppes)	6 fl. oz.	2
Bubble Up	6 fl. oz.	16
Cactus Cooler (Canada Dry)	6 fl. oz.	16
Cherry:		
(Canada Dry) wild	6 fl. oz.	16
(Shasta) black	6 fl. oz.	13
Cherry-Lime (Spree)	6 fl. oz.	1
Chocolate (Yoo-Hoo)	6 fl. oz.	87
Citrus mist (Shasta)	6 fl. oz.	9

Food and Description	Measure or Quantity	Sodium (milligrams)
Club:		
(Canada Dry)	6 fl. oz.	39
(Schweppes)	6 fl. oz.	25
(Shasta)	6 fl. oz.	23
Cola:		
(Canada Dry) *Jamaica*	6 fl. oz.	Tr.
Coca-Cola:		
Regular or caffeine free	6 fl. oz.	3
Cherry or classic	6 fl. oz.	7
Pepsi-Cola, regular or no caffeine	6 fl. oz.	1
(Royal Crown)	6 fl. oz.	<1
(Shasta) regular or cherry	6 fl. oz.	22
(Slice) cherry	6 fl. oz.	2
(Spree)	6 fl. oz.	Tr.
Cream:		
(Canada Dry)	6 fl. oz.	14
(Shasta)	6 fl. oz.	12
Dr. Diablo	6 fl. oz.	7
Dr. Nehi	6 fl. oz.	13
Dr Pepper	6 fl. oz.	9
Fruit punch:		
(Nehi)	6 fl. oz.	8
(Shasta)	6 fl. oz.	16
Ginger ale:		
(Canada Dry):		
Regular	6 fl. oz.	5
Golden	6 fl. oz.	18
(Fanta)	6 fl. oz.	13
(Nehi)	6 fl. oz.	Tr.
(Schweppes)	6 fl. oz.	10
(Shasta)	6 fl. oz.	11
(Spree)	6 fl. oz.	Tr.
Ginger beer (Schweppes)	6 fl. oz.	30
Grape:		
(Canada Dry) concord	6 fl. oz.	16
(Fanta)	6 fl. oz.	7
(Hi-C)	6 fl. oz.	6
(Nehi)	6 fl. oz.	8
(Patio)	6 fl. oz.	21

Food and Description	Measure or Quantity	Sodium (milligrams)
(Schweppes)	6 fl. oz.	15
(Shasta)	6 fl. oz.	23
Grapefruit:		
(Schwepps)	6 fl. oz.	28
(Spree)	6 fl. oz.	Tr.
Half & half (Canada Dry)	6 fl. oz.	13
Hi Spot (Canada Dry)	6 fl. oz.	19
Island Lime (Canada Dry)	6 fl. oz.	14
Kick (Royal Crown)	6 fl.oz.	25
Lemon (Hi-C)	6 fl. oz.	6
Lemon-Lime (Shasta)	6 fl. oz.	9
Lemon sour (Spree)	6 fl. oz.	12
Lemon tangerine (Spree)	6 fl. oz.	Tr.
Mandarin lime (Spree)	6 fl. oz.	Tr.
Mello Yello	6 fl. oz.	13
Mr. PiBB	6 fl. oz.	11
Mt. Dew	6 fl. oz.	16
Orange:		
(Canada Dry) *Sunripe*	6 fl. oz.	16
(Fanta)	6 fl. oz.	7
(Hi-C)	6 fl. oz.	7
(Minute Maid)	6 fl. oz.	Tr.
(Nehi)	6 fl. oz.	11
(Patio)	6 fl. oz.	21
(Schweppes) sparkling	6 fl. oz.	17
(Shasta)	6 fl. oz.	14
(Slice)	6 fl. oz.	11
Peach (Nehi)	6 fl. oz.	16
Pineapple (Canada Dry)	6 fl. oz.	16
Punch (Hi-C)	6 fl. oz.	6
Purple Passion (Canada Dry)	6 fl. oz.	14
Quinine or tonic water:		
(Canada Dry)	6 fl. oz.	5
(Schweppes)	6 fl. oz.	8
Red berry (Shasta)	6 fl. oz.	10
Red Pop (Shasta)	6 fl. oz.	10
Root beer:		
Barrelhead (Canada Dry)	6 fl. oz.	13
(Dad's)	6 fl. oz.	14
(Fanta)	6 fl. oz.	10

Food and Description	Measure or Quantity	Sodium (milligrams)
(Nehi)	6 fl. oz.	9
On Tap	6 fl. oz.	9
(Patio)	6 fl. oz.	2
Ramblin'	6 fl. oz.	10
Rooti (Canada Dry)	6 fl. oz.	13
(Schweppes)	6 fl. oz.	17
(Shasta) draft	6 fl. oz.	15
(Spree)	6 fl. oz.	1
7-UP	6 fl. oz.	10
Slice	6 fl. oz.	5
Sprite	6 fl. oz.	22
Strawberry:		
(Canada Dry)	6 fl. oz.	16
(Nehi) can	6 fl. oz.	7
(Shasta)	6 fl. oz.	23
Tahitian Treat (Canada Dry)	6 fl. oz.	16
Teem	6 fl. oz.	16
Tom Collins or collins mix		
(Canada Dry)	6 fl. oz.	13
Tropical blend (Spree)	6 fl. oz.	1
Upper 10 (Royal Crown)	6 fl. oz.	20
Whiskey Sour (Canada Dry)	6 fl. oz.	13
Wink (Canada Dry)	6 fl. oz.	14
Dietetic or low calorie:		
Apple (Slice)	6 fl. oz.	2
Birch beer (Shasta)	6 fl. oz.	17
Bubble Up:		
Diet	6 fl. oz.	16
Sugar free	6 fl. oz.	48
Cherry:		
(No-Cal)	6 fl. oz.	44
(Shasta) black	6 fl. oz.	20
Chocolate (No-Cal)	6 fl. oz.	33
Coffee (No-Cal)	6 fl. oz.	45
Cola:		
(Canada Dry)	6 fl. oz.	20
Coca-Cola	6 fl. oz.	4
Diet Rite	6 fl. oz.	<1
(No-Cal)	6 fl. oz.	18
Pepsi, diet, light or free	6 fl. oz.	2

Food and Description	Measure or Quantity	Sodium (milligrams)
(Shasta) regular or cherry	6 fl. oz.	18
(Slice) cherry	6 fl. oz.	2
Cream:		
(No-Cal)	6 fl. oz.	33
(Shasta)	6 fl. oz.	21
Dr. Pepper	6 fl. oz.	Tr.
Fresca	6 fl. oz.	Tr.
Ginger ale:		
(Canada Dry)	6 fl. oz.	22
(No-Cal)	6 fl. oz.	30
(Shasta)	6 fl. oz.	20
Grape (Shasta)	6 fl. oz.	18
Grapefruit (Shasta)	6 fl. oz.	18
Lemon-lime:		
(Minute Maid)	6 fl. oz.	1
(No-Cal)	6 fl. oz.	29
(Shasta)	6 fl. oz.	23
Mr. PiBB	6 fl. oz.	19
Orange:		
(Canada Dry)	6 fl. oz.	19
(Fanta)	6 fl. oz.	24
(Minute Maid)	6 fl. oz.	Tr.
(No-Cal)	6 fl. oz.	19
(Shasta)	6 fl. oz.	19
(Slice)	6 fl. oz.	11
Quinine or tonic water:		
(Canada Dry)	6 fl. oz.	18
(No-Cal)	6 fl. oz.	15
RC 100 (Royal Crown)	6 fl. oz.	19
Red Pop (Shasta)	6 fl. oz.	23
Root beer:		
Barrelhead (Canada Dry)	6 fl. oz.	19
(Dad's):		
Diet	6 fl. oz.	14
Sugar free	6 fl. oz.	41
(No-Cal)	6 fl. oz.	30
(Shasta) draft	6 fl. oz.	18
7-UP	6 fl. oz.	16
Slice	6 fl. oz.	5
Sprite	6 fl. oz.	Tr.

Food and Description	Measure or Quantity	Sodium (milligrams)
Strawberry (Shasta)	6 fl. oz.	18
SOLE:		
Raw (USDA):		
Whole	1 lb. (weighed whole)	117
Meat only	4 oz.	88
Frozen:		
(Frionor) *Norway Gourmet*	4-oz. fillet	350
(Gorton's):		
Fishmarket Fresh	4 oz.	110
Light Recipe, with lemon butter sauce	1 pkg.	730
(Mrs. Paul's) fillets, breaded & fried	6-oz. fillet	700
(Van de Kamp's) batter dipped, french fried	2-oz. piece	289
(Weight Watchers) in lemon sauce, 2-compartment meal	9⅛-oz. pkg.	810
SOUFFLE:		
(USDA) home recipe		
Frozen (Stouffer's):	¼ of 7″ souffle (3.9 oz.)	400
Cheese	6 oz.	1260
Corn	4 oz.	510
SOUP:		
Canned, regular pack:		
*Asparagus (Campbell), condensed, cream of	8-oz. serving	900
Bean (Campbell):		
Chunky, with ham, old fashioned	11-oz. can	1150
*Condensed, with bacon	8-oz. serving	860
Bean, black:		
*(Campbell) condensed	8-oz. serving	980
(Crosse & Blackwell)	6½-oz. serving	757
Beef:		
(Campbell):		
Chunky:		
Regular	10¾-oz. can	1110
Stroganoff	10¾-oz. can	1290

Food and Description	Measure or Quantity	Sodium (milligrams)
*Condensed:		
Regular	8-oz. serving	855
Broth	8-oz. serving	875
Consommé	8-oz. serving	785
Noodle, regular	8-oz. serving	875
(Swanson) broth	7¼-oz. can	750
Celery:		
*(Campbell) condensed, cream of	8-oz. serving	860
*(Rokeach):		
Prepared with milk	10-oz. serving	1020
Prepared with water	10-oz. serving	950
*Cheddar cheese (Campbell)	8-oz. serving	800
Chicken:		
(Campbell):		
Chunky:		
Old fashioned	10¾-oz. can	1340
& rice	19-oz. can	2160
Vegetable	19-oz. can	2200
*Condensed):		
Alphabet	8-oz. serving	870
Broth:		
Plain	8-oz. serving	890
& rice	8-oz. serving	880
Cream of	8-oz. serving	850
Mushroom, creamy	8-oz. serving	940
NoodleOs	8-oz. serving	840
& rice	8-oz. serving	840
Vegetable	8-oz. serving	870
*Semi-condensed, *Soup For One*, vegetable, full flavored	11-oz. serving	1500
(Swanson) broth	7¼-oz. can	910
Chili beef (Campbell) *Chunky*	11-oz. can	1150
Chowder:		
Clam:		
Manhattan style:		
(Campbell):		
Chunky	19-oz. can	2260
*Condensed	8-oz. serving	860

Food and Description	Measure or Quantity	Sodium (milligrams)
(Crosse & Blackwell)	6½-oz. serving	803
*(Snow's) condensed	7½-oz. serving	630
New England style:		
*(Campbell):		
Condensed:		
Made with milk	8-oz. serving	930
Made with water	8-oz. serving	880
Semi-condensed, *Soup for One:*		
Made with milk	11-oz. serving	1410
Made with water	11-oz. serving	1360
(Crosse & Blackwell)	6½-oz. serving	637
*(Gorton's)	1 can	2960
*(Snow's) condensed	7½-oz. serving	670
*Corn (Snow's) New England, condensed, made with milk	7½-oz. serving	640
*Fish (Snow's) New England, condensed, made with milk	7½-oz. serving	620
*Seafood (Snow's) New England, condensed, made with milk	7½-oz. serving	690
Consomme madrilene (Crosse & Blackwell)	6½-oz. serving	609
Crab (Crosse & Blackwell)	6½-oz. serving	933
Gazpacho (Crosse & Blackwell)	6½-oz. serving	600
Ham'n butter bean (Campbell) *Chunky*	10¾-oz. serving	1180
Lentil (Crosse & Blackwell) with ham	6½-oz. serving	979
*Meatball alphabet (Campbell) condensed	8-oz. serving	970
Minestrone:		
(Campbell):		
Chunky	19-oz. can	1880
*Condensed	8-oz. serving	930
(Crosse & Blackwell)	6½-oz. serving	720
Mushroom:		
*(Campbell), condensed:		

Food and Description	Measure or Quantity	Sodium (milligrams)
Cream of	8-oz. serving	820
Golden	8-oz. serving	900
(Crosse & Blackwell) cream of bisque	6½-oz. serving	923
*(Rokeach) cream of, prepared with water	10-oz. serving	1050
*Noodle (Campbell) & ground beef	8-oz. serving	840
*Onion (Campbell):		
Regular	8-oz. serving	950
Cream of:		
Made with water	8-oz. serving	830
Made with water & milk	8-oz. serving	860
*Oyster stew (Campbell):		
Made with milk	8-oz. serving	900
Made with water	8-oz. serving	850
*Pea, green (Campbell)	8-oz. serving	840
Pea, split (Campbell):		
Chunky, with ham	19-oz. can	1900
*Condensed, with ham & bacon	8-oz. serving	800
*Pepper pot (Campbell)	8-oz. serving	960
*Potato (Campbell) cream of:		
Made with water	8-oz. serving	930
Made with water & milk	8-oz. serving	960
Shrimp:		
*(Campbell) condensed, cream of:		
Made with milk	8-oz. serving	850
Made with water	8-oz. serving	790
(Crosse & Blackwell)	6½-oz. serving	1459
Steak & potato (Campbell) *Chunky*	19-oz. can	2220
Tomato:		
(Campbell):		
Condensed:		
Regular:		
Made with milk	8-oz. serving	770
Made with water	8-oz. serving	720
& rice, old fashioned	8-oz. serving	760

Food and Description	Measure or Quantity	Sodium (milligrams)
Semi-condensed, *Soup For One*, Royale	11-oz. serving	1080
*(Rokeach), made with water	10-oz. serving	980
Turkey (Campbell) *Chunky*, & vegetable	18¾-oz. can	2160
Vegetable:		
(Campbell):		
Chunky:		
Regular	19-oz. can	1940
Beef, old fashioned	19-oz. serving	2140
*Condensed:		
Regular	8-oz. serving	770
Beef	8-oz. serving	820
*Semi-condensed, *Soup For One*, old world	11-oz. serving	1470
*(Rokeach) vegetarian	10-oz. serving	1055
Vichyssoise (Crosse & Blackwell)	6½-oz. serving	702
*Won ton (Campbell)	8-oz. serving	870
Canned, dietetic pack:		
Bean (Pritikin) navy	½ of 14¾-oz. can	170
Beef (Campbell) chunky & mushroom, low sodium	10¾-oz. can	65
Chicken:		
(Campbell) low sodium:		
Broth	10½-oz. can	70
Chunky	10¾-oz. can	95
*(Dia-Mel) & noodle	8-oz. serving	15
(Pritikin):		
Broth, defatted	½ of 13¾-oz. can	175
Gumbo	½ of 14¾-oz. can	180
& ribbon pasta or vegetable	½ of 14½-oz. can	175
Chowder (Pritikin) any style	½ of 14¾-oz. can	170
Lentil (Pritikin)	½ of 14¾-oz. can	170
Minestrone:		
(Estee)	7½-oz. can	30
(Pritikin)	½ of 14¾-oz. can	130
Mushroom (Campbell) cream of, low sodium	10½-oz. can	55

Food and Description	Measure or Quantity	Sodium (milligrams)
Pea, split (Campbell) low sodium	10¾-oz. can	25
Tomato:		
(Campbell) low sodium, with tomato pieces	10½-oz. can	40
(Pritikin)	½ of 14½-oz. can	125
Turkey (Pritikin) vegetable, with ribbon pasta	½ of 14¾-oz. can	160
Vegetable:		
(Campbell) Chunky	10¾-oz. can	60
(Estee) & beef	7½-oz. can	130
(Pritikin)	½ of 14¾-oz. can	150
Vegetable (Campbell) low sodium, Chunky	10¾-oz. can	60
Frozen:		
*Barley & mushroom:		
(Mother's Own)	8-oz. serving	490
(Tabatchnick)	8-oz. serving	759
Bean (Kettle Ready)	8-oz. serving	1606
Bean & barley (Tabatchnick)	8-oz. serving	493
Beef (Kettle Ready) vegetable	8-oz. serving	1034
Broccoli (Tabatchnick) cream of	7½-oz. serving	507
Cauliflower (Kettle Ready) cream of	8-oz. serving	1011
Cheddar cheese (Kettle Ready)	8-oz. serving	994
Chicken (Kettle Ready):		
Cream of	8-oz. serving	1163
Gumbo	8-oz. serving	1097
Noodle	8-oz. serving	1150
Chowder, clam:		
Boston (Kettle Ready)	8-oz. serving	1215
Manhattan (Kettle Ready)	8-oz. serving	847
New England:		
(Kettle Ready)	8-oz. serving	745
(Stouffer's)	8-oz. serving	510
Lentil (Tabatchnick)	8-oz. serving	636
Minstrone:		
(Kettle Ready)	8-oz. serving	1118
(Tabatchnick)	8-oz. serving	561

Food and Description	Measure or Quantity	Sodium (milligrams)
Mushroom (Kettle Ready)		
cream of	8-oz. serving	950
Onion (Kettle Ready) french	8-oz. serving	1330
Pea, split:		
(Kettle Ready) & ham	8-oz. serving	1043
*(Mother's Own)	8-oz. serving	575
(Stouffer's) & ham	8¼-oz. serving	695
Potato:		
(Kettle Ready) cream of	8-oz. serving	834
(Tabatchnick)	8-oz. serving	607
Spinach, cream of:		
(Kettle Ready)	8-oz. serving	855
(Stouffer's)	8-oz. serving	885
(Tabatchnick)	7½-oz. serving	697
Tomato (Kettle Ready)	8-oz. serving	1940
Vegetable:		
(Kettle Ready):		
Hearty	8-oz. serving	970
Nacho	8-oz. serving	981
*(Mother's Own)	8-oz. serving	560
(Tabatchnick)	8-oz. serving	514
*Won ton (La Choy)	½ of 15-oz. pkg.	1050
*Mix (Lipton):		
Regular:		
Beef:		
Cup-A-Soup:		
Regular:		
Noodle	6 fl. oz.	830
Vegetable	6 fl. oz.	820
Lots-A-Noodles	7 fl. oz.	780
Chicken:		
Regular	8 fl. oz.	900
Cup-A-Broth	6 fl. oz.	780
Cup-A-Soup:		
Regular:		
Cream of	6 fl. oz.	840
Rice	6 fl. oz.	750
Country style,		
supreme	6 fl. oz.	870
Hearty, noodle	8 fl. oz.	695

Food and Description	Measure or Quantity	Sodium (milligrams)
Lots-A-Noodle, cream of	7 fl. oz.	755
Mushroom:		
Regular, beef	8 fl. oz.	995
Cup-A-Soup, cream of	6 fl. oz.	830
Noodle:		
Regular:		
With chicken broth	8 fl. oz.	785
Ring-O-Noodle	8 fl. oz.	855
Cup-A-Soup, beef flavored	6 fl. oz.	830
Onion, regular, beefy	8 fl. oz.	640
Pea, *Cup-A-Soup*, green	6 fl. oz.	710
Tomato, *Cup-A-Soup*, regular	6 fl. oz.	650
Vegetable:		
Regular, country	8 fl. oz.	995
Cup-A-Soup, spring	6 fl. oz.	865
Dietetic, *Cup-A-Soup-Trim:*		
Beef	6 fl. oz.	695
Chicken	6 fl. oz.	560
Herb vegetable	6 fl. oz.	560
SOUP GREENS, canned (Durkee)	2½-oz. jar	408
SOURSOP, raw (USDA):		
Whole	1 lb. (weighed with skin & seeds)	43
Flesh only	4 oz.	16
SOYBEAN: (USDA):		
Young seeds, canned:		
Solids & liq.	4 oz.	268
Drained solids	4 oz.	268
Mature seeds:		
Raw	1 lb.	23
Raw	1 cup (7.4 oz.)	10
Cooked	4 oz.	2
Oil roasted:		
(Soy Ahoy) regular, barbecue or garlic	1 oz.	6
(Soytown)	1 oz.	6

Food and Description	Measure or Quantity	Sodium (milligrams)
SOYBEAN CURD or TOFU (USDA):		
Regular	4 oz.	8
Cake	4.2-oz. cake	8
SOYBEAN FLOUR (See FLOUR)		
SOYBEAN GRITS, high fat (USDA)	1 cup (4.9 oz.)	1
SOYBEAN PROTEIN (USDA)	1 oz.	60
SOYBEAN PROTEINATE (USDA)	1 oz.	340
SOYBEAN SPROUT (See BEAN SPROUT)		
SOY SAUCE (See SAUCE, Soy)		
SPAGHETTI (plain spaghetti products are essentially the same in caloric value and carbohydrate content on the same weight basis. The longer the cooking, the more water is absorbed and this affects the nutritive value):		
Dry (USDA):		
Whole	1 oz.	<1
Broken	1 cup (2.5 oz.)	1
Cooked:		
8–10 minutes, "al dente"	1 cup (5.1 oz.)	1
8–10 minutes, "al dente"	4 oz.	1
14–20 minutes, tender	1 cup (4.9 oz.)	1
14–20 minutes, tender	4 oz.	1
Canned, regular pack:		
(Franco-American):		
Regular:		
With meatballs in tomato sauce	7⅜-oz. can	820
In meat sauce	7½-oz. serving	1110
In tomato sauce with cheese	7⅜-oz. serving	810
SpaghettiOs:		
With meatballs in tomato sauce	7⅜-oz. serving	910

Food and Description	Measure or Quantity	Sodium (milligrams)
With sliced franks in tomato sauce	7⅜-oz. serving	990
In tomato & cheese sauce	7⅜-oz. serving	910
(Hormel) & beef, *Short Orders*,	7½-oz. can	1091
(Libby's) & meatballs in tomato sauce	7½-oz. serving	1359
Canned, dietetic pack (Dia-Mel) & meatballs in tomato sauce	8-oz. can	55
Frozen:		
(Armour) *Dinner Classics*, with meatballs	11-oz. meal	1130
(Banquet) with meat sauce	8-oz. casserole	1242
(Blue Star) *Dining Lite*, with beef & mushrooms	11-oz. meal	1550
(Conagra) *Light & Elegant*, & meat sauce	10¼-oz. entree	700
(Green Giant) & meatballs in tomato sauce, twin pouch	10-oz. entree	989
(Morton):		
Casserole	8-oz. casserole	700
Dinner	11½-oz. dinner	1300
(Stouffer's):		
Regular, & meat sauce	14-oz. meal	1970
Lean Cuisine, with beef & mushroom sauce	11½-oz. meal	1455
(Swanson) entree, in tomato sauce with breaded veal	8¼-oz. entree	810
SPAGHETTI SAUCE (See also SPAGHETTI SAUCE MIX and SAUCE, Italian:		
Regular:		
Gardenstyle (Ragú) chunky	¼ of 15½-oz. jar	400
Home style (Ragú)	4 oz.	400
Marinara:		
(Prince)	4 oz.	590
(Ragú)	4 oz.	740
Meat flavored:		
(Hunt's)	4 oz.	520

Food and Description	Measure or Quantity	Sodium (milligrams)
(Prego)	4 oz.	680
(Ragú)	4 oz.	740
Meatless or plain:		
(Prego)	4 oz.	670
(Ragú)	4 oz.	740
Mushroom:		
(Hunt's)	4 oz.	520
(Prego)	4 oz.	640
(Prince)	4 oz.	580
(Ragú)	4 oz.	740
Sausage & green peppers (Prego Plus)	4 oz.	480
Veal (Prego Plus) & sliced mushrooms	4 oz.	380
Dietetic:		
(Featherweight)	⅔ cup	<10
(Furman's)	½ cup	<10
(Prego) no salt added	4 oz.	25
(Pritikin) plain or mushroom	4 oz.	35
*SPAGHETTI SAUCE MIX:		
(Durkee):		
Regular	½ cup	747
Mushroom	1⅓ cups	1553
(French's):		
Italian style	⅝ cup	900
Mushroom	⅝ cup	1045
Thick homemade style	⅞ cup	1455
(Spatini)	½ cup	546
SPAM (Hormel):		
Regular	1-oz. serving	432
& cheese chunks	1-oz. serving	405
Deviled	1 T.	125
Smoke flavored	1 oz.	387
SPANISH MACKEREL, raw (USDA):		
Whole	1 lb.	188
Meat only	4 oz.	77
SPECIAL K, cereal (Kellogg's)	1 cup (1 oz.)	220

Food and Description	Measure or Quantity	Sodium (milligrams)
SPINACH:		
Raw (USDA):		
Untrimmed	1 lb. (weighed with stems & roots)	232
Trimmed or packaged	1 lb.	322
Trimmed, whole leaves	1 cup (1.2 oz.)	23
Trimmed, chopped	1 cup (1.8 oz.)	37
Boiled (USDA) whole leaves, drained	1 cup (5.5 oz.)	78
Canned, regular pack:		
(USDA):		
Solids & liq.	½ cup (4.1 oz.)	274
Drained solids	½ cup	264
(Del Monte) solids & liq.	½ cup (4.1 oz.)	355
(Larsen) *Freshlike,* solids & liq.	½ cup	340
(Sunshine) whole leaf, solids & liq.	½ cup (4.1 oz.)	300
Canned, dietetic or low calorie:		
(USDA) low sodium:		
Solids & liq.	4 oz.	39
Drained solids	4 oz.	36
(Del Monte) no salt added	½ cup	57
(Larsen) *Fresh-Lite,* no salt added	½ cup	20
Frozen:		
(USDA) chopped, boiled, drained	4 oz.	59
(Birds Eye):		
Chopped or leaf	⅓ of 10-oz. pkg.	82
Creamed	⅓ of 9-oz. pkg.	277
& water chestnuts, with selected seasonings	⅓ of 10-oz. pkg.	239
(Green Giant):		
In butter sauce	½ cup	465
Creamed	½ cup	395
Harvest Fresh	½ cup	350
(Stouffer's):		
Creamed	4½ oz.	855
Souffle	4 oz.	600

Food and Description	Measure or Quantity	Sodium (milligrams)
SQUASH, SUMMER:		
Fresh (USDA):		
Crookneck & straightneck, yellow:		
Whole	1 lb. (weighed untrimmed)	4
Boiled, drained:		
Diced	½ cup (3.6 oz.)	1
Slices	½ cup (3.1 oz.)	<1
Scallop, white & pale green:		
Whole	1 lb. (weighed untrimmed)	4
Boiled, drained, mashed	½ cup (4.2 oz.)	1
Zucchini & cocazelle, green:		
Whole	1 lb. (weighed untrimmed)	4
Boiled, drained slices	½ cup (2.7 oz.)	<1
Canned (Del Monte) zucchini, in tomato sauce	½ cup (4.2 oz.)	485
Frozen:		
(USDA):		
Unthawed	4 oz.	3
Boiled, drained	4 oz.	3
(Birds Eye):		
Sliced	⅓ of 10-oz. pkg.	2
Zucchini	⅓ of 10-oz. pkg.	3
(Larsen)	3.3 oz.	0
(McKenzie)	3.3 oz.	19
(Mrs. Paul's) zucchini sticks, batter fried	⅓ of 9-oz. pkg.	630
(Southland) Crookneck	⅕ of 16-oz. pkg.	0
SQUASH, WINTER:		
Fresh (USDA):		
Acorn:		
Whole	1 lb. (weighed with skin & seeds)	3
Baked, flesh only, mashed	½ cup (3.6 oz.)	1
Boiled, mashed	½ cup (4.1 oz.)	1
Butternut:		
Whole	1 lb. (weighed with skin & seeds)	3

Food and Description	Measure or Quantity	Sodium (milligrams)
Baked, flesh only	4 oz.	1
Boiled, flesh only	4 oz.	1
Hubbard:		
Whole	1 lb. (weighed with skin & seeds)	3
Baked, flesh only	4 oz.	1
Boiled, flesh only, diced	½ cup (4.2 oz.)	1
Boiled, flesh only, mashed	½ cup (4.3 oz.)	1
Frozen:		
(USDA) heated	½ cup (4.2 oz.)	1
(Birds Eye)	⅓ of pkg.	2
(Southland) butternut	⅕ of 20-oz. pkg.	0
START, instant breakfast drink	½ cup	7
STEAK & GREEN PEPPERS, frozen (Swanson) in oriental-style sauce	8½-oz. entree	1111
STIR-FRY SEASONING MIX (Kikkoman)	1-oz. pkg.	3
STOCK BASE (French's):		
Beef	1 tsp. (4 g.)	470
Chicken	1 tsp. (3.2 g.)	480
STRAINED FOOD (See **BABY FOOD**)		
STRAWBERRY:		
Fresh (USDA):		
Whole	1 lb. (weighed with caps & stems)	4
Whole, capped	1 cup (5.1 oz.)	1
Canned (USDA) unsweetened or low calorie, water pack, solids & liq.	4 oz.	1
Frozen (Birds Eye):		
Halves	⅓ of 16-oz. pkg.	1
Whole	¼ of 16-oz. pkg.	<1
Whole, quick thaw, in lite syrup	½ of 10-oz. pkg.	5
STRAWBERRY DRINK (Hi-C):		
Canned	6 fl. oz.	<1

Food and Description	Measure or Quantity	Sodium (milligrams)
*Mix	6 fl. oz.	43
STRAWBERRY JELLY,		
sweetened (Home Brands)	1 T.	7
STRAWBERRY NECTAR,		
canned (Libby's)	6 fl. oz.	5
STRAWBERRY PRESERVES or JAM:		
Sweetened (Smucker's)	1 T.	2
Dietetic or low calorie:		
(Dia-Mel)	1 T.	<3
(Diet Delight)	1 T.	30
(Estee)	1 T. (.6 oz.)	Tr.
(Featherweight)	1 T.	40–50
(Louis Sherry) wild	1 T.	<3
STRAWBERRY SHORTCAKE,		
cereal (General Mills)	1 cup	190
STUFFING MIX:		
*Beef (Stove Top)	½ cup	582
Chicken:		
(Pepperidge Farm) pan style	1 oz.	420
*(Stove Top):		
Regular	½ cup	640
Reduced salt	½ cup	559
*Cornbread (Stove Top)	½ cup	666
Cube (Pepperidge Farm) regular or unseasoned	1 oz.	430
Herb seasoned (Pepperidge Farm)	1 oz.	410
*New England Style (Stove Top)	½ cup	636
*Pork (Stove Top)	½ cup	621
*With rice (Stove Top)	½ cup	505
*San Francisco Style (Stove Top)	½ cup	638
*Turkey (Stove Top)	½ cup	634
White bread (Mrs. Cubbison's)	1 oz.	480
STURGEON (USDA) steamed	4 oz.	122
SUCCOTASH:		
Canned solids & liq.:		
(Comstock):		
Cream style	½ cup	350

Food and Description	Measure or Quantity	Sodium (milligrams)
Whole kernel	½ cup	500
(Larsen) *Freshlike*	½ cup (4.5 oz.)	330
(Libby's):		
Cream style	½ cup (4.6 oz.)	317
Whole kernel	¼ of 16-oz. can	262
(Stokely-Van Camp)	½ cup (4.5 oz.)	275
Frozen:		
(USDA) boiled, drained	½ cup (3.4 oz.)	36
(Birds Eye)	⅓ of 10-oz. pkg.	33
(Frosty Acres)	3.3 oz.	47
SUCKER, including **WHITE MULLET** (USDA) raw:		
Whole	1 lb. (weighed whole)	109
Meat only	4 oz.	64
SUGAR, beet or cane (there are no differences in calories and carbohydrates among brands) (USDA):		
Brown:		
Regular	1 lb.	136
Brownulated	1 cup (5.4 oz.)	46
Firm-packed	1 cup (7.5 oz.)	64
Firm-packed	1 T. (.5 oz.)	4
Confectioners':		
Unsifted	1 cup (4.3 oz.)	1
Unsifted	1 T. (8 g.)	<1
Sifted	1 cup (3.4 oz.)	<1
Sifted	1 T. (6 g.)	<1
Stirred	1 cup (4.2 oz.)	1
Stirred	1 T. (8 g.)	<1
Granulated	1 lb.	5
Granulated	1 cup (6.9 oz.)	2
Granulated	1 T. (.4 oz.)	<1
Granulated	1 lump (1⅛" × ¾" × ⅜", 6 g.)	<1
Maple	1 lb.	64
Maple	1¾" × 1¼" × ½" piece (1.2 oz.)	4

Food and Description	Measure or Quantity	Sodium (milligrams)
SUGAR APPLE, raw (USDA):		
Whole	1 lb. (weighed with skin & seeds)	22
Flesh only	4 oz.	12
SUGAR CORN POPS, cereal (Kellogg's)	1 cup (1 oz.)	95
SUGAR CRIPS, cereal (Post)	⅞ cup (1 oz.)	25
SUGAR PUFFS, cereal (Malt-O-Meal)	⅞ cup (1 oz.)	26
SUGAR SMACKS, cereal (Kellogg's)	¾ cup (1 oz.)	70
SUGAR SUBSTITUTE:		
(Estee)	1 tsp.	0
(Featherweight):		
Liquid	3 drops	5
Tablet, half grain Saccharin	1 tablet	4
Tablet, quarter grain Saccharin	1 tablet	2
Sprinkle Sweet (Pillsbury)	1 tsp.	1
Spoon for Spoon	1 tsp.	0
Sweet 'N Low:		
Brown	1 tsp.	19
Granulated	1-g. packet	3
Liquid	1 drop	0
Sweet*10 (Pillsbury)	⅛ tsp.	2
***SUKIYAKI DINNER,** canned:		
(Chun King) stir fry	6 oz.	405
(La Choy) bi-pack	¾ cup	990
SUNFLOWER SEED:		
(USDA):		
In hulls	4 oz. (weighed in hull)	18
Hulled	1 oz.	9
(Fisher):		
In hull, roasted, salted	1 oz.	58
Hulled, roasted:		
Dry, salted	1 oz.	160
Oil, salted	1 oz.	180
(Frito-Lay's)	1 oz.	171

Food and Description	Measure or Quantity	Sodium (milligrams)
(Planters):		
Dry roasted	1 oz.	260
Unsalted	1 oz.	Tr.
SUNSHINE PUNCH DRINK,		
canned, *Ssips* (Johanna Farms)	8.45-fl.-oz. container	10
SURIMI, *Crab Delights* (Louis		
Kemp) chunks, flakes or legs	2 oz.	550
SUZY Q (Hostess):		
Banana	2¼-oz. cake	195
Chocolate	2½-oz. cake	313
SWEETBREADS (USDA) beef:		
Raw	1 lb.	435
Braised	4 oz.	132
SWEET POTATO:		
Raw (USDA):		
All kinds, unpared	1 lb. (weighed whole)	37
All kinds, pared	4 oz.	11
Firm-fleshed, Jersey types, pared	4 oz.	11
Soft-fleshed, Puerto Rico variety, pared	4 oz.	11
Baked (USDA) peeled after baking	3.9-oz. sweet potato (5″ × 2″)	13
Baked (USDA) peeled after boiling	5-oz. sweet potato) 5″ × 2″)	15
Candied (USDA) home recipe	6.2-oz. sweet potato (3½″ × 2¼″)	74
Canned, regular pack (USDA):		
In syrup, solids & liq.	4 oz.	54
Vacuum or solid pack	4 oz.	52
Canned, dietetic or low calorie, without added sugar & salt (USDA)	4 oz.	14
Dehydrated flakes (USDA):		
Dry	½ cup (2 oz.)	105

Food and Description	Measure or Quantity	Sodium (milligrams)
*Prepared with water	½ cup (4.4 oz.)	57
Frozen (Mrs. Paul's) regular	⅓ of 12-oz. pkg.	105
SWEET POTATO PIE (USDA)		
home recipe, made with lard	⅙ of 9″ pie (5.4 oz.)	331
SWEET & SOUR CHICKEN (La Choy):		
*Canned	¾ cup	440
Frozen	12-oz. entree	2010
SWEET & SOUR ORIENTAL, canned (La Choy):		
With chicken	½ of 15-oz. can	1420
With pork	½ of 15-oz. can	1540
SWEET & SOUR PORK, frozen (La Choy)	12-oz. entree	2200
SWISS STEAK, frozen (Swanson)	10-oz. dinner	830
SYRUP:		
Sweetened:		
Apricot (Smucker's)	1 T.	4
Blackberry (Smucker's)	1 T.	2
Chocolate:		
(USDA):		
Fudge type	1 T. (.7 oz.)	17
Thin type	1 T. (.7 oz.)	10
Bosco	1 T. (.7 oz.)	25
(Hersey's)	1 T. (.7 oz.)	15
(Nestlé) *Quik*	1 T. (.7 oz.)	24
Corn:		
(USDA) light & dark blend	1 T. (.7 oz.)	14
Karo:		
Dark	1 T. (.7 oz.)	37
Light	1 T. (.7 oz.)	29
Maple:		
(USDA)	1 T. (.7 oz.)	2
(Home Brands)	1 T.	13
Karo, imitation	1 T. (.7 oz.)	32
Pancake & waffle:		
(USDA) cane & maple	1 T. (.7 oz.)	<1
Aunt Jemima	1 T. (.7 oz.)	15
Golden Griddle	1 T. (.7 oz.)	20

Food and Description	Measure or Quantity	Sodium (milligrams)
Karo	1 T. (.7 oz.)	32
Log Cabin:		
Regular	1 T. (.7 oz.)	6
Buttered	1 T. (.7 oz.)	38
Country kitchen	1 T. (.7 oz.)	10
Maple-honey	1 T. (.7 oz.)	4
Mrs. Butterworth's	1 T. (.7 oz.)	24
Raspberry (Smucker's) red	1 T. (.7 oz.)	5
Strawberry (Smucker's)	1 T. (.6 oz.)	2
Dietetic or low calorie:		
Blueberry:		
(Dia-Mel)	1 T. (.5 oz.)	15
(Estee)	1 T. (.5 oz.)	0
(Featherweight)	1 T.	<25
Chocolate:		
(Estee) *Choco-Syp*	1 T. (.5 oz.)	3
(Diet Delight)	1 T. (.6 oz.)	10
Maple (Cary's)	1 T.	15
Pancake or waffle:		
(Aunt Jemima)	1 T. (.6 oz.)	29
(Dia-Mel)	1 T. (.5 oz.)	10
(Diet Delight)	1 T.	30
(Estee)	1 T.	0
(Featherweight)	1 T.	30

T

*TACO (Ortega)	1 oz.	104
TACO SEASONING MIX:		
*(Durkee)	1 cup	1115
(French's)	1¼-oz. pkg.	2190
(Old El Paso)	1 pkg.	3569
TACO SHELL:		
(Gebhardt)	.4-oz. shell	0

Food and Description	Measure or Quantity	Sodium (milligrams)
Old El Paso	.4-oz. shell	47
(Ortega)	.4-oz. shell	55
(Rosarita)	.4-oz. shell	0
TACO BELL RESTAURANT:		
Bellbeefer:		
Regular	5-oz. serving	710
With cheese & tomato	5½-oz. serving	670
Burrito:		
Bean	7.2-oz. serving	935
Beef	6.7-oz. serving	989
Combination	8.4-oz. serving	777
Supreme	5.6-oz. serving	855
Crispas, cinnamon	2.2-oz. serving	158
Enchirito	6.5-oz. serving	1030
Nachos:		
Regular	3.3-oz. serving	319
Bellgrande	10.6-oz. serving	1140
Pintos & cheese	5.1-oz. serving	732
Taco:		
Regular	3.1-oz. serving	279
Bellgrande	5.2-oz. serving	353
Light	5.0-oz. serving	426
Taco salad	18.3-oz. serving	1455
Tostada:		
Regular	5.7-oz. serving	534
Beefy	7.4-oz. serving	714
TAMALE:		
Canned:		
(Hormel) beef:		
Regular:		
Plain	1 tamale	275
Hot & spicy	1 tamale	306
Short Orders	7½-oz. can	1140
(Old El Paso) with chili gravy	1 tamale	189
(Pride of Mexico)	2-oz. tamale	310
Frozen (Hormel) beef	1 tamale	555
TAMARIND, fresh (USDA):		
Whole	1 lb. (weighed with pods & seeds)	111
Flesh only	4 oz.	58

Food and Description	Measure or Quantity	Sodium (milligrams)
*TANG, instant breakfast drink:		
Grape	6 fl. oz.	5
Orange, regular or diet	6 fl. oz.	1
TANGERINE or MANDARIN ORANGE:		
Fresh (USDA):		
Whole	1 lb. (weighed with peel)	7
Whole tangerine	4.1 oz. (2⅜" dia.)	2
Sections (without membranes)	1 cup (6.8 oz.)	4
Canned, regular pack (Del Monte) solids & liq.	5½ oz.	<10
Canned, dietetic or low calorie, solids & liq.:	¼ of 22-oz. can	9
(Diet Delight) juice pack	½ cup (4.3 oz.)	5
(Featherweight) water pack	½ cup	<10
TANGERINE DRINK, canned (Hi-C)	6 fl. oz.	<1
TANGERINE JUICE:		
Fresh (USDA)	½ cup (4.4 oz.)	1
Canned (USDA):		
Unsweetened	½ cup (4.4 oz.)	1
Sweetened	½ cup (4.4 oz.)	1
*Frozen:		
(USDA)	½ cup (4.4 oz.)	1
(Minute Maid) sweetened	6 fl. oz.	2
TAPIOCA, dry, quick cooking, granulated:		
(USDA)	1 cup (5.4 oz.)	5
(USDA)	1 T. (10 g.)	<1
(Minute)	1 T.	<1
TAQUITO, BEEF, frozen (Van de Kamp's) shredded	8 oz.	990
TARO, raw (USDA):		
Tubers, whole	1 lb. (weighed with skin)	27
Tubers, skin removed	4 oz.	8
TARRAGON (French's)	1 tsp.	1
TASTEEOS, cereal (Ralston-Purina)	1¼ cups (1 oz.)	210

Food and Description	Measure or Quantity	Sodium (milligrams)
TEA (See also TEA, ICED):		
Bag:		
(Celestial Seasonings):		
After dinner:		
Amaretto Nights,		
Cinnamon Vienna or		
Swiss Mint	1 bag	<1
Bavarian Chocolate		
Orange		
Caffeine free	1 bag	5
Fruit & tea	1 bag	<1
Herb:		
Almond Sunset,		
Emperor's Choice,		
Mandarin Orange		
Spice, Red Zinger		
or *Sleepy Time*	1 bag	2
Chamomile	1 bag	5
Cranberry Cove or		
Spearmint	1 bag	6
Mellow Mint, Mo's		
24 or *Roastaroma*	1 bag	4
Premium black tea, any		
flavor	1 bag	<1
(Lipton)	1 bag	0
(Tender Leaf)	1 bag	0
*Nestea	1 tsp.	0
(Tender Leaf)	1 tsp.	Tr.
TEA, ICED:		
Canned, sweetened (Lipton)		
lemon flavored	6 fl. oz.	20
*Mix:		
Pre-sweetened, lemon flavored:		
Country Time	8 fl. oz.	Tr.
(Lipton)	8 fl. oz.	Tr.
Nestea	8 fl. oz.	<10
Unsweetened, dietetic or low		
calorie:		
(Crystal Light)	8 fl. oz.	<1
(Lipton) lemon flavored	1 cup (8 fl. oz.)	0

Food and Description	Measure or Quantity	Sodium (milligrams)
Nestea:		
Plain free	6 fl. oz.	0
Lemon flavored	8 fl. oz.	0
TERIYAKI, frozen:		
(Armour) *Dinner Classics*:		
Chicken	10½-oz. meal	1520
Steak	10-oz. meal	1550
(Conagra) *Light & Elegant*, beef	8-oz. entree	625
(Stouffer's) beef	10-oz. meal	1450
TERIYAKI MARINADE & SAUCE (La Choy)	1 oz.	1640
***TEXTURED VEGETABLE PROTEIN** (Morningstar Farms):		
Breakfast links	¾-oz. link	225
Breakfast patties	1.3-oz. pattie	470
Breakfast strips	.3-oz. strip	124
Grillers, hamburger-like patties	2.1-oz. pattie	334
THURINGER, sausage:		
(Eckrich):		
Sliced	1-oz. slice	380
Smoky Tang	1 oz.	350
(Hormel):		
Packaged, sliced	1 slice	353
Whole:		
Regular	1 oz.	332
Beefy	1 oz.	313
Old Smokehouse	1 oz.	328
Tangy, chub	1 oz.	317
(Ohse):		
Regular	1 oz.	340
Beef	1 oz.	330
(Oscar Mayer) summer sausage:		
Regular	.8-oz. slice	269
Beef	.8-oz. slice	316
THYME, dried (French's)	1 tsp.	1
TIGER TAIL (Hostess)	2¼-oz. piece	249
TOASTER CAKE or PASTRY:		
Pop-Tarts (Kellogg's):		
Regular:		
Blueberry	1 piece (1.83 oz.)	220

Food and Description	Measure or Quantity	Sodium (milligrams)
Brown sugar cinnamon	1 piece (1¾ oz.)	215
Cherry	1 piece (1.83 oz.)	230
Strawberry	1 piece (1.83 oz.)	225
Frosted:		
Blueberry	1 piece (1.83 oz.)	220
Brown sugar cinnamon	1 piece (1¾ oz.)	205
Cherry	1 piece (1.83 oz.)	230
Chocolate fudge	1 piece (1.83 oz.)	230
Chocolate-vanilla creme	1 piece (1.83 oz.)	220
Concord grape, Dutch apple, raspberry & strawberry	1 piece (1.83 oz.)	215
Toaster Streudel (Pillsbury):		
Blueberry, raspberry or strawberry	1 piece	205
Cinnamon	1 piece	200
Toastettes (Nabisco)		
Regular:		
Apple	1 piece	170
Blueberry, cherry or strawberry	1 piece	200
Frosted:		
Brown sugar cinnamon	1 piece	170
Fudge	1 piece	210
Strawberry	1 piece	200
Toast-r-Cake (Thomas'):		
Blueberry	1.2-oz. piece	180
Bran	1.2-oz. piece	225
Corn	1.2-oz. piece	191
TOASTIES, cereal (Post)	1¼ cups	298
TOASTY O's, cereal (Malt-O-Meal)	1¼ cups (1 oz.)	281
TODDLER BABY FOOD (See BABY FOOD)		
TOFU (See SOYBEAN CURD)		
TOFUTTI		
Frozen:		
Regular:		
Chocolate supreme	4 fl. oz.	130

Food and Description	Measure or Quantity	Sodium (milligrams)
Maple walnut or vanilla almond bark	4 fl. oz.	95
Vanilla	4 fl. oz.	90
Wildberry supreme	4 fl. oz.	100
Cuties:		
Chocolate	1 piece	130
Vanilla	1 piece	110
Lite Lite	4 fl. oz.	80
Love Drops:		
Cappuccino	4 fl. oz.	120
Chocolate vanilla	4 fl. oz.	100
Soft-serve:		
Regular	4 fl. oz.	65
Hi-Lite	4 fl. oz.	75
TOMATO:		
Fresh (USDA):		
Green:		
Whole, untrimmed	1 lb. (weighed with core & stem end)	12
Trimmed, unpeeled	4 oz.	3
Ripe:		
Whole:		
Eaten with skin	1 lb.	14
Peeled	1 lb. (weighed with skin, stem ends & hard core)	12
Peeled	1 med. (2″ × 2½″, 5.3 oz.)	4
Peeled	1 small (1¾″ × 2½″, 3.9 oz.)	3
Sliced, peeled	½ cup (3.2 oz.)	3
Boiled (USDA)	½ cup (4.3 oz.)	5
Canned, regular pack:		
(USDA) whole, solids & liq.	½ cup (4.2 oz.)	155
(Contadina):		
Sliced, baby	4 oz.	465
Stewed	4 oz.	405
Whole, round & pear	1 cup	390

Food and Description	Measure or Quantity	Sodium (milligrams)
(Del Monte) solids & liq.:		
Stewed	½ cup (4 oz.)	355
Wedges	½ cup (4 oz.)	355
Whole, peeled	½ cup (4 oz.)	220
(Hunt's):		
Crushed	½ cup	300
Italian style	4 oz.	415
Stewed	4 oz.	460
Whole	4 oz.	415
(Libby's)		
Stewed	½ of 16-oz. can	567
Whole, peeled, solids & liq.	½ of 16-oz. can	386
(Stokely-Van Camp) solids & liq.:		
Stewed	½ cup (4.2 oz.)	223
Whole	½ cup (4.3 oz.)	190
Canned, dietetic or low calorie:		
(USDA) low sodium	4 oz.	3
(Del Monte) no salt added	½ cup	45
(Diet Delight) whole, peeled, solids & liq.	½ cup (4.3 oz.)	15
(Featherweight)	½ cup	<10
(Furman's) crushed	½ cup	<10
(Hunt's) whole "No-Salt-Added" whole	4 oz.	15
(S&W) *Nutradiet*	½ cup	15
TOMATO JUICE:		
Canned, regular pack:		
(USDA)	½ cup (4.3 oz.)	244
(USDA)	6 fl. oz. (6.4 oz.)	364
(Campbell)	6 fl. oz.	570
(Hunt's)	6 fl. oz.	550
(Libby's)	6 fl. oz.	455
(Ocean Spray)	6 fl. oz.	550
Canned, dietetic or low calorie:		
(USDA)	4 oz. (by wt.)	3
(Diet Delight)	6 fl. oz.(6.4 oz.)	20
(Featherweight)	6 fl. oz.	<20
(Hunt's) "No-Salt-Added"	6 fl. oz.	20

Food and Description	Measure or Quantity	Sodium (milligrams)
(S&W) *Nutradiet*	6 fl. oz.	20
Concentrate (USDA):		
Canned	4 oz. (by wt.)	896
*Canned, diluted with 3 parts water by volume	4 oz. (by wt.)	237
*Dehydrated (USDA)	½ cup (4.3 oz.)	312
TOMATO JUICE COCKTAIL:		
(USDA)	4 oz. (by wt.)	227
(Ocean Spray) *Firehouse Jubilee*	6 fl. oz.	599
Snap-E-Tom	6 fl. oz. (6.5 oz.)	980
TOMATO PASTE, canned:		
Regular pack:		
(USDA) no salt added	6-oz. can	65
(USDA) no salt added	½ cup (4.6 oz.)	50
(USDA) no salt added	1 T. (.6 oz.)	6
(USDA) salt added	6-oz. can	1343
(Contadina):		
Regular	6 oz.	135
Italian	6 oz.	2130
Italian with mushroom	6 oz.	2205
(Del Monte)	6 oz.	110
(Hunt's):		
Regular	6 oz.	900
Italian Style	6 oz.	1575
Dietetic:		
(Del Monte)	6 oz.	110
(Featherweight) low sodium	6 oz.	70
(Hunt's) no salt added	6 oz.	75
TOMATO & PEPPERS, hot chili:		
(Old El Paso)	¼ cup	273
(Ortega) Jalapeno	1-oz. serving	22
TOMATO, PICKLED, canned		
(Claussen) Kosher, green, halves	1-oz. piece	326
TOMATO PUREE:		
Canned, regular pack:		
(USDA)	1 cup (8.8 oz.)	998
(Contadina)	1 cup (8.8 oz.)	180
(Hunt's)	1 cup (8 oz.)	360

Food and Description	Measure or Quantity	Sodium (milligrams)
Canned, dietetic or low calorie:		
(USDA)	8 oz. (by wt.)	14
(Featherweight)	1 cup	<20
TOMATO SAUCE, canned:		
Regular pack:		
(Contadina):		
Regular	½ cup	510
Italian style	½ cup	620
(Del Monte):		
Regular	½ cup (4 oz.)	665
With onions	½ cup (4 oz.)	575
(Hunt's):		
Regular	4 oz.	665
With bits	4 oz.	695
With cheese	4 oz.	795
Herb	4 oz.	495
Italian	4 oz.	515
With mushroom	4 oz.	710
With onions	4 oz.	670
Special	4 oz.	315
(Libby's)	½ of 8-oz. can	697
(Stokely-Van Camp)	½ cup (4.5 oz.)	850
Dietetic (Hunt's) "no-salt-added"	4 oz.	25
TOMATO SOUP (see **SOUP, Tomato**)		
TOM COLLINS (Mr. Boston)	3 fl. oz.	39
TONGUE (USDA) beef, medium fat, braised	4 oz.	69
TONGUE, CANNED, PORK (Hormel) cured	3 oz.	966
TOPPING:		
Sweetened:		
Butterscotch (Smucker's)	1 T.	37
Chocolate:		
(Hershey's) fudge	1 T.	16
(Smucker's):		
Fudge	1 T.	22
Fudge nut	1 T.	27
Marshmallow (see *MARSH MALLOW FLUFF*)		

Food and Description	Measure or Quantity	Sodium (milligrams)
Pecan (Smucker's) in syrup	1 T.	0
Walnuts, in syrup (Smucker's)	1 T.	0
Dietetic or low calorie, chocolate (Diet Delight)	1 T. (.6 oz.)	9
TOPPING, WHIPPED:		
Canned or aerosol:		
Cool Whip (Birds Eye) frozen, non-dairy	1 T. (.2 oz.)	1
(Dover Farms) dairy	1 T.	3
(Johanna) aerosol	1 T.	2
Lucky Whip, aerosol	1 T. (.2 oz.)	4
Spoon'N Serve (Rich's) frozen, non-dairy	1 T. (.14 oz.)	9
Whip Topping (Rich's) aerosol	¼-oz. serving	5
*Mix:		
Regular (Dream Whip)	1 T. (.2 oz.)	4
Dietetic (D-Zerta)	1 T.	4
TORTELLINI, frozen (Buitoni):		
Cheese:		
Regular	2.6 oz.	262
Tricolor	2.6 oz.	259
Verdi	2.6 oz.	228
Meat	2.4 oz.	297
TORTILLA, CORN (Old El Paso)	1 oz.	193
TOSTADA, BEEF, frozen (Van de Kamp's)	8½ oz.	720
TOSTADA SHELL (Old El Paso)	1 shell	66
TOTAL, cereal (General Mills)	1 cup (1 oz.)	310
TRIPE:		
Beef (USDA):		
Commercial	4 oz.	82
Pickled	4 oz.	52
Canned (Libby's)	¼ of 24-oz. can	147
TRIX, cereal (General Mills)	1 cup (1 oz.)	170

Food and Description	Measure or Quantity	Sodium (milligrams)
TUNA:		
Raw (USDA) Yellowfin, meat only	4 oz.	42
Canned, in oil:		
(USDA) solids & liq.	6½-oz. can	1472
(Bumble Bee) undrained:		
Chunk, light	½ cup	327
Solid white	½ cup	414
(Chicken of the Sea) chunk, light:		
Solids & liq.	6½-oz. can	1196
Drained solids	6½-oz. can	1072
Canned in water, solids & liq.:		
(USDA) no salt added	6½-oz. can	75
(USDA) salt added	6½-oz. can	1610
(Featherweight) low sodium	6½-oz. can	93
(Star Kist) chunk, white	6½-oz. can	92
TUNA HELPER (General Mills):		
Country dumplings	⅕ of pkg.	1020
Creamy noodles	⅕ of pkg.	880
Noodles & cheese sauce	⅕ of pkg.	745
TUNA-NOODLE CASSEROLE, frozen (Stouffer's)	5¾ oz.	670
TUNA PIE, frozen:		
(Banquet)	8-oz. pie	565
(Morton)	8-oz. pie	1120
TUNA SALAD, canned		
(Swanson) *Spreadable*	1½-oz. serving	270
TURBOT, GREENLAND		
(USDA) raw, meat only	4 oz.	64
TURF & SURF DINNER, frozen		
(Armour) *Classic Lites*	10-oz. meal	890
TURKEY:		
Raw (USDA):		
Dark meat	4 oz.	92
Light meat	4 oz.	58
Meat only:		
Chopped	1 cup (5 oz.)	183
Diced	1 cup (4.8 oz.)	176
Light	4 oz.	93

Food and Description	Measure or Quantity	Sodium (milligrams)
Light	1 slice (4″ × 2″ × ¼″, 3 oz.)	35
Dark	4 oz.	112
Dark	1 slice (2½″ × 1⅝″ × ¼″, .7 oz.)	21
Canned, boned, (Swanson) chunk	2½-oz. serving	380
Packaged:		
(Carl Buddig) smoked:		
Regular	1 oz.	400
Ham	1 oz.	435
Salami	1 oz.	400
(Hormel) breast:		
Regular	1 slice	242
Smoked	1 slice	270
(Ohse):		
Oven cooked	1 oz.	190
Smoked, breast	1 oz.	340
Turkey bologna	1 oz.	300
Turkey salami	1 oz.	260
(Oscar Mayer) breast, sliced	¾-oz. slice	294
Roasted, meat only (USDA):		
Dark	4 oz.	112
Light	4 oz.	93
TURKEY DINNER or ENTREE, frozen:		
(USDA) sliced turkey, mashed potatoes & peas	12-oz. dinner	1360
(Armour) *Classic Lites*, parmesan	11-oz. meal	480
(Banquet):		
American Favorites	11-oz. dinner	1416
Extra Helping	19-oz. dinner	2165
(Conagra) *Light & Elegant*, sliced	8-oz. entree	1020
(Stouffer's) casserole with gravy & dressing	9¾-oz. meal	1125
(Swanson):		
Dinner, 4-compartment	11½-oz. dinner	1260
Entree	8¾-oz. entree	1090

Food and Description	Measure or Quantity	Sodium (milligrams)
Hungry Man:		
Dinner	18½-oz. dinner	2150
Entree	13¼-oz. entree	1740
Main Course	9¼-oz. entree	1120
TURKEY GIZZARD (USDA):		
Raw	4 oz.	66
Simmered	4 oz.	58
TURKEY PIE:		
Home recipe (USDA) baked	⅓ of 9″ pie	633
Frozen:		
(USDA) unheated	8-oz. pie	837
(Banquet):		
Regular	8-oz. pie	1111
Supreme	8-oz. pie	1370
(Stouffer's)	10-oz. pie	1735
(Swanson):		
Regular	8-oz. pie	800
Chunky	10-oz. pie	950
Hungry Man	16-oz. pie	1590
TURKEY SALAD, canned		
(Carnation) *Spreadable*	1-oz. serving	129
TURKEY TETRAZZINI,		
frozen (Stouffer's)	6 oz.	620
TURMERIC (French's)	1 tsp.	Tr.
TURNIP (USDA):		
Fresh:		
Without tops	1 lb. (weighed with skins)	191
Pared, diced	½ cup (2.4 oz.)	33
Pared, slices	½ cup (2.3 oz.)	31
Boiled, drained:		
Diced	½ cup (2.8 oz.)	27
Mashed	½ cup (4 oz.)	39
TURNIP GREENS, leaves & stems:		
Canned:		
(USDA) solids & liq.	½ cup (4.1 oz.)	274
(Stokely-Van Camp) chopped	½ cup (4.1 oz.)	335
(Sunshine) solids & liq.:		
Chopped	½ cup (4.1 oz.)	252

Food and Description	Measure or Quantity	Sodium (milligrams)
& diced turnips	½ cup (4.1 oz.)	391
Frozen:		
(Birds Eye):		
Chopped	⅓ of 10-oz. pkg.	11
Chopped, with diced turnips	⅓ of 10-oz. pkg.	15
(Frosty Acres)	3.3 oz.	10
(McKenzie) chopped	3.3 oz.	66
(Southland):		
chopped	⅕ of 16-oz. pkg.	10
With diced turnips	⅕ of 16-oz. pkg.	35
Mashed	⅓ of 11-oz. pkg.	60
TURNOVER:		
Frozen (Pepperidge Farm):		
Apple	1 turnover	220
Blueberry	1 turnover	240
Cherry	1 turnover	290
Peach	1 turnover	260
Raspberry	1 turnover	270
Refrigerated (Pillsbury):		
Apple	1 turnover	320
Blueberry or cherry	1 turnover	310
TWINKIE (Hostess):		
Regular	1½-oz. cake	149
Devil's food	1½-oz. cake	213

U

UFO'S, canned (Franco-American):		
Regular	7½ oz.	790
With meteors	7½ oz.	780

Food and Description	Measure or Quantity	Sodium (milligrams)

V

VEAL, medium fat (USDA):
  Chunk:
    Raw

    Braised, lean & fat
  Flank:
    Raw

    Stewed, lean & fat
  Foreshank:
    Raw

    Stewed, lean & fat
  Loin:
    Raw

    Broiled, medium done, chop, lean & fat
  Plate:
    Raw

    Stewed, lean & fat
  Rib:
    Raw, lean & fat

    Roasted, medium done, lean & fat
  Round & rump:
    Raw

Food	Measure	Sodium
Chunk Raw	1 lb. (weighed with bone)	327
Braised, lean & fat	4 oz.	91
Flank Raw	1 lb. (weighed with bone)	404
Stewed, lean & fat	4 oz.	91
Foreshank Raw	1 lb. (weighed with bone)	212
Stewed, lean & fat	4 oz.	91
Loin Raw	1 lb. (weighed with bone)	338
Broiled chop, lean & fat	4 oz.	91
Plate Raw	1 lb. (weighed with bone)	322
Stewed, lean & fat	4 oz.	91
Rib Raw, lean & fat	1 lb. (weighed with bone)	314
Roasted, lean & fat	4 oz.	91
Round & rump Raw	1 lb. (weighed with bone)	314

Food and Description	Measure or Quantity	Sodium (milligrams)
Broiled, steak or cutlet, lean & fat	4 oz. (weighed without bone)	91
VEAL DINNER or ENTREE, frozen:		
(Armour) *Dinner Classics*, parmigiana	10¾-oz. meal	1430
(Banquet) parmigiana:		
Dinner	11-oz. dinner	1310
Entree, family	32-oz. pkg.	4805
Entree, for one, breaded	5-oz. serving	842
(Morton) dinner:		
Regular	12-oz. dinner	1300
Regular	20-oz. dinner	2300
Light	11-oz. dinner	1300
(Swanson) parmigiana:		
Regular	12¾-oz. dinner	1120
Hungry Man	20-oz. dinner	2010
(Weight Watchers) parmigiana, patty, 2-compartment	8¹⁄₁₆-oz. meal	1040
VEGETABLE BOUILLON:		
(Herb-Ox):		
Cube	1 cube	920
Packet	1 packet	880
MBT	6-g. packet	780
(Wyler's) instant	1 tsp.	910
VEGETABLE FAT (See FAT)		
VEGETABLE FLAKES, dehydrated (French's)	1 T.	20
VEGETABLE JUICE COCKTAIL:		
Canned, regular pack:		
(USDA)	4 oz. (by wt.)	227
V-8 (Campbell):		
Regular or spicy hot	6 fl. oz.	625
Canned, low sodium:		
(Featherweight)	6 fl. oz.	25
(S&W) *Nutradiet*	6 fl. oz.	25
V-8 (Campbell)	6 fl. oz.	50

Food and Description	Measure or Quantity	Sodium (milligrams)
VEGETABLES, MIXED:		
Canned, regular pack:		
(Chun King) chow mein, drained solids	½ of 8-oz. can	20
(Del Monte) solids & liq.	½ cup	355
(La Choy) Chinese style, drained	⅓ of 14-oz. can	35
(Libby's) solids & liq.	½ cup (4.2 oz.)	345
(Stokely-Van Camp) solids & liq.	½ cup (4.3 oz.)	123
(Veg-All) solids & liq.:		
Regular	½ cup	320
For stew	½ cup	380
Canned, dietetic or low calorie:		
(Featherweight)	½ cup	25
(Larsen) *Fresh-Lite*	½ cup	25
Frozen:		
(USDA) boiled, drained	½ cup (3.2 oz.)	48
(Birds Eye):		
Regular:		
Broccoli, cauliflower & carrots in cheese sauce	5 oz.	380
Carrots, peas & pearl onions	⅓ of 10-oz. pkg.	60
Mixed	⅓ of 10-oz. pkg.	10
With onion sauce	⅓ of 8-oz. pkg.	340
Farm Fresh:		
Broccoli, baby carrots & water chestnuts	⅕ of 16-oz. pkg.	25
Broccoli, cauliflower & carrots	⅕ of 16-oz. pkg.	25
Broccoli, corn & red pepper dices	⅕ of 16-oz. pkg.	15
Broccoli, green beans, onion & red pepper	⅕ of 16-oz. pkg.	15
Brussels sprouts, cauliflower & carrots	⅕ of 16-oz. pkg.	20
International Style:		
Bavarian style beans & spaetzle	⅓ of 10-oz. pkg.	420

Food and Description	Measure or Quantity	Sodium (milligrams)
Chinese style	⅓ of 10-oz. pkg.	370
Italian style	⅓ of 10-oz. pkg.	570
Japanese style	⅓ of 10-oz. pkg.	490
New England style	⅓ of 10-oz. pkg.	410
San Francisco style	⅓ of 10-oz. pkg.	400
Stir Fry:		
Chinese	⅓ of 10-oz. pkg.	540
Japanese	⅓ of 10-oz. pkg.	510
(Frosty Acres):		
Regular	3.3 oz.	50
Dutch style or rancho fiesta	3.2 oz.	30
Italian style	3.2 oz.	20
Oriental style	3.2 oz.	15
Soup mix	3 oz.	35
Stew	3 oz.	21
Swiss mix	3 oz.	36
(Green Giant):		
Regular:		
Broccoli, carrots fanfare	½ cup	20
Broccoli, cauliflower & carrots in cheese sauce	½ cup	465
Broccoli, cauliflower supreme	½ cup	30
Cauliflower, green bean festival	½ cup	30
Corn, broccoli bounty	½ cup	10
Mixed, in butter sauce	½ cup	345
Mixed, polybag	½ cup	35
Pea, pea pod & water chestnuts, in butter sauce	½ cup	410
Pea, sweet, & cauliflower medley	½ cup	35
Harvest Fresh, mixed	½ cup	220
Harvest Get Together:		
Broccoli, cauliflower medley	½ cup	470
Broccoli fanfare	½ cup	455

Food and Description	Measure or Quantity	Sodium (milligrams)
Cauliflower-carrot bonanza	½ cup	295
Chinese style	½ cup	280
Japanese style	½ cup	155
(La Choy) Chinese	⅓ of 12-oz. pkg.	540
(Larsen):		
Regular	3.3 oz.	45
California or Italian blend	3.3 oz.	20
Chuckwagon blend	3.3 oz.	5
Midwestern or Scandinavian blend	3.3 oz.	30
Oriental blend	3.3 oz.	10
Soup or stew	3.3 oz.	40
Winter blend	3.3 oz.	25
Wisconsin blend	3.3 oz.	15
(Le Seuer) pea, onion & carrots in butter sauce	½ cup	100
(McKenzie)	3.3 oz.	56
(Southland):		
Gumbo	⅕ of 16-oz. pkg.	10
Soup	⅕ of 16-oz. pkg.	40
Stew	⅕ of 20-oz. pkg.	30
VEGETABLES IN PASTRY, frozen (Pepperidge Farm):		
Asparagus with mornay sauce	½ of 7½-oz. pkg.	245
Broccoli with cheese	½ of 7½-oz. pkg.	455
Cauliflower & cheese sauce	½ of 7½-oz. pkg.	465
Mushrooms dijon	½ of 7½-oz. pkg.	415
Spinach almondine	½ of 7½-oz. pkg.	325
Zucchini provençal	½ of 7½-oz. pkg.	290
VEGETABLE SOUP (See **SOUP**, Vegetable)		
VEGETABLE STEW, canned, *Dinty Moore* (Hormel)	⅓ of 24-oz. can	1047
"VEGETARIAN FOODS":		
Canned or dry:		
Chicken, fried (Loma Linda) with gravy	1½-oz. piece	170
Chili (Worthington)	½ cup (4.9 oz.)	695
Choplet (Worthington)	1.6-oz. slice	263

Food and Description	Measure or Quantity	Sodium (milligrams)
Cutlet (Worthington)	2.2-oz. slice	434
Dinner cuts (Loma Linda):		
Regular	2.1-oz. piece	330
No salt added	1.8-oz. piece	15
Franks (Loma Linda):		
Big	1.9-oz. piece	220
Sizzle	1.2-oz. piece	170
FriChik (Worthington)	1.6-oz. piece	277
Granburger (Worthington)	6 T. (1.2 oz.)	933
Linketts (Loma Linda)	1.3-oz. link	170
Little links (Loma Linda)	.8-oz. link	105
Numete (Worthington)	½" slice (2.4 oz.)	370
Nuteena (Loma Linda)	½" slice (2.4 oz.)	120
Proteena (Loma Linda)	½" slice (2.5 oz.)	460
Protose (Worthington)	½" slice (2.7 oz.)	476
Redi-burger (Loma Linda)	½" slice (2.4 oz.)	370
Sandwich spread (Loma Linda)	1 T. (.6 oz.)	100
Saucettes (Worthington)	1 link	190
Skallops (Worthington) drained	½ cup (3 oz.)	315
Soyameat (Worthington):		
Beef-like slices	1-oz. slice	183
Chicken-like slices	1-oz. slice	167
Stew pac (Loma Linda)	2-oz.	220
Super links (Worthington)	1.9-oz. link	449
Swiss steak & gravy (Loma Linda)	2.6-oz. steak	350
Tender bits (Loma Linda)	.6-oz. piece	85
VegeBurger (Loma Linda):		
Regular	½ cup (3.8 oz.)	190
No salt added	½ cup (3.8 oz.)	55
Vegelona (Loma Linda)	½" slice (2.4 oz.)	210
Vegetable steak (Worthington)	1.3-oz. piece	148
Vegetarian burger (Worthington)	⅓ cup (3.3 oz.)	545
Veja-links (Worthington)	1.1-oz. link	169
Vita-Burger (Loma Linda)	1 T. (¼ oz.)	50
Worthington 209, turkey-like flavor	1.1-oz. slice	229

Food and Description	Measure or Quantity	Sodium (milligrams)
Frozen:		
Beeflike-pie (Worthington)	8-oz. pie	1109
Bologna (Loma Linda)	1-oz. slice	245
Bolono (Worthington)	.7-oz. slice	206
Chicken, fried (Loma Linda)	2-oz. piece	510
Chicken-like pie (Worthington)	8-oz. pie	930
Chicken-like slices (Worthington)	.1-oz. slice	288
Corned beef-like, sliced (Worthington)	.5-oz. slice	155
Fillets (Worthington)	1.5-oz. piece	368
FriPats (Worthington)	2.5-oz. piece	379
Meatballs (Loma Linda)	.3-oz. piece	53
Meatless salami (Worthington)	.7-oz. slice	300
Prosage (Worthington):		
Links	.8-oz. link	140
Patties	1.3-oz. piece	297
Roll	⅜" slice (1.2 oz.)	254
Sizzle burger (Loma Linda)	2½-oz. piece	320
Smoked turkey-like slices (Worthington)	1 slice (.7-oz.)	200
Stakelets (Worthington)	3-oz. piece	604
Stripples (Worthington)	.3-oz. strip	123
Tuno (Worthington)	2-oz. serving	343
Wham (Worthington) sliced	.8-oz. slice	261
VERMOUTH:		
Dry (Great Western) 16% alcohol	3 fl. oz.	20
Sweet (Great Western) 16% alcohol	3 fl. oz.	20
VICHY WATER (Schweppes)	6 fl. oz.	76
VIENNA SAUSAGE, (See SAUSAGE)		
VINEGAR:		
Cider:		
(USDA)	1 T. (.5 oz.)	<1
(USDA)	½ cup (4.2 oz.)	<1
(White House) apple	1 T.	2

Food and Description	Measure or Quantity	Sodium (milligrams)
Distilled:		
(USDA)	1 T. (.5 oz.)	<1
(USDA)	½ cup (4.2 oz.)	1
(White House) white	1 T.	2
Red wine or red wine with garlic (Regina)	1 T. (.5 oz.)	20
White wine (Regina)	1 T. (.5 oz.)	10
VODKA (See **DISTILLED LIQUOR**)		

W

WAFER (See **COOKIE or CRACKER**)		
WAFFELOS, cereal (Ralston Purina)	1 cup (1 oz.)	116
WAFFLE:		
Home recipe (USDA)	7″ waffle (2.6 oz.)	356
Frozen:		
(USDA)	1.6-oz. waffle (8 in 13-oz. pkg.)	296
(USDA)	.8-oz. waffle (6 in 5-oz. pkg.)	155
(Aunt Jemima) jumbo:		
Regular	1¼-oz. waffle	261
Apple-cinnamon or blueberry	1¼-oz. waffle	243
Buttermilk	1¼-oz. waffle	267
(Eggo):		
Regular or strawberry	1.4-oz. waffle	265
Blueberry	1.4-oz. waffle	260
Roman Meal:		
Regular	1½-oz. waffle	325
Golden Delights	1.4-oz. piece	252

Food and Description	Measure or Quantity	Sodium (milligrams)
WAFFLE MIX (See also **PANCAKE & WAFFLE MIX**) (USDA):		
Complete mix:		
Dry	1 oz.	291
*Prepared with water	2.6-oz. waffle	420
Incomplete mix:		
Dry	1 oz.	406
*Prepared with egg & milk	2.6-oz. waffle	514
*Prepared with egg & milk	7.1-oz. waffle	1372
WAFFLE SYRUP (See **SYRUP**)		
WALNUT:		
(USDA):		
Black, in shell, whole	1 lb. (weighed in shell)	3
Black, shelled, whole	4 oz. (weighed whole)	3
Black, chopped	½ cup (2.1 oz.)	2
English or Persian, in shell, whole	1 lb. (weighed in shell)	4
English or Persian, shelled, whole	4 oz.	2
English or Persian chopped	½ cup (2.1 oz.)	1
English or Persian, halves	½ cup (1.8 oz.)	1
(Fisher) black or English	1 oz.	0
WATER CHESTNUT, CHINESE:		
Raw (USDA):		
Whole	1 lb. (weighed unpeeled)	70
Peeled	4 oz.	23
Canned:		
(Chun King) drained solids:		
Sliced	½ of 8-oz. can	22
Whole	½ of 8½-oz. can	24
(La Choy) sliced, drained solids	¼ cup	Tr.
WATERCRESS, raw (USDA):		
Untrimmed	½ lb. (weighed untrimmed)	108

Food and Description	Measure or Quantity	Sodium (milligrams)
Trimmed	½ cup (.6 oz.)	8
WATERMELON, fresh (USDA):		
Whole	1 lb. (weighed with rind)	2
Wedge	2-lb. wedge (4″ × 8″ measured with rind)	4
Diced	1 cup (5.6 oz.)	2
WATERMELON DRINK, canned, *Capri Sun*	6¾ fl. oz.	1
WAX GOURD, raw (USDA):		
Whole	1 lb. (weighed with skin & cavity contents)	19
Flesh only	4 oz.	7
WEAKFISH (USDA):		
Raw, whole	1 lb. (weighed whole)	163
Broiled, meat only	4 oz.	635
WEINER WRAP, refrigerated (Pillsbury):		
Plain	1 wrap	430
Cheese	1 wrap	395
WELSH RAREBIT, home recipe (USDA)	1 cup (8.2 oz.)	770
WENDY'S		
Bacon, breakfast	1 strip	223
Bacon cheeseburger on white bun	1 burger	860
Breakfast sandwich	1 sandwich	770
Buns:		
Wheat, multi-grain	1 bun	220
White	1 bun	266
Chicken sandwich on wheat bun	1 sandwich	500
Chili:		
Small order	8 oz.	1070
Large order	12 oz.	1605
Condiments:		
Bacon	½ strip	112

Food and Description	Measure or Quantity	Sodium (milligrams)
Cheese, American	1 slice	260
Ketchup	1 tsp.	65
Lettuce	1 piece	0
Mayonnaise	1 T.	80
Mustard	1 tsp.	50
Onion rings	1 piece (.3 oz.)	0
Pickle, dill	4 slices (.3 oz.)	125
Relish	.3-oz. serving	70
Tomatoes	1 slice (.5 oz.)	0
Danish	1 piece (3 oz.)	340
Drinks:		
Coffee	6 fl. oz.	0
Cola:		
Regular	12 fl. oz.	15
Dietetic or low calorie	12 fl. oz.	20
Fruit flavored drink	12 fl. oz.	10
Hot chocolate	6 fl. oz.	145
Milk:		
Regular	8 fl. oz.	120
Chocolate	8 fl. oz.	150
Non-cola soft drink	12 fl. oz.	35
Orange juice	6 fl. oz.	0
Tea:		
Hot	6 fl. oz.	15
Iced	12 fl. oz.	20
Egg, scrambled	1 order	160
Frosty dairy dessert:		
Small	12 fl. oz.	220
Medium	16 fl. oz.	293
Large	20 fl. oz.	367
Hamburger:		
Double on white bun	1 burger	575
Kids Meal	1 burger	265
Single:		
On wheat bun	1 burger	290
On white bun	1 burger	410
Omelets:		
Ham & cheese	1 omelet	405
Ham, cheese & mushroom	1 omelet	570

Food and Description	Measure or Quantity	Sodium (milligrams)
Ham, cheese, onion & green pepper	1 omelet	485
Mushroom, onion & green pepper	1 omelet	200
Potatoes:		
Baked, hot stuffed:		
Plain	1 potato	60
Bacon & cheese	1 potato	1180
Broccoli & cheese	1 potato	430
Cheese	1 potato	450
Chicken a la King	1 potato	820
Chili & cheese	1 potato	610
Sour cream & chives	1 potato	230
Stroganoff & sour cream	1 potato	910
French fries	1 regular order	95
Home fries	1 order	745
Salad Bar, *Garden Spot*:		
Alfalfa sprouts	2 oz.	DNA
Bacon bits	3.5 grams	95
Blueberries, fresh	1 T. (.5 oz.)	0
Breadsticks	1 piece	DNA
Broccoli	½ cup (1.6 oz.)	10
Cataloupe	2 pieces (2 oz.)	35
Carrot	¼ cup (1 oz.)	15
Cauliflower	½ cup (1.8 oz.)	5
Cheese:		
American, imitation	1 oz.	DNA
Cheddar, imitation	1 oz.	450
Cottage	½ cup	425
Mozzarella, imitation	1 oz.	320
Swiss, imitation	1 oz.	450
Chow mein noodles	¼ cup (.4 oz.)	80
Cole slaw	½ cup	70
Cracker, saltine	1 piece	37
Croutons	1 piece	5
Cucumber	1/4 cup (.9 oz.)	0
Eggs	1 T. (.3 oz.)	10
Lettuce:		
Iceberg	1 cup	5
Romaine	1 cup	5

Food and Description	Measure or Quantity	Sodium (milligrams)
Mushroom	¼ cup	5
Onions, red	1 T.	0
Oranges, fresh	1 piece	0
Pasta salad	½ cup	400
Pea, green	½ cup	90
Peaches, in syrup	1 piece	0
Peppers:		
Banana or milk pepperocini	1 T.	DNA
Bell	¼ cup	5
Jalapeno	1 T.	4
Pineapple chunks in juice	½ cup	0
Sunflower seeds & raisins	½ cup	10
Tomato	1 oz.	0
Watermelon, fresh	1 piece (1 oz.)	0
Salad dressings:		
Regular:		
Blue cheese	1 T.	85
Celery seed	1 T.	65
French, red	1 T.	130
Italian, golden	1 T.	260
Oil	1 T.	0
Ranch	1 T.	155
Thousand Island	1 T.	115
Dietetic or low calories:		
Bacon & tomato	1 T.	160
Cucumber, creamy	1 T.	140
Italian	1 T.	180
Thousand Island	1 T.	125
Wine vinegar	1 T.	5
Salad, side, pick-up window	1 order	540
Salad, taco	1 order	1100
Sausage	1 patty (1.6 oz.)	410
Toast:		
Regular, with margarine	1 slice	205
French	1 slice	425
WESTERN DINNER, frozen:		
(Banquet) American Favorites	11-oz. dinner	1518
(Morton):		
Regular	11⅛-oz. dinner	1400
Light	11-oz. dinner	1010

Food and Description	Measure or Quantity	Sodium (milligrams)
(Swanson):		
Regular	12¼ oz. dinner	1040
Hungry Man	17½ oz. dinner	1900
WHALE MEAT, raw (USDA)	4 oz.	88
WHEAT CEREAL (Elam's)		
cooked	1 oz.	190
WHEAT CEREAL, CRACKED		
(Elam's)	1 oz.	4
WHEATENA, dry	¼ cup (1.1 oz.)	5
WHEAT FLAKES, cereal		
(Featherweight)	1¼ cups	5
WHEAT GERM:		
(USDA) crude, commercial,		
milled	1 oz.	<1
(Elam's) raw	1 oz.	<5
(Kretschmer)	1 oz.	0
WHEAT GERM CEREAL:		
(USDA)	¼ cup (1 oz.)	<1
(Kretschmer):		
Regular	¼ cup (1 oz.)	<5
Brown sugar & honey	¼ cup (1 oz.)	0
WHEAT HEARTS, cereal		
(General Mills)	¾ cup	410
WHEATIES, cereal (General		
Mills)	1 cup (1 oz.)	370
WHEAT & OATMEAL		
CEREAL, hot (Elam's)	1-oz. serving	11
WHEAT, ROLLED (USDA):		
Uncooked	1 cup (3.1 oz.)	2
Cooked	1 cup (7.7 oz.)	640
WHEAT, SHREDDED, cereal		
(See **SHREDDED WHEAT**)		
WHEAT, WHOLE-GRAIN		
(USDA) hard red spring	1 oz.	<1
WHEAT, WHOLE-MEAL,		
cereal (USDA):		
Dry	1 oz.	<1
Cooked	4 oz.	240
WHISKEY or WHISKY (See		
DISTILLED LIQUOR)		

Note: *WHEAT HEARTS is preceded by an asterisk (★).

Food and Description	Measure or Quantity	Sodium (milligrams)
WHISKEY SOUR COCKTAIL MIX:		
*(Bar-Tender's) (Holland House):	3½ fl. oz.	50
Instant	.56-oz. packet	4
Liquid	1 oz.	105
WHITE CASTLE:		
Bun only	1 bun	131
Cheese only	.3-oz. piece	154
Cheeseburger	2.3-oz. sandwich	361
Chicken sandwich	2¼-oz. sandwich	497
Fish sandwich, without tartar sauce	1 sandwich	201
French fries	3.4-oz. serving	193
Hamburger	2.1-oz. sandwich	266
Onion chips	3.3-oz. order	823
Onion rings	1 order	566
Sausage & egg sandwich	3.4-oz. sandwich	698
Sausage sandwich	1.7-oz. sandwich	488
WHITEFISH, LAKE (USDA):		
Raw:		
Whole	1 lb. (weighed whole)	111
Meat only	4 oz.	59
Baked, stuffed, made with bacon, butter, onion, celery & bread crumbs, home recipe	4 oz.	221
WHITEFISH & PIKE (See **GELFILTE FISH**)		
WIENER (See **FRANKFURTER**)		
WIENER WRAP (Pillsbury)	1 wrap	430
WILD BERRY, fruit drink (Hi-C)	6 fl. oz.	5
WILD RICE, raw (USDA)	½ cup (2.9 oz.)	6
WINE (most wines are listed by kind, brand, vineyard, region or grape name):		
Cooking (Regina):		
Burgundy or sauterne	¼ cup (1 fl. oz.)	365
Sherry	¼ cup (1 fl. oz.)	370

Food and Description	Measure or Quantity	Sodium (milligrams)
Dessert (USDA) 18.8% alcohol	3 fl. oz.	4
Table (USDA) 12.2% alcohol	3 fl. oz.	4
WORCHESTERSHIRE SAUCE (See **SAUCE**)		

Y

YEAST:
  Baker's:
    Compressed:

(USDA)	1 oz.	5
(Fleishmann's)	⅗-oz. cake	7

    Dry:

(USDA)	1 oz.	15
(USDA)	7-g. pkg.	4
(Fleischmann's)	¼ oz. (pkg. or jar)	10

    Brewer's dry, debittered:

(USDA)	1 oz.	34
(USDA)	1 T. (8 g.)	10

YOGURT:
  Regular:
    Plain:
      (Colombo):

Regular	8-oz. container	160
Natural Lite	8-oz. container	182
(Dannon)	8-oz. container	160
(Johanna)	8-oz. container	140
(La Yogurt)	6-oz. serving	140
Lite-Line (Borden)	8-oz. container	150
(Meadow Gold)	8-oz. container	160
(Mountain High)	8-oz. container	140
(Whitney's)	6-oz. container	140

    Apple:
      (Dannon) Dutch, Fruit

on the bottom	8-oz. container	120

Food and Description	Measure or Quantity	Sodium (milligrams)
(Sweet 'n Low) Dutch	8-oz. container	170
Apple & raisins (Whitney's)	6-oz. container	95
Banana (Dannon) fruit on the bottom	8-oz. container	120
Blueberry:		
(Breyer's)	8-oz. container	125
(Dannon):		
Fresh flavor	8-oz. container	160
Fruit on the bottom	4.4-oz. container	65
Fruit on the bottom	8-oz. container	120
(Mountain High)	8-oz. container	140
(Sweet 'n Low)	8-oz. container	170
(Whitney's)	6-oz. container	95
Boysenberry:		
(Dannon) fruit on the bottom	8-oz. container	120
(Sweet'n Low)	8-oz. container	170
(Whitney's)	6-oz. container	95
Cherry:		
(Breyer's) black	8-oz. container	125
(Dannon) fruit on the bottom	8-oz. container	120
(Sweet 'n Low)	8-oz. container	170
(Whitney's)	6-oz. container	95
Cherry vanilla, *Lite-Line* (Borden)	8-oz. container	150
Coffee:		
(Dannon) fresh flavors	8-oz. container	140
(Johanna)	8-oz. container	140
(Whitney's)	6-oz. container	125
Exotic fruit (Dannon) fruit on the bottom	8-oz. container	120
Lemon:		
(Dannon) fresh flavors	8-oz. container	140
(Johanna)	8-oz. container	140
(Sweet 'n Low)	8-oz. container	170
(Whitney's)	6-oz. container	125
Mixed berries (Dannon):		
Extra smooth	4.4-oz. container	80
Fruit-on-the-bottom	4.4-oz. container	65

Food and Description	Measure or Quantity	Sodium (milligrams)
Fruit-on-the-bottom	8-oz. container	120
Hearty nuts & raisins	8-oz. container	120
Peach:		
(Breyer's)	8-oz. container	120
(Dannon) fruit on the bottom	8-oz. container	120
Lite-Line (Borden)	8-oz. container	150
(Sweet 'n Low)	8-oz. container	170
(Whitney's)	6-oz. container	95
Pineapple:		
(Breyer's)	8-oz. container	125
Light 'N Lively	8-oz. container	120
Raspberry:		
(Breyer's)	8-oz. container	125
(Dannon):		
Extra smooth	4.4-oz. container	80
Fresh flavors	8-oz. container	160
Fruit-on-the-bottom	8-oz. container	120
Light 'N Lively	8-oz. container	130
(Meadow Gold)	8-oz. container	160
(Sweet 'n Low)	8-oz. container	170
(Whitney's)	6-oz. container	95
Strawberry:		
(Breyer's)	8-oz. container	120
(Dannon):		
Extra smooth	4.4-oz. container	80
Fresh flavors	8-oz. container	160
Fruit-on-the-bottom	4.4-oz. container	65
Fruit-on-the-bottom	8-oz.container	120
Light 'N Lively	8-oz. container	130
Lite-Line (Borden)	8-oz. container	150
(Sweet 'n Low)	8-oz. container	170
(Whitney's)	6-oz. container	95
Strawberry banana:		
(Dannon):		
Fresh flavors	8-oz. container	160
Fruit-on-the-bottom	4.4-oz. container	65
Fruit-on-the-bottom	8-oz. container	120
Light 'N Lively	8-oz. container	120
(Sweet 'n Low)	6-oz. container	170

Food and Description	Measure or Quantity	Sodium (milligrams)
(Whitney's)	6-oz. container	95
Tropical Fruit (Sweet'n Low)	8-oz. container	170
Vanilla:		
(Breyer's)		
(Dannon):		
Fresh flavors	4.4-oz. container	90
Hearty nuts & raisins	8-oz. container	120
(La Yogurt)	6-oz. container	100
(Whitney's)	6-oz. container	125
Frozen, hard (Dannon):		
Boysenberry, *Danny-On-A-Stick,* carob coated	2½-fl.-oz. bar	15
Chocolate, *Danny-On-A-Stick,* chocolate coated	2½-fl.-oz. bar	15
Raspberry, red, *Danny-On-A-Stick,* chocolate coated	2½-fl.-oz. bar	15
YOGURT DRINK (Dannon)		
Dan up	8-oz. container	110

Z

ZITI, frozen:		
(Morton) light	11-oz. dinner	790
(Weight Watchers)	11¼-oz. serving	1387
ZWIEBACK:		
(Gerber)	1 piece	16
(Nabisco)	1 piece	10

CANADIAN SUPPLEMENT

Food and Description	Measure or Quantity	Sodium (milligrams)

A

AWAKE (General Foods) orange 4 fl. oz.   23

B

BARLEY (Ogilvie), pearl	1 cup	2
BEAN, BAKED, canned		
(Campbell) in tomato sauce	8-oz. serving	784
BEAN, GREEN, frozen (McCain):		
French style	⅓ of 10-oz. pkg.	2
Whole	3.3-oz. serving	1
BEAN, LIMA, frozen (McCain)	3.3-oz. serving	1
BEAN, YELLOW OR WAX, frozen (McCain)	⅓ of 10.6-oz. pkg.	1
BEEF DINNER OR ENTREE, frozen (Swanson):		
Regular, sliced	8½-oz. entree	757
Hungry Man, sliced	17-oz. dinner (482 g.)	1335
TV Brand:		
Chopped sirloin	10-oz. dinner (283 gms.)	974
Sliced	11½-oz. dinner	1044
BEEF PIE, frozen (Swanson):		
Regular	8-oz. pie (227 g.)	1008
Hungry Man	16-oz. pie (454 g.)	1952
BEEF STEW:		
Canned, regular pack (Bounty)	8-oz. serving	884
Frozen (EfficienC)	8-oz. entree (227 g.)	953

Food and Description	Measure or Quantity	Sodium (milligrams)
BEET, canned (Habitant) pickled:		
Cubed	3–4 pieces (30 g.)	12
Sliced	4 slices (30 g.)	15
Whole, baby	2 beets (70 g.)	28
BROCCOLI, frozen (McCain):		
Chopped	⅓ of 10.6-oz. pkg.	3
Spears	⅓ of 10.6-oz. pkg.	3
BRUSSELS SPROUT, frozen (McCain)	⅓ of 10.6-oz. pkg.	10
BUTTERSCOTCH CHIPS (Baker's)	6.2-oz. pkg.	243

C

Food and Description	Measure or Quantity	Sodium (milligrams)
CABBAGE, STUFFED, frozen (Stouffer's) *Lean Cuisine*	305-g. entree	990
CAFIX	1 cup	3
CAKE, frozen:		
Banana (McCain)	⅛ of 19-oz. cake	306
Chocolate:		
(McCain):		
Regular	⅛ of 19-oz. cake	306
Fiesta	⅛ of 19-oz. cake	128
(Pepperidge Farm)	⅙ of 13-oz. cake	231
Coconut (Pepperidge Farm)	⅙ of 13-oz. cake	106
Devil's food (Pepperidge Farm)	⅙ of 13-oz. cake	204
Maple spice (Pepperidge Farm)	⅙ of 13-oz. cake	151
Marble (McCain)	⅛ of 19-oz. cake	303
Neapolitan Fiesta (McCain)	⅛ of 19-oz. cake	126
Shortcake (McCain):		
Raspberry	⅛ of 25-oz. cake	164
Strawberry	⅛ of 25-oz. cake	217
Vanilla:		
(McCain)	⅛ of 18-oz. cake	287
(Pepperidge Farm) layer	⅙ of 13-oz. cake	199

Food and Description	Measure or Quantity	Sodium (milligrams)
CAKE ICING, regular (General Mills):		
Chocolate	¹⁄₁₂ of container	113
Vanilla	¹⁄₁₂ of container	96
CAKE ICING MIX, regular (General Mills):		
Chocolate, fudge	¹⁄₁₂ pkg.	41
White:		
Fluffy	¹⁄₁₂ pkg.	29
Traditional	¹⁄₁₂ pkg.	66
*CAKE MIX, regular (General Mills):		
Angel food:		
Regular	¹⁄₁₆ of cake	172
Confetti	¹⁄₁₆ of cake	136
Cherry chip, layer	¹⁄₁₂ of cake	278
Chocolate, layer:		
German	¹⁄₁₂ of cake	286
Milk	¹⁄₁₂ of cake	281
Sour cream, fudge	¹⁄₁₂ of cake	293
Devil's food, layer	¹⁄₁₂ of cake	320
Lemon, layer	¹⁄₁₂ of cake	271
Orange, layer	¹⁄₁₂ of cake	269
Pound, golden	¹⁄₁₂ of cake	171
White, layer:		
Regular	¹⁄₁₂ of cake	273
Sour cream	¹⁄₁₂ of cake	274
CARROT, frozen (McCain):		
Diced, sticks or whole	3½-oz. serving	33
Sliced	3½-oz. serving	26
CATSUP, FRUIT (Habitant)	1 T.	45
CAULIFLOWER, frozen (McCain)	3½-oz. serving	31
CEREAL:		
Bran (Quaker):		
Corn	1 cup	259
Oat	⅓ cup	1
Harvest Crunch (Quaker):		
Regular, apple & cinnamon or raisins & dates	⅓ cup	16

Food and Description	Measure or Quantity	Sodium (milligrams)
Bran & raisins	⅓ cup	19
Muffets (Quaker)	2 pieces	3
Oat (Ogilvie)	¾ cup	Tr.
Wheat Hearts (Ogilvie)	¾ cup (3 T.)	<1
Vita B (Ogilvie)	¾ cup	<1
CHICKEN A LA KING, frozen (EfficienC)	7-oz. entree (198 g.)	739
CHICKEN DINNER OR ENTREE, frozen:		
(Stouffer's):		
Regular, escalloped	326 g. meal	1440
Lean Cuisine:		
a l'orange	228-g. meal	520
Cacciatore	308 g. meal	1170
& vegetables	361-g. meal	1325
(Swanson):		
Regular, fried	7-oz. entree	890
Hungry Man:		
Boneless	19-oz. dinner	1709
Fried	15-oz. dinner	1097
TV Brand, fried	11½-oz. entree	1126
CHICKEN PIE, frozen (Swanson):		
Regular	8-oz. pie (227 g.)	863
Hungry Man	16-oz. pie (454 g.)	2093
CHICKEN STEW:		
Canned (Bounty)	8-oz. serving	968
Frozen (EfficienC)	8-oz. entree	765
CHILI OR CHILI CON CARNE, canned, with beans (Bounty)	8-oz. serving	1043
CHOCOLATE, BAKING (Baker's):		
Unsweetened	1-oz. square	1
Milk, chips	6.2-oz. pkg.	89
Semi-sweet:		
Regular	1-oz. square	1
Chips	6.2-oz. pkg.	4
Sweet	1-oz. square	<1

Food and Description	Measure or Quantity	Sodium (milligrams)
CHOW CHOW (Habitant):		
Green tomato	2 T. (25 mL)	117
Red tomato	2 T. (25 mL)	165
CLAMATO JUICE DRINK,		
canned (Mott's)	4 fl. oz.	520
COCOA:		
Dry, unsweetened (Fry's)	1 T. (5 g.)	38
*Mix, regular (Cadbury's) instant	6 fl. oz. (1 pouch)	160
COCONUT, packaged (Baker's):		
Angel Flake	½ of 7-oz. pkg.	242
Premium Shred	½ of 7-oz. pkg.	246
***COFFEE,** instant, *General Foods International Coffee:*		
Irish Mocha Mint	6 fl. oz.	18
Orange Cappucino	6 fl. oz.	101
Suisse Mocha	6 fl. oz.	25
Vienna Royale	6 fl. oz.	101
CORN, frozen (McCain) whole kernel	¼ of 12.4-oz. pkg.	1
CRANAPPLE JUICE DRINK (Ocean Spray)	8 fl. oz.	8
CRANBERRY JUICE COCKTAIL, canned (Ocean Spray)	8 fl. oz.	45
CRANBERRY SAUCE, canned (Ocean Spray) jellied or whole	2-fl.-oz. serving	16
CREAM, canned (Nestlé) pure, thick	1 T. (15 ml.)	4
CROUSTINES (Catelli)	1 slice	28

D

DOUGHNUT, frozen (McCain) chocolate iced	¼ of 9-oz. pkg.	150

Food and Description	Measure or Quantity	Sodium (milligrams)

FIDDLEHEAD GREENS, frozen (McCain) — ⅓ of 10½-oz. pkg. — 2

FISH DINNER OR ENTREE, frozen (Stouffer's) *Lean Cuisine:*

Divan	351-g. meal	780
Florentine	255-g. meal	810
Jardiniere	319-g. meal	930

FLOUR:

Bisquick (General Mills)	¼ cup	369
Five Roses:		
All-purpose or unbleached	¼ cup	<1
Whole wheat	¼ cup	<1
(Swansdown) cake	½ cup (2 oz.)	1

G

*GELATIN DESSERT MIX:

Regular (Jell-O):		
All flavors except cherry & lime	½ cup	69
Cherry	½ cup	71
Lime	½ cup	57
Dietetic (D-Zerta):		
Lemon	½ cup	73
Orange, strawberry or raspberry	½ cup	74

GRAPE DRINK, canned, *Welch's* — 8 fl. oz. (8.4 oz.) — 24

GRAPEFRUIT JUICE, canned (Ocean Spray) — 8 fl. oz. — 10

Food and Description	Measure or Quantity	Sodium (milligrams)
GRAPE JUICE, canned, *Welch's,* purple or white	8 fl. oz.	8
GRAVY, canned (Franco-American):		
Beef	2-oz. serving	279
Chicken	2-oz. serving	285
Mushroom	2-oz. serving	307
Onion	2-oz. serving	348

H

HAM DINNER OR ENTREE, frozen (Swanson) *TV Brand*	10½-oz. dinner	1254

I

ICE MAGIC (General Foods) chocolate or chocolate mint	.6-oz. serving	10

J

JAM:		
(Habitant)	1 T. (15 mL)	<1
(Laura Secord)	1 T. (15 mL)	<1
JELL-O PUDDING POPS (General Foods):		
Chocolate	2.1-oz. pop	92
All other flavors	2.1-oz. pop	57

Food and Description	Measure or Quantity	Sodium (milligrams)

K

*KOOL-AID (General Foods):
  Regular, sugar added after
    bought | 8 fl. oz. | 1
  Pre-sweetened, with sugar:
    All except orange and
      sunshine punch | 8 fl. oz. | 1
    Orange or sunshine punch | 8 fl. oz. | 0
  Dietetic, sugar free:
    Cherry, grape or tropical
      punch | 8 fl. oz. | 2
    Orange | 8 fl. oz. | 0
    Strawberry | 8 fl. oz. | 1

L

LASAGNA, frozen (EfficienC) | 9.2-oz. entree | 1350
LEMONADE, canned, *Country Time* | 10 fl. oz. | 53
LINGUINI, frozen (Stouffer's)
  Lean Cuisine | 273-g. meal | 990

M

MACARONI:
  Dry (Catelli) | 3 oz. | 2
  Canned (Franco-American) and
    beef | 8-oz. serving | 1386
  Frozen (Swanson) and beef | 8-oz. casserole | 1307

Food and Description	Measure or Quantity	Sodium (milligrams)
MACARONI & CHEESE:		
Canned (Franco-American)	8 oz.	1000
Frozen:		
(EfficienC)	8-oz. entree	1157
(Swanson)	8-oz. casserole	1110
Mix (Catelli)	3 oz.	582
MARMALADE, sweet (Laura Secord)	1 T.	<1
MEATBALL, frozen (Swanson) and gravy	9-oz. entree	1029
MEATBALL STEW, frozen (Stouffer's) *Lean Cuisine*	283-g. meal	1250
MINERAL WATER (Montclair)	100 mL.	9
***MUFFIN MIX** (General Mills):		
Apple cinnamon	1 muffin	189
Blueberry	1 muffin	124
Butter pecan	1 muffin	150
Corn	1 muffin	322
Honey bran	1 muffin	165

N

NOODLE, dry (Catelli):		
Egg	3 oz.	5
Lasagna, spinach	3 oz.	14

O

OLIVE (Habitant)	.2 oz.	143
ONION, PICKLED (Habitant):		
Sour	4 onions	155
Sweet	4 onions	140

Food and Description	Measure or Quantity	Sodium (milligrams)

P

Food and Description	Measure or Quantity	Sodium (milligrams)
PANCAKE, frozen (EfficienC)	1.7-oz. pancake	232
PATTY SHELL, frozen		
(Pepperidge Farm) regular	1.7-oz. shell (47.2 g.)	194
PEA, green, frozen (McCain)	¼ of 12.4-oz. pkg.	72
PEA & CARROT, frozen (McCain)	⅓ of 10½-oz. pkg.	55
PICKLE (Habitant):		
Bread & butter	4 slices (30 g.)	163
Dill, with or without garlic:		
Regular	1 piece	480
Baby	1 piece	240
Polskie Ogorki	1 piece	480
Sour:		
Gherkins	2 pieces	310
Mixed	3–4 pieces (30 g.)	500
Sweet:		
Gherkins	2 pieces	175
Mixed:		
Regular	3–4 pieces	279
Mustard	2–3 pieces	267
PIE, frozen (McCain):		
Banana cream	⅙ of 14-oz. pie	129
Chocolate cream	⅙ of 14-oz. pie	132
Coconut cream	⅙ of 14-oz. pie	132
Lemon cream	⅙ of 14-oz. pie	168
Mincemeat	⅛ of 24-oz. pie	243
Pecan	⅛ of 20-oz. pie	157
Pumpkin	⅛ of 22-oz. pie	167
Raisin	3½-oz. serving	283
*PIE CRUST MIX		
(General Mills)	⅙ of double-crust shell	389

Food and Description	Measure or Quantity	Sodium (milligrams)
*PIE MIX (General Mills)		
Boston cream	⅛ of pie	451
PIZZA SAUCE (Catelli) *Pizza Pronto:*		
Mild	2 T.	186
Spicy	1 T.	182
PORK DINNER or ENTREE, frozen (Swanson) *TV Brand,* loin of	11-oz. dinner	901
POTATO, frozen (McCain):		
Country style	2-oz. serving	15
Diced, all-purpose	2-oz. serving	4
French fries	2-oz. serving	15
Hashbrowns, western style	2-oz. serving	170
Puffs	⅓ of 8.8-oz. pkg.	27
Superfries	2-oz. serving	17
PRUNE NECTAR, canned, *Welch's*	8 fl. oz. (8.6 oz.)	15
PUDDING OR PIE FILLING:		
Canned, regular pack (Laura Secord):		
Banana	5-oz. serving	156
Butter pecan	5-oz. serving	212
Butterscotch	5-oz. serving	156
Chocolate:		
Regular	5-oz. serving	169
Fudge	5-oz. serving	179
Mint	5-oz. serving	187
Maple	5-oz. serving	158
Mocha	5-oz. serving	165
Rice	5-oz. serving	206
Tapioca	5-oz. serving	149
Vanilla	5-oz. serving	234
*Mix:		
Regular:		
Banana cream (Jell-O):		
Regular	½ cup	194
Instant	½ cup	463
Butter pecan (Jell-O):		
Regular	½ cup	190

Food and Description	Measure or Quantity	Sodium (milligrams)
Instant	½ cup	398
Butterscotch (Jell-O):		
Regular	½ cup	246
Instant	½ cup	436
Caramel (Jell-O):		
Regular	½ cup	246
Instant	½ cup	453
Chocolate (Jell-O):		
Plain:		
Regular	½ cup	219
Instant	½ cup	748
Cream, regular	½ cup	198
Fudge, instant	½ cup	429
Coconut cream (Jell-O)		
regular	½ cup	212
Custard (Bird's)	½ cup	74
Lemon (Jell-O) instant	½ cup	350
Pistachio (Jell-O) instant	½ cup	399
Tapioca:		
(Jell-O) instant	½ cup	179
Minit (General Foods)	½ cup	135
Vanilla (Jell-O):		
Regular	½ cup	194
Instant	½ cup	423
Dietetic (D-Zerta):		
Butterscotch	½ cup	248
Chocolate	½ cup	221
Vanilla	½ cup	196

Q

QUENCH (General Foods):
Canned
Regular:

Fruit punch	9.5 fl. oz.	36
Grape	9.5 fl. oz.	86
Lemonade	9.5 fl. oz.	58

Food and Description	Measure or Quantity	Sodium (milligrams)
Orange	9.5 fl. oz.	55
Dietetic:		
Fruit punch, grape or orange	8½ fl. oz.	1
Lemonade	8½ fl. oz.	0
*Mix, regular:		
Fruit punch	8½ fl. oz.	3
Grape	8½ fl. oz.	2
Lemonade or orange	8½ fl. oz.	1
QUIK (Nestlé):		
Powder:		
Chocolate	2 heaping tsps.	25
Strawberry	2 heaping tsps.	15
Ready-to-serve	170 mL	95

R

RAVIOLI, canned (Catelli)	1 cup (250 mL)	1112
RELISH (Habitant):		
Cubed	1 T.	57
Hamburger	1 T.	167
Hot dog	1 T.	182
Sweet	1 T.	88
ROLL OR BUN, frozen (McCain):		
Danish, iced	2-oz. serving	208
Honey	2-oz. serving	221

S

SALISBURY STEAK, frozen:		
(EfficienC)	5¾-oz. entree	722
(Swanson):		
Regular	5½-oz. entree	537
Hungry Man	17-oz. dinner	1393

Food and Description	Measure or Quantity	Sodium (milligrams)
TV Brand	11½-oz. dinner	1496
SAUCE, canned (Habitant):		
Barbecue	2 T.	170
Chicken, hot	2 T.	171
SCALLOP DINNER, OR ENTREE, frozen (Stouffer's)		
Lean Cuisine	312-g. entree	1200
*SOUP, canned, regular pack:		
Asparagus (Campbell) condensed, cream of	7-oz. serving	824
Bean (Campbell) condensed, with bacon	7-oz. serving	746
Beef (Campbell) condensed:		
Broth	7-oz. serving	666
Mushroom	7-oz. serving	830
Noodle	7-oz. serving	685
With vegetables & barley	7-oz. serving	697
Cabbage (Habitant)	1 cup	881
Celery (Campbell) condensed, cream of	7-oz. serving	815
Cheddar cheese (Campbell) condensed	7-oz. serving	776
Chicken (Campbell) condensed:		
Broth	7-oz. serving	588
Cream of:		
Made with milk	7-oz. serving	796
Made with water	7-oz. serving	746
Creamy, & mushroom	7-oz. serving	790
Gumbo	7-oz. serving	805
Noodle	7-oz. serving	815
NoodleOs	7-oz. serving	750
With rice	7-oz. serving	656
& stars	7-oz. serving	921
Vegetable	7-oz. serving	799
Chicken (Habitant):		
Cream of	1 cup	717
Noodle	1 cup	901
Rice	1 cup	807
Chowder, clam (Campbell) condensed:		
Manhattan style	7-oz. serving	769

Food and Description	Measure or Quantity	Sodium (milligrams)
New England style	7-oz. serving	766
Consomme (Campbell) condensed	7-oz. serving	563
Minnestrone:		
(Campbell)	7-oz. serving	793
(Habitant)	1 cup	1105
Mushroom:		
(Campbell) golden	7-oz. serving	847
(Habitant) cream of	1 cup	508
Noodle (Campbell) condensed, & ground beef	7-oz. serving	705
Onion (Campbell) condensed:		
Regular	7-oz. serving	815
Cream of, made with water	7-oz. serving	577
Ox Tail (Campbell) condensed	7-oz. serving	885
Oyster stew (Campbell) condensed	7-oz. serving	626
Pea, French Canadian style (Campbell) condensed	7-oz. serving	626
Pea, green:		
(Campbell) condensed	7-oz. serving	823
(Habitant):		
Regular	1 cup	907
With ham	1 cup	926
Potato (Campbell) condensed, cream of, made with water	7-oz. serving	895
Scotch broth (Campbell) condensed	7-oz. serving	885
Shrimp (Campbell) condensed	7-oz. serving	815
Tomato:		
(Campbell):		
Regular	7-oz. serving	702
Bisque	7-oz. serving	865
& rice, old fashioned	7-oz. serving	658
(Habitant):		
Cream of	1 cup	750
Vermicelli	1 cup	935
Turkey (Campbell) condensed:		
Noodle	7-oz. serving	714
Vegetable	7-oz. serving	749

Food and Description	Measure or Quantity	Sodium (milligrams)
Vegetable:		
(Campbell) condensed:		
Regular	7-oz. serving	680
Beef	7-oz. serving	751
Country style	7-oz. serving	835
Cream of, made with water	7-oz. serving	895
Old fashioned	7-oz. serving	711
Vegetarian	7-oz. serving	513
(Habitant)	1 cup (9 oz.)	1118
SPINACH, frozen (McCain)	⅓ of 12-oz. pkg.	22
SPAGHETTI, canned:		
(Catelli) in tomato & cheese sauce	1 cup	1291
(Franco-American) & ground beef	8-oz. serving	936
In tomato sauce	8-oz. serving	779
SpaghettiOs	8-oz. serving	902
SPAGHETTI SAUCE, canned (Catelli):		
Garlic	5.3 fl. oz. (150 mL)	811
Hot & spicy	5.3 fl. oz. (150 mL)	827
Mild	5.3 fl. oz. (150 mL)	827
SQUASH, frozen (McCain)	¼ of 14-oz. pkg.	3
STRUDEL, frozen (Pepperidge Farm):		
Apple	⅙ of strudel (2.3 oz.)	56
Blueberry	⅙ of strudel (2.3 oz.)	60
SWISS STEAK DINNER OR ENTREE, frozen (Swanson) *TV Brand*	11¼-oz. dinner	682
SYRUP, sweetened:		
Banana (Milk Mate)	1½ T. (25 mL)	811
Butter pecan (Habitant)	1 T.	<1

Food and Description	Measure or Quantity	Sodium (milligrams)
Chocolate (Milk Mate):		
Regular	1½ T. (25 mL)	70
Fudge	1½ T. (25 mL)	67
Strawberry (Milk Mate)	1½ T. (25 mL)	9
Table (Habitant)	1 T. (15 mL)	<1

T

*TANG (General Foods):		
Grapefruit	4.2 fl. oz.	87
Orange	4.2 fl. oz.	1
Orange & grapefruit	4.2 fl. oz.	42
Pineapple & grapefruit	4.2 fl. oz.	51
TOMATO PASTE, canned (Catelli)	1 T.	7
TOMATO SAUCE, canned, regular pack (Catelli):		
Plain	½ cup (80 g.)	536
Marinara	½ cup	469
With meat	½ cup (80.5 g.)	547
Mushroom	½ cup	608
TOPPING, WHIPPED, frozen, Cool Whip (General Foods)	1 T. (.1 oz.)	1
TURKEY DINNER OR ENTREE, frozen:		
(EfficienC) sliced	5.2-oz. entree	521
(Swanson):		
Regular	8¾-oz. entree	995
Hungry Man	19-oz. dinner	1552
TV Brand	11½-oz. dinner	1048
TURKEY PIE, frozen (Swanson):		
Regular	8-oz. pie	864
Hungry Man	16-oz. pie	2193
TURNOVER, frozen:		
Apple:		
(McCain)	2-oz. serving	101

Food and Description	Measure or Quantity	Sodium (milligrams)
(Pepperidge Farm)	2.7-oz. piece	202
Blueberry (Pepperidge Farm)	2.7-oz. piece	214
Blueberry/raspberry (McCain)	2-oz. serving	102
Raspberry (Pepperidge Farm)	2.7-oz. piece	214
Strawberry (Pepperidge Farm)	2.7-oz. piece	208

V

VEGETABLES, MIXED, frozen		
(McCain)	⅓ of 10.6-oz. pkg.	42
V-8 JUICE:		
Regular	6 fl. oz.	650
Spicy hot	6 fl. oz.	630

W

*WHIP'N CHILL (Jell-O):		
Chocolate	½ cup	93
Lemon	½ cup	91
Strawberry	½ cup	140
Vanilla	½ cup	60

Y

YOGURT, regular (Laura Secord):		
Blueberry	4.5-oz. serving	65
Peach	4.5-oz. serving	65
Raspberry	4.5-oz. serving	65
Strawberry	4.5-oz. serving	89

PLUME (0452)

TAKE CARE OF YOURSELF WITH PLUME

PLUME

FEELING GOOD

☐ **LIFE PRINTS: New Patterns of Love and Work for Today's Women. G. B**
R. Barnett, and C. Rivers. Provides a role model for young women, a supp
confirmation for women in midlife, and a guide for all women who are lool
satisfy their needs for self-esteem and pleasure but don't know where t
(138600—

☐ **DARE TO CHANGE: How to Program Yourself for Success, by Joe Alex**
Most people never come close to fulfilling their potential for achievemer
happiness. They are held back not by outside forces—but by the "inner sabc
that have been programmed into them since childhood and that cripple
ability to see, think, and act. This innvoative guide to discovery and grow
prove that you have the power to direct your own life—and make your
better than your past (158547—

☐ **THE COMPLETE GUIDE TO WOMEN'S HEALTH by Bruce D. Shephard**
and Carroll A. Shephard, R.N., Ph.D. The most comprehensive, up-to-d.
source available for making vital health decisions . . . advice on diet fitnes
common symptoms from A to Z, explained and referenced . . . "Excellent, in
tive . . . beautifully organized"—Jane Brody, *The New York Times.* (259800—$

☐ **SMART KIDS WITH SCHOOL PROBLEMS by Priscilla L. Vail.** Effective me
to turn school failure into school success . . . "A hallmark work!"—*Library Jou*
(262429—

Prices slightly higher in Canada.

Buy them at your local bookstore or use this convenient
coupon for ordering.

NEW AMERICAN LIBRARY
P.O. Box 999, Bergenfield, New Jersey 07621

Please send me the PLUME BOOKS I have checked above. I am enclosing $____
(please add $1.50 to this order to cover postage and handling). Send check or r
order—no cash or C.O.D.'s. Prices and numbers are subject to change without r

Name _____

Address _____

City _____ State _____ Zip Code _____
Allow 4-6 weeks for delivery.
This offer subject to withdrawal without notice.